Anaphylaxis

Chemical Immunology and Allergy

Vol. 95

Series Editors

Johannes Ring Munich
Kurt Blaser Davos
Monique Capron Lille
Judah A. Denburg Hamilton
Stephen T. Holgate Southampton
Gianni Marone Naples
Hirohisa Saito Tokyo

Anaphylaxis

Volume Editor

Johannes Ring Munich

32 figures, 1 in color, and 37 tables, 2010

KARGER

Basel · Freiburg · Paris · London · New York · Bangalore · Bangkok · Shanghai · Singapore · Tokyo · Sydney

Chemical Immunology and Allergy
Formerly published as 'Progress in Allergy' (Founded 1939),
continued 1990–2002 as 'Chemical Immunology'
Edited by Paul Kallós 1939–1988, Byron H. Waksman 1962–2002

Prof. Dr. med. Dr. phil. Johannes Ring
Klinik und Poliklinik für Dermatologie und
Allergologie am Biederstein
Technische Universität München
Christine Kühne Center for Allergy
Research and Education (CK-CARE)
Biedersteiner Strasse 29
DE–80802 München (Germany)
E-Mail johannes.ring@lrz.tum.de

Bibliographic Indices. This publication is listed in bibliographic services, including Current Contents® and PubMed/MEDLINE.

© Copyright 2010 by S. Karger AG, P.O. Box, CH–4009 Basel (Switzerland)
www.karger.com
Printed in Switzerland on acid-free and non-aging paper (ISO 9706) by Reinhardt Druck, Basel
ISSN 1660–2242
ISBN 978–3–8055–9441–7
e-ISBN 978–3–8055–9442–4

Contents

Allergens and Elicitors

Preface

Among several emergencies in allergy, anaphylaxis is probably the most dramatic and life-threatening reaction giving rise to a considerable number of fatalities, some of which often go unrecognized. It is important to stress this life-threatening character of an allergic reaction in a time when allergic diseases are regarded by some as minor complaints or just 'impairment of feeling well'. The dangerous character of this type of allergy is based not only upon the dramatic clinical symptomatology when it occurs, but also on the fact that affected individuals – once having survived an episode – are seemingly healthy and tend to neglect the risk of a future episode. Furthermore, there is the problem of 'hidden allergens' which makes it almost impossible for a person suffering from food anaphylaxis for example to avoid the allergen in daily life since declaration rules are leaky but also inadvertent or false contaminations may occur or even transfer of allergen from another individual to the patient – for example by a kiss!

As spectacular as these events are sometimes referred to in the yellow press, as negligent many doctors and also scientists as well as patients are behaving in spite of this potentially life-threatening risk. I would like to tell a very personal episode: When I came back from my post-doctoral fellowship at Scripps Clinical Research Foundation in La Jolla to the Munich Dermatology Department in 1978, I started the allergen-specific immunotherapy with purified insect venom extracts which had just been so successfully tried in the historic double-blind, placebo-controlled trial by the group of Lawrence Lichtenstein in Baltimore. Since then, I have treated several thousand patients successfully and given many lectures on the topic, sometimes *ad meam nauseam* – I felt I can no longer listen to myself telling the same story. In spite of this, in my rather close circle of acquaintances, one day a 35-year-old young man who was aware of the problem he had with insect stings with minor flush episodes or itching palms, but had not taken this seriously, died when he was mountain climbing in the Karwendel mountains in Bavaria. This 'shock' motivated me to continue to 'preach' like the voice in the wilderness. It just shows you that it is important to bring the message and the scientific progress to the people.

This was also the main motivation to put together this book, because for some time – since the last Novartis Foundation Symposium volume 2004 – not so much has been comprehensively compiled on this topic.

I am very grateful to the excellent group of authors who have contributed to this book, to Dr. Franz and Dr. Grosber, as well as to Mr. Nold, Ms. Smit and Mr. Jappert from Karger Publishers who were of tremendous help in the editing process. May this book be widely distributed not only among allergists but among all doctors dealing with patients potentially affected in order to prevent anaphylactic reactions, but also in order to correctly treat these patients both in the acute phase as well as in the long-term management.

Johannes Ring

Charles M. Richet on Anaphylaxis

A Facsimile (1904)

Richet CM: De l'anaphylaxie ou sensibilité croissante des organismes à des doses successives de poison. Arch Fisiol 1904;1:129–142.[1]

DE L'ANAPHYLAXIE
OU SENSIBILITÉ CROISSANTE DES ORGANISMES
À DES DOSES SUCCESSIVES DE POISON

par M. Charles Richet.

(Laboratoire de Physiologie de la Faculté de Médecine de Paris)

J'ai appelé *anaphylaxie* (ανα, *en arrière*, φυλαξις, *protection*) la propriété curieuse que possèdent certains poisons d'augmenter, au lieu de diminuer, la sensibilité de l'organisme à leur action. On peut en effet concevoir, dans les effets successifs d'un poison, trois modalités différentes :

1º Sensibilité égale ;

2º Sensibilité moindre ;

3º Sensibilité plus grande.

Lorsque l'organisme est de moins en moins sensible au poison, on dit qu'il y a immunité ; et on peut appeler *prophylactique* ou *immunisante* l'action des injections antérieures, puisque elle a eu pour effet de diminuer la sensibilité organique.

De fait la plupart des auteurs ont étudié, à cause de son grand intérêt pratique — et peut être aussi parce qu'elle est plus fréquente — l'action prophylactique des poisons ; et d'innombrables travaux ont été faits sur l'immunité.

Mais quant aux effets anaphylactiques des poisons, on ne possède jusque à présent que peu de données ; et cependant, au point de vue théorique, comme au point de vue pratique, l'importance du phénomène parait considérable (*).

(*) Avant la publication de mon travail (P. Portier et Ch. Richet. De l'action anaphylactique de certains venins. *Bull. de la Soc. de Biol.*, 1902, 170-72 ; et *Trav. du Lab. de Physiologie,* V, 1902, 506-509) on ne trouve dans la science que des documents épars, et des faits isolés, très rares, attribuables à l'anaphylaxie.

Knorr (Experimentelle Untersuchungen über die Grenzen der Heilungsmöglichkeit des Tetanus. Marburg, 1895, 18) a vu que les cobayes supportent mal les injections de toxine tétanique, et qu'ils deviennent de plus en plus sensibles ; de sorte qu'il a du renoncer à les vacciner par ces injections réitérées de toxine. Mais il n'a pas insisté sur ce phénomène, d'autant plus que cette même toxine agit comme immunisante chez certains animaux, si elle est anaphylactisante chez d'autres.

En étudiant avec J. Héricourt la sensibilité des chiens aux injections de sérum d'anguille, non seulement nous n'avons pas pu obtenir l'immunisation ; mais nous avons

9

I. Effets du venin des Actinies.

Si l'on coupe les tentacules des Actinies au ras du corps, on peut séparer l'animal en deux parties; d'une part le pédicule et la cavité gastro-intestinale; d'autre part les tentacules. La section est facile à faire; car les Actinies avec lesquelles j'opérais (*Anemonia sulcata*) n'ont pas les tentacules rétractiles. Alors je plaçais ces tentacules dans la glycérine pure, à proportions égales, soit un volume de tentacules pour un volume de glycérine. Dans ces conditions il n'y a pas de putréfaction, et on peut conserver des solutions intactes pendant assez longtemps.

Mais dans la masse il se produit des effets de digestion, et, au bout de cinq ou six jours, une grande partie des éléments constituants des tentacules sont entrés en dissolution dans ce liquide glycériné, formant une masse épaisse, mucilagineuse, de consistance visqueuse.

Pour dissoudre toutes les substances solubles, il faut broyer la masse avec du sable fin bien propre; on obtient alors un liquide plus épais encore, qui, par sa densité et sa consistance épaisse, parait impossible à filtrer.

Cependant, à force de patience, la filtration n'est pas impossible; car, si l'on place le mélange sur de grands entonnoirs munis d'un bon filtre Chardin, on a à la longue un liquide assez trouble qu'on obtient en quantités notables; et sur le papier filtre se dépose un produit

---

vu le contraire de l'immunisation, c'est à dire la sensibilité croissante: « à la suite de plusieurs injections, ces animaux (chiens) ont fini par dépérir, devenir étiques, et finalement mourir dans la cachexie. » (Effets lointains des injections de sérum d'anguille, par J. Héricourt et Ch. Richet; *Bull. de la Soc. de Biol.*, 29 janvier 1898, 137).

Plus tard, Behring et Kitashima (*Berl. klin. Woch.*, 1901, 157), reprenant les expériences de Knorr, ont retrouvé la sensibilité croissante des cobayes aux injections de toxine tétanique. Ils admettent qu'il y a une hyperesthésie spécifique acquise de certains organes au poison diphtéritique; mais, comme Knorr, ils ont vu là quelque chose de tout à fait particulier à l'organisme du cobaye.

Plus récemment, M. Arthus (Injections répétées de sérum de cheval chez le lapin; *Bull. de la Soc. de Biol.*, 16 juin 1903, p. 817-821), à la suite de nos expériences d'anaphylaxie par le poison des Actinies, a donné des faits extrêmement intéressants sur la sensibilité croissante du lapin aux injections de sérum de cheval; et il a pu montrer que l'anaphylaxie est probablement un phénomène d'ordre général.

C'est d'ailleurs ce que j'avais indiqué en disant, à propos du venin des Actinies dont les effets sont si nettement anaphylactiques: « il est probable que beaucoup de venins, ou de toxines, sont dans ce cas. »

insoluble, noir brunâtre, qui adhère au papier, tandis que la majeure partie du liquide, presque limpide, surnage ; on décante ce qui est resté sur l'entonnoir ; on l'ajoute au liquide qui a filtré, et on finit par avoir ainsi un liquide épais, extrêmement trouble, qu'on filtre de nouveau deux fois ou trois fois encore, et qui enfin devient tout à fait transparent, surtout si l'on ne prend que les parties qui filtrent les 2e, 3e et 4e jour.

Pour éviter toute altération, il est bon que ces filtrations se fassent dans la glacière, ou tout au moins à basse température.

Ce liquide glycériné est très toxique. Cependant, au fur et à mesure des filtrations, sa toxicité diminue quelque peu. Pour donner une idée de la puissance toxique du liquide primitif, contenant à peu près 50 % de glycérine, et 50 % de tentacules actiniques ; je mentionnerai l'expérience suivante :

Un chien (*Amphitryon*) de 31 Kil. reçoit le 8 mars 1902, cc. 1,6 de liquide (soit cc. 0,8 de tentacule), et il meurt le troisième jour. Or on doit admettre qu'il y a à peine 10 % d'éléments solides dans le tentacule; de sorte qu'il a suffi de gr. 0,08 pour empoisonner 31 Kil. de chien, soit la minime quantité pour 1 Kil. de chien, de 0,0025 de la totalité des substances solides du tentacule.

Mais, avec les liquides bien filtrés, probablement parce que toutes les matières toxiques n'ont pas été dissoutes, la toxicité est moindre, et il faut environ cc. 0,15 de l'extrait glycériné (volumes égaux de glycérine et de tentacules) par Kil. de chien pour déterminer la mort.

Voici les chiffres relatifs à la dose toxique : (*)

N. de l'expérience	Noms des Chiens	Dose de toxine en cc. par Kil.	Durée de la survie	
I	*Mascarelle*	0,5	10 heures	
II	*Lindor*	0,4	10 »	
III	*Muscadin*	0,3	36 »	24 heures
IV	*Toto*	0,3	10 »	
V	*Polyphème*	0,25	4 jours	
VI	*Enée*	0,25	17 »	8 jours
VII	*Matamore*	0,25	4 »	
VIII	*Sganarelle*	0,24	4 »	
IX	*Araminte*	0,21	10 »	
X	*Marton*	0,20	3 »	5 jours
XI	*Polichinelle*	0,20	4 »	
XII	*Hernani*	0,20	2 »	
XIII	*Pancrace*	0,18	1 »	
XIV	*Lycidas*	0,18	survit	

(*) L'injection était faite dans la veine saphène tibiale ; et, au moment de l'injection, le liquide était dilué dans 10 fois son volume d'eau distillée.

N. de l'expérience	Noms des Chiens	Dose de toxine en cc. par Kil.	Durée de la survie
XV	*Lubin*	0,18	survit
XVI	*Chrysale*	0 16	4 jours
XVII	*Moutonne*	0,16	5 »
XVIII	*Flipote*	0,16	survit
XIX	*Doña Sol*	0,15	3 jours
XX	*Don Luis*	0,15	4 »
XXI	*Circé*	0,15	survit
XXII	*Angélique*	0,15	»
XXIII	*Gubetta*	0,15	»
XXIV	*Bobino*	0,14	6 jours
XXV	*Philaminte*	0,14	survit
XXVI	*Gorgibus*	0,13	9 jours
XXVII	*Anemonio*	0,13	survit
XXIX	*X....*	0,125	5 jours
XXX à XXXVI	*Sept chiens*	0,12	survivent
XXXVII	*Antiochus*	0,12	5 jours
XXXVIII	*Blanchette*	0,12	6 »
XXXIX	*Géronte*	0,10	5 »
XL	*Dandin*	0,10	8 »
XLI	*Bobèche*	0,10	17 »
de XLI à L	*Neuf chiens*	0,10	survivent
LI	*Isabelle*	0,08	7 jours
LII	*Sottenville*	0,08	survit
LIII à LVIII	*Cinq chiens*	0,05	survivent

De ces chiffres se déduisent les moyennes suivantes, centésimales, de mortalité :

Nombre d'expériences	Doses de toxine	Mortalité pour 100	Durée de la survie chez les animaux qui meurent
II	de 0,5 à 0,3	100	10 heures
II	0,3	100	1 jour
VIII	de 0,25 à 0,20	100	6 jours
XI	de 0,18 à 0,15	55	4 »
XII	de 0,14 à 0,12	36	6 »
XIV	de 0,10 à 0,08	28	9 »
V	0,05	0	

Ces nombreuses expériences nous permettent de déduire des conclusions fermes sur la toxicité de l'extrait glycérique des tentacules actiniens: et nous pouvons dire, en résumé:

1.º Pour des doses supérieures à 0,25, la mort survient en quelques heures, mais dix heures au moins, quand la dose n'est pas supérieure à 0,50.

2.º Pour des doses dépassant 0,18, et inférieures ou égales à 0,25, la mort est fatale, survenant au bout de deux, trois, quatre ou cinq jours.

3.º Pour des doses allant de cc. 0,125 à cc. 0,18, il y a incertitude : tantôt survie, tantôt mort, en 5 ou 6 jours.

4.º Pour des doses de cc. 0,12 et au dessous, la mort ne survient qu'exceptionnellement et au bout d'une semaine au moins.

Les effets toxiques de ce venin des Actinies sont caractéristiques ; ils semblent dus à deux poisons bien distincts, et que j'ai réussi à isoler.

L'un, que j'ai appelé *thalassine*, et que j'ai pu obtenir à l'état de pureté parfaite, sous la forme d'un corps cristallisable (une phénylcarbylamine propionique??) produit des démangeaisons intenses, un prurit violent, et de l'urticaire ; mais, même à des doses cent fois plus fortes que la dose minime (gr. 0,0005) qui produit l'urticaire, il n'est pas mortel.

Je n'étudie pas dans ce mémoire les effets de la thalassine.

L'autre poison, insoluble dans l'alcool, se coagulant par la chaleur, est une toxo-albumine que j'ai appelée *congestine* ; car sa propriété caractéristique est d'amener une congestion intense de tout l'appareil circulatoire intestinal. Ce sont les effets de cette congestine qui déterminent les formes du processus toxique par l'action de l'extrait glycériné.

Trois à quatre minutes après que l'injection a été faite, le chien est pris de vomissements qui deviennent de plus en plus violents, incoercibles, et probablement très douloureux, à cause de la violence des efforts qui sont faits pour l'expulsion du contenu stomacal. Puis la diarrhée survient, avec selles liquides, mêlées à du sang, et ténesme rectal très intense. Dans les intervalles de ces efforts désespérés de défécation, l'animal semble souffrir de coliques très violentes. Il se retire dans un coin aussi obscur que possible, se couche, sans qu'on puisse le décider à marcher. Parfois la respiration est comme gênée (peut être par les vives douleurs abdominales). Dans les cas graves, dès le début, il y a des phénomènes nerveux caractérisés par quelques troubles de la démarche, sorte de paraplégie avec contracture. Surtout on note de l'insensibilité. Dans les cas moins graves, la sensibilité est conservée ; mais on observe un état de prostration qui, au bout d'une heure ou deux, si la dose n'a pas été très forte, se dissipe.

Si la dose a été de 0,15 à 0,25, l'animal meurt le deuxième, le troisième ou le quatrième jour, avec un affaiblissement général de plus en plus marqué, dans un état de prostration et de demi coma, presque d'insensibilité complète. L'urine est rare et albumineuse. Il ne prend pas de nourriture; mais la soif est intense. La respiration est laborieuse, plutôt lente; il n'y a pas d'accélération notable du cœur. Le sang est coagulable.

A l'autopsie les lésions sont caractéristiques; *toute la muqueuse gastro-intestinale est hémorrhagique.* Souvent il y a du sang liquide dans l'estomac, dans l'intestin, voire même dans la cavité péritonéale. Les *plèvres* sont injectées de sang; il y a des suffusions sanguines dans le péricarde. La muqueuse intestinale est tapissée par la couche épaisse d'une mucosité jaune brune, sanguinolente, sorte d'exsudat muqueux, qui, étant râclé avec le dos du scalpel, laisse voir la muqueuse de l'intestin dans un état de congestion extraordinaire.

II. Effets anaphylactiques.

Tels sont les effets d'une première injection; et telles sont les doses toxiques. Mais, si l'animal a reçu précédemment une dose, même faible, de poison, l'action est toute différente.

Voici un premier tableau qui indiquera bien l'accroissement énorme de l'action toxique (ou anaphylaxie) par l'effet d'injections antécédents.

Nom du Chien	Dose d'actinotoxine antérieurement injectée	Temps écoulé entre les deux injections (en jours)	Dose d'actinotoxine injectée en cc.	Durée de la survie (en heures)
Mathurin	0,10	23	0,25	0,75
Epagneul	?	15	0,25	2,00
Pierrot	0,08	15	0,16	0,50
Bassette	0,10	32	0,15	6,00
Galatée	0,12	16	0,12	6,00
Chloralosa	0,06	14	0,10	1,50
Arlequine	0,10 (quatre fois)	?	0,11	4,00
Neptune	0,10	22	0,10	0,40
Diane	?	18	0,08	1,50
Fracasse	deux fois injecté	74	0,15	2,50
Angélique	trois fois injectée	72	0,15	6,00
MOYENNE			0,15	2,75

Ainsi la différence est éclatante entre la sensibilité des chiens ayant reçu une injection antérieure, et la sensibilité des chiens normaux.

A une dose faible, les animaux meurent en quelques heures, alors que cette même dose, injectée à un animal non injecté précédemment, est à peu près inoffensive.

Je prendrai notamment pour exemple le chien *Neptune,* gros mâtin, à poil ras, très vigoureux, qui, après avoir reçu, 22 jours auparavant, la dose de 0,10 qui ne l'avait presque pas rendu malade, reçoit du même liquide la même dose de 0,10. Alors aussitôt, quelques secondes après que l'injection a été terminée, il est extrêmement malade : la respiration devient angoissée, haletante. Il peut à peine se trainer ; se couche sur le flanc, est pris de diarrhée et de vomissements sanguinolents. La sensibilité est abolie, et il meurt en vingt cinq minutes.

Or, chez des chiens non injectés antérieurement, des doses dix fois plus fortes, 1 cc. par Kilogramme, ne tuent pas les animaux avec cette même rapidité.

On ne peut assurément invoquer l'état défectueux de santé, au moins apparent, de l'animal. Car ces chiens anaphylactisés paraissent dans un état excellent. Leur poids a augmenté (après avoir baissé pendant la première semaine). Ils sont vifs, gais, le poil luisant, et on ne les distinguerait en rien des autres chiens normaux, non injectés.

On ne peut pas invoquer le fait de la non élimination du poison ; de sorte qu'il y aurait une action cumulative ; car, même en faisant la somme des quantités injectées, et en supposant, ce qui est absurde, qu'en 22 jours ou 15 jours il n'y a pas eu une seule parcelle de la toxine qui ait été éliminée, on ne peut pas expliquer ces effets foudroyants, intenses, que détermine l'injection de toxine chez des animaux sensibilisés.

Ainsi la chienne *Chloralosa,* qui n'avait reçu que 0,06, reçoit, 14 jours après, la dose de 0,10, et elle meurt en une heure et demie. Or les chiens qui reçoivent en une seule fois 0,16 ne meurent que tardivement, et quelquefois même survivent. Je n'ai jamais vu de mort déterminée en deux ou trois heures, chez des chiens intacts, par des doses d'actinotoxine inférieures à 1,5 (par Kilogramme).

L'hypothèse d'une rétention de la toxine avec accumulation dans l'organisme est d'autant plus improbable que, même au bout d'un très long temps, l'anaphylaxie se produit encore. Pour diverses raison, et surtout parce que je n'emploie plus l'extrait glycérique, mais la congestine pure, qui donne des résultats un peu différents, je n'ai pas fait beaucoup d'expériences sur des chiens ayant reçu la première injection plus de trois mois et demi auparavant. Mais, même au bout de trois mois et demi, il y a encore anaphylaxie.

Le 26 mai, on injecte cinq chiens à la dose de 0,22. (Par suite d'une lente altération l'extrait glycérique est moins actif, et la dose toxique différente de la dose toxique pour les animaux normaux). Quatre chiens neufs sont, le premier jour, à peine malades. Mais *Pierrette,* injectée 105 jours auparavant, et dont l'état de santé est florissant,
est tout de suite extrêmement malade. Pendant la durée même de l'injection elle fait
des efforts de vomissement. Détachée, elle tombe sur le flanc, paraplégique. La respiration est anxieuse, et, au bout de quinze minutes à peine, s'arrête. Le cœur bat mal. On
fait la respiration artificielle par compression du thorax ; mais le cœur cesse de battre.
La mort est survenue en moins de vingt cinq minutes (un peu plus de vingt minutes)
après le début de l'injection.

A l'autopsie il n'y a pas de caillots dans le cœur; mais une suffusion sanguine
considérable sous-endocardique dans le ventricule gauche. Rien au ventricule droit. L'estomac est rouge, violacé, avec une congestion intense. Le péritoine est hémorrhagié. Il
n'y a rien au cerveau.

Voici la marche des poids de l'animal, marche qui indique qu'il était dans un
excellent état de santé au 26 mai.

Le	16	janvier	12	K.	(Première injection de 0,05)
	27	»	11,2		
	10	février	11,3		(Seconde injection de 0,11)
	21	»	10,6		
	23	mars	13,0		
	26	mai	16,0		

Sur les quatre autres chiens injectés avec la même solution et à la même dose,
trois survivent ; un quatrième ne meurt que le septième jour.

Une autre expérience, qui devra être répétée, semble prouver que,
même au bout d'une année, l'anaphylaxie existe encore.

Le 12 février 1902, *Lubin,* chien loulou noir, reçoit 0,18 de toxine.

12	février	K.	7,3	
13	»		7,3	
18	»		7,0	
22	»		6,5	
4	mars		7,4	
9	mai		7,2	(seconde injection de 0,14)
16	»		7,0	
28	»		7,8	

Le 28 février 1903 il pèse 8 Kil. et l'état de santé est excellent. Alors on lui
injecte gr. 0,06 par Kil. de congestine (partie active du venin des actinies). Il meurt
en quinze minutes, avec asphyxie, vomissements, diarrhée sanguinolente. Le même jour
un autre chien de même poids reçoit la même dose de congestine, et meurt en quatre
heures et demie.

Dans ce cas évidemment la dose était trop forte, et pour *Lubin* et pour le chien témoin ; mais c'en est assez cependant pour prouver que même au bout de neuf mois il y a encore de l'anaphylaxie. Je poursuis en ce moment des expériences dans ce sens, afin de juger quel est le maximum de cette durée. J'ai lieu de croire qu'elle est beaucoup plus considérable qu'on ne serait tenté d'abord de le supposer.

Plus récemment j'ai fait l'expérience suivante. Cinq chiens recoivent des doses variables de congestine.

	Massillonne	0,032
	Mérovée	0,032
(le 24 Novembre 1903)	*Chilpéric*	0,042
	Dagobert	0,042
	Chapelaine	0,047

Les deux chiens anaphylactisés, *Massillonne* et *Chapelaine,* sont tout de suite extremement malades. Les trois autres chiens ont des vomissements, quelques défécations, mais ne paraissent pas dans un état grave. *Mérovée* meurt cependant au bout de cinq jours. *Chilpéric* et *Dagobert* survivent. Quant à *Massillonne* et *Chapelaine,* elles meurent quelques heures après l'injection. Or *Chapelaine* avait reçu l'injection anaphylactisante le 24 Juin, et *Massillonne* ver le 11 juin ; ce qui montre à quel point se prolongent les effets de l'anaphylaxie. — Ells n'étaient malades ni l'une ni l'autre. Le poids de *Massillonne* avait monté de 5,5 k. à 6,5 k. au 24 Novembre ; le poids de *Chapelaine,* de 5 k., à 5 k., n'avait pas changé.

Non seulement au bout d'un long temps l'anaphylaxie n'a pas disparu ; mais encore un certain temps est nécessaire pour qu'elle apparaisse ; car, si l'on fait la seconde injection deux ou trois jours après la première, on n'observe pas d'effet de toxicité augmentée, et les chiens se comportent comme des chiens normaux. Souvent j'ai injecté à des chiens des doses de 0,12 quelques jours après une première injection de 0,12, et je n'ai pas observé d'accidents.

A vrai dire je ne saurais préciser encore à quel moment l'anaphylaxie est à son maximum. C'est un point que je me propose d'étudier avec plus de détails lorsque j'aurai réussi à préparer à l'état sec l'élément actif du poison, ou *congestine*, débarrassé de son antitoxine, ou *thalassine* (*).

(*) Voyez sur les détails de préparation, que je ne puis pas aborder ici, le mémoire présenté à la *Société de Biologie de Paris*. De la thalassine considérée comme antitoxine cristallisée ; 25 juillet 1903, p. 1071-1073.

III. Des effets antitoxiques
parallèles aux effets anaphylactiques.

Ce qui complique singulièrement le problème, c'est que la puissance anaphylactique du venin des Actinies est associée à une autre action antagoniste qui produit l'immunité.

On a donc dans le même liquide deux effets tout opposés, dus probablement, ainsi que je le dirai tout à l'heure, à deux substances distinctes. Il y a immunité de l'animal d'une part, et d'autre part sensibilité plus grande ; *prophylaxie* et *anaphylaxie* tout à la fois.

Ce qui frappe d'abord dans les effets anaphylactiques, c'est leur soudaineté. A peine l'injection est elle terminée, comme nous l'avons vu pour *Neptune* et *Pierrette*, les accidents éclatent, formidables, irrésistibles.

Le 29 avril on injecte à 4 chiens les doses suivantes

Fracasse	0,15	anaphylactisé au 74e jour
Angélique	0,15	» au 72e jour
Hernani	0,20	chien témoin
Doña Sol	0,15	»

Hernani et *Doña Sol* sont à peine malades. *Hernani* est un peu engourdi et endormi. *Doña Sol* a des démangeaisons modérées et une soif vive; elle est à peine malade.

Au contraire, tout de suite après l'injection, *Fracasse* et *Angélique* sont mourants. *Fracasse*, une minute après l'injection, a des vomissements intenses. La respiration est difficile, anhélante, mêlée d'écume. Il s'étend sur le flanc, immobile et insensible, sans réactions ni réflexes. Il urine sous lui, et parait mourant. Un quart d'heure après l'injection, il se relève pour déféquer des matières liquides, muqueuses, sanguinolentes, avec un ténesme rectal intense. Il meurt trois heures et demie après l'injection.

Pour *Angélique* les symptômes sont les mêmes que pour *Fracasse*, aussi immédiats et aussi intenses. Une demi heure après l'injection, elle est mourante, sur le flanc, avec des tremblements demi-convulsifs et une diarrhée sanguinolente profuse ; ténesme rectal intense. Elle meurt dans la nuit, et n'a probablement survécu que quelques heures.

Les doses de 0,20 (pour *Hernani*, et 0,15 (pour *Doña Sol*) ont été cependant mortelles pour ces deux animaux; mais la mort n'est survenue que tardivement, de sorte que ce qui caractérise surtout l'anaphylaxie, c'est la soudaineté et la violence des accidents, plus que la diminution de la dose mortelle. Le 30 avril, *Doña Sol* parait bien portante. Son poids, de K. 5,4 le 24 avril, est de 5,0 le premier mai ; elle ne parait pas trop malade ; elle meurt le 4 mai. Quant à *Hernani*, qui avait reçu une dose plus forte que *Fracasse* et *Angélique,* le 30 avril, il est un peu engourdi, comme fatigué, mais ne parait pas malade. Le premier mai cependant il est assez malade, titubant, ne mangeant plus, ayant une soif très vive (T=37°,5). Le 2 mai il est mourant, inerte, et il meurt dans la nuit du 2 ou 3 mai.

L'expérience la plus caractéristique est la suivante. Le 21 mars 1902 on injecte quatre chiens, dont deux témoins et deux injectés antérieurement.

Gorgibus	chien témoin	0,13
Don Luis	»	0,15
Arlequine	injectée 4 fois	0,11
Colombine	»	0,14

Immédiatement après l'injection *Arlequine* et *Colombine* sont extrêmement malades, et de la même manière. Elles sont couchées par terre, ne se relevant que pour défécations sanglantes, avec ténesme rectal intense, et vomissements réitérés. Au contraire *Gorgibus* et *Don Luis* sont à peine malades. *Gorgibus* n'a que des démangeaisons sans vomissements. *Don Luis,* après une courte période de vomissements alimentaires, parait tranquille et nullement malade. Mais, malgré cette apparente immunité, *Don Luis* et *Gorgibus* meurent les jours suivants (*Don Luis* le quatrième jour ; *Gorgibus* le neuvième jour). Quant à *Arlequine* et à *Colombine, Arlequine* meurt au bout de quatre heures ; mais *Colombine* survit.

Voici encore un autre cas dans lequel il y a eu à la fois anaphylaxie et prophylaxie.

Deux chiens, *Argante* et *Anemonio,* ont reçu des injections antérieures (non pas tout à fait de l'extrait glycérique, mais d'un virus actinique un peu diversement préparé ; (*Argante,* 67 jours auparavant ; *Anemonio,* 58 jours auparavant). Ils reçoivent les mêmes doses 0,15 du même liquide qui a été injecté à *Fracasse* et *Angélique, Doña Sol* et *Hernani*; mais le 30 avril au lieu du 29 avril. Ils sont tout de suite très malades. *Argante,* immédiatement après l'injection, est comme foudroyé. Insensibilité presque complète. Il tombe sur le flanc. Défécation, diarrhée, ténesme. Il n'a pas la force de se traîner, et va sous lui. L'urine, les vomissements et la défécation se mélangent. Dix minutes après l'injection, il est mourant. Cependant il se relève en titubant, dans une attitude de demi hypnose et de demi contracture. Le lendemain il est à peine malade. (30 avril, K.13,5 — 2 mai, K. 12,8 — 6 mai, K. 12,3 — 16 mai, K. 13,0) finalement il survit. *Anemonio* est presque aussi malade qu'*Argante*. Il tombe sur le flanc, immédiatement après l'injection. Respiration anhélante, difficile. Mais il survit.

Ainsi, voici deux chiens dont l'état a été tout de suite absolument grave, mais qui se sont remis, alors que *Doña Sol* et *Hernani,* qui avaient reçu la même dose de toxine et qui n'étaient presque pas malades, sont morts. *Argante* et *Anemonio* étaient *anaphylactisés,* ce qui est évident par l'intensité et la soudaineté des accidents immédiats ; mais ils étaient aussi *prophylactisés,* comme cela apparait par leur survie.

Avant de tenter l'explication de ces faits, d'apparence paradoxale, je dois mentionner une autre expérience, dans laquelle il est prouvé que des doses différentes ont une même action anaphylactique, mais n'ont pas la même action prophylactique.

Le 15 mai on injecte à trois chiens témoins (*) 0,15 d'actinotoxine pour chacun, et 0,15 aussi à deux chiens ; *Caro,* ayant reçu antérieurement le 30 avril 0,15 d'actinotoxine, et *Bassette,* ayant reçu le 15 avril 0,10 d'actinotoxine. *Caro* et *Bassette* sont tout de suite très malades, tandis que les trois autres, sauf quelques vomissements, paraissent indemnes. *Caro* tombe sur le flanc, vomit, est presque insensible, et ne peut se relever. *Bassette* est encore plus malade ; elle est mourante, respirant à peine, si bien qu'on peut la croire morte. Cependant, un quart d'heure après l'injection, elle se relève avec diarrhée profuse, sanguinolente, et ténesme rectal. Elle meurt dans la nuit. Au contraire *Caro* survit ; et on peut se demander si, après ces effets anaphylactiques éclatants, la survie ne serait pas due à ce que la dose antérieure d'actinotoxine a été plus forte pour lui que pour *Bassette*. Peut être est ce aussi dû à un intervalle de temps moins considérable ; trente jours d'anaphylaxie pour *Bassette,* et quinze jours pour *Caro*.

IV. CONCLUSIONS ET THÉORIE.

Il n'est pas difficile d'expliquer le double effet, anaphylactique et prophylactique de la toxine actinienne, si l'on suppose que les tentacules des Actinies cèdent à la glycérine deux poisons différents ; l'un anaphylactique, l'autre, prophylactique.

J'ai été assez heureux pour séparer ces deux poisons et reconnaître à l'un et à l'autre des propriétés chimiques et physiologiques très différentes. Les physiologistes auraient probablement, bien avant moi, réussi à faire cette même séparation pour les autres virus et venins, s'ils avaient eu à leur disposition des quantités suffisantes ; mais je ne sache pas qu'on ait eu encore 40 Kilogrammes d'un venin (dans la glycérine) assez actif pour tuer un chien à la dose de cc. 0,05 par Kilogrs. Aussi suis-je convaincu que, jusque à présent, on ne possède pas de produit plus avantageux que le virus des Actinies pour faire l'étude méthodique des venins.

Les deux substances qui s'y trouvent (parmi plusieurs autres que je n'ai pas réussi à isoler) sont la *thalassine* et la *congestine*.

(*) Deux de ces chiens témoins avaient antérieurement reçu en injection un liquide organique, que nous savons maintenant être inactif (corps des *Velella*) (cœlentéré) — *Loustica* et *Jaunet*.

La *thalassine,* que j'ai pu extraire cristallisée, est une amine complexe, soluble dans l'alcool à 60 o/o; insoluble dans l'alcool absolu, résistant à l'ébullition, assez peu toxique, mais provoquant, à la très faible dose de 0,0003 par Kil. des démangeaisons intenses, quelquefois même, chez certains chiens sensibles, elle agit à la dose de 0,0001 par Kil. Elle est *prophylactique ;* c'est à dire qu'elle confère aux animaux une immunité relative. Elle contient 10 o/o d'azote.

La *congestine,* insoluble dans l'alcool à 50 o/o, est détruite par la chaleur. C'est une albumine qui a les réactions des albumines (16 o/o d'azote). Injectée à des chiens, elle tue à la dose de 0,008 (environ) par Kilogr. et provoque des congestions intenses de tout l'appareil vasculaire intestinal. C'est très probablement la substance qui produit l'anaphylaxie.

Nous avons donc dans le virus des Actinies à la fois la toxine (c'est à dire la *congestine*) et l'antitoxine (c'est à dire la *thalassine*).

Il est inutile, semble-t-il, d'insister sur l'importance de ce fait; car jusque à présent on n'avait pas pu obtenir d'antitoxine cristallisée; et, malgré tous les travaux faits sur les propriétés des antitoxines, il est permis de dire qu'on n'en avait jamais vu encore.

Peut être alors, quand on aura chimiquement séparé la toxine de l'antitoxine, pourra-t-on constater dans toutes les toxines des effets nettement anaphylactiques ; car, tant que l'antitoxine est mélangée à la toxine, c'est un mélange de deux actions antagonistes qu'on observe.

Quant à l'explication de l'anaphylaxie, elle n'est probablement pas simple. Pour le moment nous devons nous borner à en constater les modalités, sans oser en donner une explication satisfaisante. Deux mois ou trois mois après l'injection d'un virus, l'organisme est devenu sans défense. L'injection antérieure a modifié les cellules nerveuses de telle sorte qu'elles ne peuvent plus résister à l'action de ce même poison, précédemment presque inoffensif. Comment cette sensibilité est elle survenue ? Est ce par la destruction d'une antitoxine naturelle existant à l'état normal dans la cellule ? Est ce par la production de substances qui forment avec la toxine des combinaisons très toxiques ? Est ce, comme cela est plus vraisemblable, par un autre mécanisme encore inconnu ? Voilà ce que nous ne savons pas.

Il est inutile d'essayer l'explication par une néphrite; d'abord parce que les animaux anaphylactisés n'ont pas d'albumine dans l'urine; ensuite parce que la sondaineté des accidents est telle — survenant quelques minutes après l'injection — que la non élimination par les reins n'explique par du tout pourquoi en quelques minutes le système nerveux a été si profondément intoxiqué.

A vrai dire, quoique l'anaphylaxie soit un phénomène nouveau qui n'avait pas encore été dénommé ni décrit ; il faut sans doute la rattacher à un fait très connu, étudié en tous ses détails, à savoir l'étrange propriété de la tuberculine, qui, injectée à des animaux sains, est sans effet, alors qu'elle tue rapidement les animaux tuberculeux. En réalité les animaux tuberculeux sont anaphylactisés contre la tuberculine.

Il y avait donc lieu de mettre bien en relief cette propriété des venins d'exalter la sensibilité organique, quel que soit le mécanisme de cette sensibilité accrue.

Ring J (ed): Anaphylaxis. Chem Immunol Allergy. Basel, Karger, 2010, vol 95, pp 1–11

History and Classification of Anaphylaxis

Johannes Ring · Heidrun Behrendt · Alain de Weck

Department of Dermatology and Allergy Biederstein, ZAUM – Zentrum Allergie und Umwelt, Helmholtz Zentrum München/Technische Universität München, Munich, Germany, and Universidad de Navarra, Pamplona, Spain

Abstract

Anaphylaxis as the maximal variant of an acute systemic hypersensitivity reaction can involve several organ systems, particularly the skin, respiratory tract, gastrointestinal tract and the cardiovascular system. The severity of anaphylactic reaction is variable and can be classified into severity grades I–IV. Some reactions are fatal. Most frequent elicitors of anaphylaxis are foods in childhood, later insect stings and drugs. The phenomenon itself has been described in ancient medical literature, but was actually recognized and named at the beginning of the 20th century by Charles Richet and Paul Portier. In the course of experiments starting on the yacht of the Prince of Monaco and continued in the laboratory in Paris, they tried to immunize dogs with extracts of *Physalia* species in an attempt to develop an antitoxin to the venom of the Portuguese man-of-war. While Charles Richet believed that anaphylaxis was a 'lack of protection', it has become clear that an exaggerated immune reaction, especially involving immunoglobulin E antibodies, is the underlying pathomechanism in allergic anaphylaxis besides immune complex reactions. Non-immunologically mediated reactions leading to similar clinical symptomatology have been called 'anaphylactoid' or 'pseudo-allergic' – especially by Paul Kallos – and are now called 'non-immune anaphylaxis' according to a consensus of the World Allergy Organization (WAO). The distinction of different pathophysiological processes is important since non-immune anaphylaxis cannot be detected by skin test or in vitro allergy diagnostic procedures. History and provocation tests are crucial. The intensity of the reaction is not only influenced by the degree of sensitization but also by concomitant other factors as age, simultaneous exposure to other allergens, underlying infection, physical exercise or psychological stress or concomitant medication (e.g. β-blockers, NSAIDs); this phenomenon has been called *augmentation* or *summation anaphylaxis*.

In spite of the dramatic increase in prevalence of allergic diseases over the last decades, allergy is often not taken seriously because symptoms of e.g. hay fever are regarded as 'mild' or 'bagatelle' in the general public. This rather superficial opinion has to be contradicted not only due to the serious impairment in quality of life going along with many allergic diseases, but also with regard to mortality due to severe respiratory disease and a variety of life-threatening emergencies in allergy like fatal asthma attack, laryngeal edema, severe serum sickness with vasculitis and nephritis, bullous

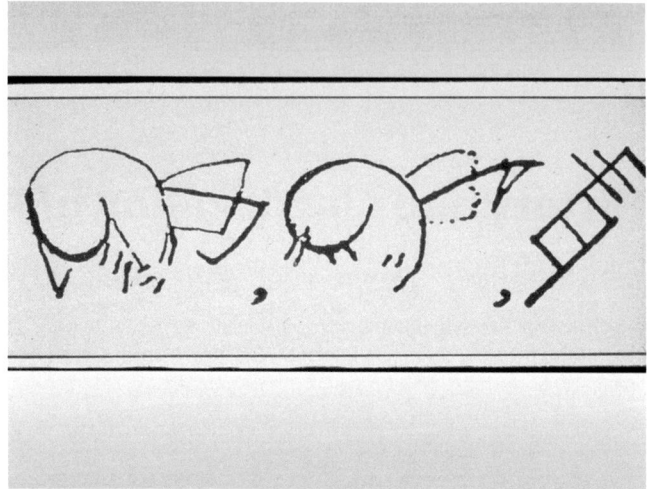

Fig. 1. Hieroglyph from the tomb of pharaoh Menes showing the sting of a 'kheb' wasp or hornet (Arenberg et al. [1]).

drug eruptions like toxic epidermal necrolysis or anaphylaxis, which undoubtedly represents the most acute life-threatening condition in allergy [2, 3, 13, 21, 31, 38].

History

The phenomenon of anaphylaxis itself is old and has been described in ancient Greek and Chinese medical literature, mostly in connection with the consumption of certain foods which was called 'idiosyncrasy' by Hippocrates or has been mentioned by Titus Aurelius Lucretius in his famous Opus *De natura rerum: Quod ali cibus est, aliis fuat acre venenum* [see 36]. The first documented anaphylactic patient might have suffered from Hymenoptera venom anaphylaxis as we can read in hieroglyphs from the tomb of pharaoh Menes in old Egypt, who supposedly died in 2641 BC on a journey in the Atlantic Ocean trying to get ashore on an island when he was stung by a 'kheb', an insect that was most likely a wasp, a hornet or honeybee (fig. 1) [41]. It has to be mentioned that there is a controversy whether the hieroglyph actually shows a hippopotamus and not a wasp [47].

The first description of an unusual reaction to bee stings can be found in a Latin article by Udalricus Staudigelius (Ulrich Staudigl), a Benedictine monk in the monastery Andechs in Bavaria, who in 1699 described long-lasting severe local reactions after bee stings which recurred after some weeks (*De curiosis post apum ictus symptomatibus*). The history of insect sting allergy has been described in a very acribic article by Ulrich Müller [*Allergo Journal* 2009;18:342–352]. The first medical case description of actual insect sting anaphylaxis comes from France by Dr. Desbrest in 1765, when a 30-year-old villager was stung during gardening by a bee in the eyelid; he collapsed and died

2   Ring · Behrendt · de Weck

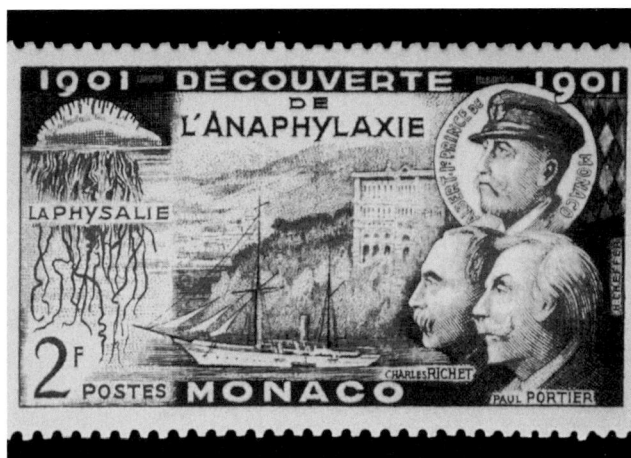

Fig. 2. Stamp from the Principality of Monaco celebrating 100 years anaphylaxis discovery.

soon thereafter. There were several case reports in the 19th century of fatal insect sting reactions in Europe and the USA [13]. The first description of experimental anaphylaxis seems to be that of François Magendie [23] who described in 1839 that rabbits injected with egg albumin often died after the second or third injection. Generally, these reactions were regarded as 'toxic' and attributed to poison of animals.

This was also the motive and opinion of Charles Richet and Paul Portier when they did their classical experiments in 1901 on the yacht 'Princess Alice II' of the Prince of Monaco and later on in the laboratory in Paris (fig. 2). Richet, who was professor of physiology and had done research in several areas including psychosomatic medicine, pulmonology and infectious diseases, had been invited by Prince Albert I of Monaco to join a cruise to the Cape Verde Islands and was accompanied by the assistant Paul Portier. They tried to isolate the toxin from actinia extracts, especially found in the tentacles of *Physalia physalis*, the Portuguese man-of-war. They immunized some pigeons and dogs either with the toxin attenuated by heat or with non-lethal smaller doses of toxin. After certain periods of incubation (one to several weeks) another injection was administered using a stronger dose in order to see whether the animal was immunized (i.e. should tolerate the toxin). The opposite occurred and was described very precisely in the 1902 notebook of Paul Portier when the dog 'Neptune' who had received a dose of 0.05 cc/kg of actinotoxin on January 14, and 0.1 cc/kg on January 22 with minor symptoms of itching and some 'dyspnoea' received 0.12 cc/kg on February 10. Already some seconds after the injection, the animal became very sick, the respiration gasping, the animal produced vomiting of mucus and blood, bloody defecation, stupor and died within 25 min. Richet, when notified by Portier, recognized immediately that this surprising phenomenon was new (*'C'est un phénomène nouveau, il faut le baptiser!'*). In trying to find a name, he wanted to express 'lack of protection' and should have used 'aphylaxis' (Greek α privativum = negation);

however, for euphonic and rhythmic reasons, he preferred 'anaphylaxis' [33], a term which rapidly spread all over the world. For its description, Richet won the Nobel Prize in 1913, although he still believed it to be a condition of 'lack of protection' against a poison. However, Richet humbly wrote in his Nobel award address: 'The discovery of anaphylaxis is not at all the result of deep thinking but of simple observation, almost accidental. It had no other merit than that of not refusing to see the facts which presented themselves before me completely evident' [41].

This discovery, describing an obvious disadvantage through immunization – since earlier immunization was only connected with a positive and desired effect of protection against pathogenic organisms by Louis Pasteur, Robert Koch or E. von Behring – subsequently led to the creation of the term 'allergy' by Clemens Freiherr von Pirquet in 1906 [29].

Later on, researchers realized that similar symptoms can be elicited in animals not immunized or by the injection of histamine and were called 'anaphylactoid reactions' (Behring 1916, Hanzlik 1920, Lorenz 1977 [quoted in 36]).

The direct histamine release evoked by several substances (e.g. codeine, dextran in certain rat strains or gelatine blood substitutes) led to the development of the concept of 'pseudo-allergic reactions' by Paul Kallos [10].

Only at the beginning of the 21st century a consensus of several task forces in Europe and in the World Allergy Organization (WAO) came to the new nomenclature, where anaphylaxis is defined by the clinical symptomatology independent of the pathophysiology; so, we have to distinguish between an allergic anaphylaxis and a non-immune anaphylaxis (formerly pseudo-allergic reaction) [18].

Pathophysiology of Anaphylaxis

After the discovery by Prausnitz and Küstner in 1921 that the individual hypersensitivity, namely an allergic reaction to fish, could be transferred by serum from one individual into another non-allergic individual [39], this activity in the serum was called reagin and in the 1960s characterized as immunoglobulin E antibodies by the groups of K. and T. Ishizaka in Baltimore and Johansson and Bennich in Uppsala [41]. IgE-mediated anaphylaxis is the major pathomechanism of allergic anaphylaxis. It has been shown that bridging of IgE molecules by bi- or plurivalent allergens (two or more IgE-binding epitopes per molecule) on the surface of basophils and mast cells is the triggering event in anaphylaxis. In the case of drugs and chemical elicitors of anaphylaxis, apparently univalent elicitors are, however, also encountered [9].

There are also other immunological mechanisms, especially via IgG or IgM antibodies with immune complex formation, which can lead to similar clinical conditions [20, 34, 42] as has been shown in dextran anaphylaxis (table 1). Triggering of mast cells and basophils leads to release of various vasoactive mediators, among which histamine was the first recognized in 1908 (fig. 3, 4) [6].

Table 1. Pathophysiology of anaphylactic reactions

Immunoglobulin E-mediated (type I)

IgG or IgM immune complex reaction

Non-immune hypersensitivity via direct mediator release or direct activation of plasma-protein systems

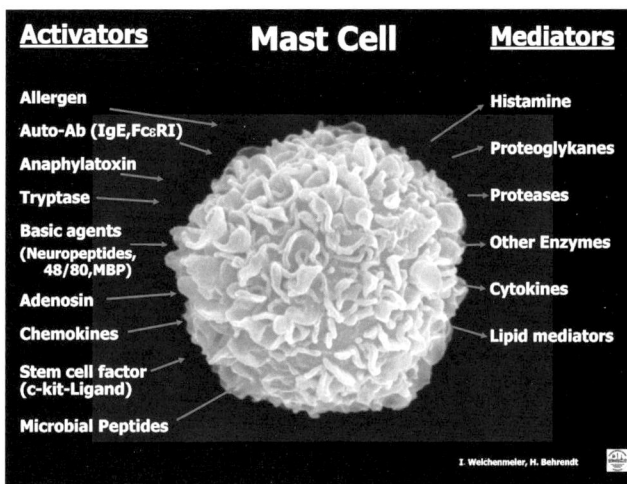

Fig. 3. Mast cell in different stages of secretion (from Heidrun Behrendt).

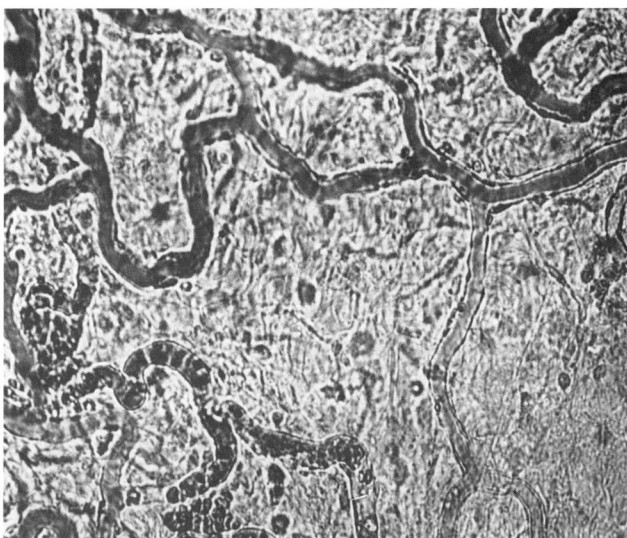

Fig. 4. Microcirculatory stasis in the rabbit omentum during anaphylactic shock (from [11]).

Table 2. Prevalence of symptoms in anaphylactic reactions according to Przybilla and Rueff [see 18]. A meta-analysis of 1,865 cases from 14 publications (Liebermann) and 865 own patients with insect venom anaphylaxis

Symptom	Percentage
Urticaria, angioedema	85–90
Flush	45–55
Dyspnea, wheezing	45–50
Swelling of upper airways	50–60
Vertigo, syncope, hypotension	30–35
Nausea, vomitus, diarrhea, cramps	25–30
Loss of conscience	22
Rhinitis	15–20
Headache	5–8
Substernal pain	4–6
Pruritus on unaltered skin	2–5
Cerebral cramps	1–2

Apart from this clear-cut immunologically mediated pattern, other mechanisms leading to release of vasoactive mediators or activation of relevant plasma protein systems (coagulation, complement, kallikrein-kinin) can elicit anaphylaxis-like or pseudo-allergic symptoms [10, 11, 36]. It always has to be kept in mind that the term 'pseudo-allergic' or 'non-immune' anaphylaxis is negatively defined, that means that it is not possible to detect immunological sensitization in the serum or at the cellular level or in the skin test. Possibly, with advanced technology these reactions may be turned from pseudo-allergic into true allergic reactions when the detection of sensitization may be successful.

Clinical Symptomatology

Anaphylaxis most commonly starts with symptoms on the skin or the respiratory tract (table 2). The symptomatology is variable; there is no obligatory involvement of all organ systems. A major characteristic of anaphylaxis is the rather rapid onset of symptoms after contact with the elicitor. The interval varies between a few seconds or minutes until 1 or 2 h, partly dependent upon the route of application (rapid onset after intravenous allergen exposure) and degree of sensitization. Experience in insect sting anaphylaxis in

Table 3. Classification of anaphylactic reactions according to severity of clinical symptoms [35]

Grade	Symptoms			
	skin	abdominal	respiratory	cardiovascular
I	pruritus flush urticaria angioedema			
II	pruritus flush urticaria angioedema (not mandatory)	nausea cramping	rhinorrhea hoarseness dyspnea	tachycardia (Δ >20 beats/min) blood pressure change (Δ >20 mm Hg systolic) arrhythmia
III	pruritus flush Urticaria angioedema (not mandatory)	vomiting defecation diarrhea	laryngeal edema bronchospasm cyanosis	shock
IV	pruritus flush urticaria angioedema (not mandatory)	vomiting defecation diarrhea	respiratory arrest	cardiac arrest

over 800 patients shows that 90% of symptoms start within the first 30 min and the more rapidly the symptoms occur, the more severe the reaction will end [31, 48].

According to the different intensity of clinical symptoms, several attempts have been made to classify anaphylaxis according to severity, the most common scales have been published by Mueller [26] and Ring and Messmer [35] (table 3).

Symptoms of anaphylaxis comprise mainly: (1) The skin (itch, flush, urticaria, angioedema) and the neighbouring mucous membranes. Itchy palms, paresthesias in the pharynx or genital mucosa are often the first symptoms. (2) The respiratory tract (sneezing, rhinorrhea, hoarseness, dysphonia, laryngeal edema, cough, bronchospasm, respiratory arrest). (3) Abdominal symptoms (nausea, cramps, vomitus, defecation, also miction and uterus cramps occur). (4) Cardiovascular symptoms (tachycardia, blood pressure changes – not necessarily hypotension, but also transient-type hypertension has been observed as first symptom – arrhythmia, shock, cardiac arrest). Primary cardiac manifestation in anaphylaxis has been observed as measured by ECG changes (T-flattening, supraventricular arrhythmia, AV block) and marked changes of central venous pressure are common. During anaphylaxis, myocardial infarction may occur [5, 7, 24, 30, 45, 49].

Prodromi of anaphylaxis comprise metallic 'fishy' taste, anxiety, sweating, headache, disorientation. Autopsy cases have shown few specific findings; sometimes there is inflation of the lung and pulmonary edema with peribronchial eosinophilic

Table 4. Differential diagnosis of anaphylactic reactions (according to Przybilla)

Cardiovascular disease
Vagovasal syncope
Other forms of shock (hemorrhagic, cardiogenic, septic)
Cardiac arrhythmia
Hypertonic crisis
Pulmonary embolus
Capillary leak syndrome

Neuropsychiatric diseases
Hyperventilation
Panic fear attacks
Globus hystericus
Anaphylaxis factitia
Hoigné syndrome
Epileptic cramps
Apoplectic insult
Other conditions of coma in patients with loss of consciousness (metabolic, traumatic)

Respiratory disease
Vocal cord dysfunction
Foreign body or tumor in tracheal or bronchial obstruction

Intoxication
Scombroid fish poisoning
Drugs
Alcohol or substances with disulfiram effect (e.g. mushrooms, griseofulvin, sulfonyl urea)

Pathological mediator secretion
Mastocytosis
Mast cell or basophil leukemia
Carcinoid syndrome
Thyroid carcinoma
Pheochromocytoma

Hereditary angioneurotic edema with C1 esterase inhibitor

---

infiltrates. Hemorrhage in the gastric mucosa as well as hepatosplenomegaly are sometimes reported [31, 49]. In immune complex anaphylaxis fibrinoid deposits in the lung have been observed [42]. Differential diagnosis of anaphylaxis includes a variety of conditions shown in table 4. Usually, the symptoms of anaphylaxis disappear within hours [12], however protracted courses or biphasic courses have been reported (a second wave of symptoms after 6–20 h) [44].

Fatal anaphylaxis occurs mostly due to bronchial obstruction or cardiac arrest, but also disseminated intervascular coagulation as well as adrenalin overdose [2, 7, 21, 31]. When anaphylactic reactions are survived, long-lasting sequels are rare. However,

Table 5. Elicitors of anaphylactic reactions

Drugs (all forms!)
Foods
Additives
Insect venoms
Occupational agents (e.g. latex)
Aeroallergens
Contact urticariogens
Seminal fluid
Echinococcal cysts
Cold, heat, UV radiation
Exercise
Summation (infection, stress, exercise, other allergen concomitant exposure, medication as β-blockers, NSAIDs, ACE inhibitors)
Idiopathic (?)

morbidity can result from myocardial or cerebral infarction or venous thrombosis [27]; anaphylaxis during pregnancy can lead to death or damage of the newborn.

Management of Anaphylaxis

Regarding the management of anaphylaxis, differentiation should be made between the acute treatment of an anaphylactic reaction [see chapter by Ring et al., section: Treatment and Prevention, p. 201] and the management of a patient who has undergone an anaphylactic episode.

All patients who have survived an anaphylaxis have to undergo allergy diagnosis! Three aspects have to be considered in the diagnostic procedure: (1) determination of the eliciting agent; (2) description of the relevant pathomechanism (e.g. IgE or non-immune), and (3) offering of a compatible alternative (especially with drug allergy).

Allergens and Elicitors

Another way to classify anaphylactic reactions regards the eliciting agents; the most common elicitors of anaphylaxis are drugs, insect venoms, foods, additives, aeroallergens (table 5). The spectrum of elicitors is very broad, e.g. anaphylaxis has been described to ethanol [cf. 36]. In a recent large series of 601 US patients, food was considered the cause in 22% and drugs in 11% but in most cases the cause of anaphylaxis remained undetermined [48]. Epidemiological reviews indicate that penicillins [17] and insect stings are still the most frequent causes of anaphylaxis [28]. Rare cases of passive transfer by IgE antibodies via blood transfusion have been described as well as attempted suicide (penicillin-allergic nurse). In belletristic literature, murder attempts by eliciting anaphylaxis can be found. Also a psychosomatic condition 'anaphylaxis factitia' exists in the sense of Münchhausen's syndrome. When no elicitor can be found, the term 'idiopathic' anaphylaxis is used [2, 16, 35, 40, 50].

The route of application can be either by oral intake, parenterally or via the air or direct skin contact (contact anaphylaxis) [37]. In spite of great progress in experimental and clinical allergology, anaphylaxis still represents a major problem both for researchers and clinicians.

References

1 Arenberg KM, Harper DS, Larsson BL: Footnotes on allergy. Uppsala, Pharmacia AB, 1980.
2 Barnard JH: Studies of 400 Hymenoptera sting deaths in the United States. J Allergy Clin Immunol 1973;52:259–264.
3 Bochner BS, Lichtenstein LM: Anaphylaxis. N Engl J Med 1991;324:81–88.
4 Brockow K, Kiehn M, Riethmüller C, Vieluf D, Berger J, Ring J: Efficacy of antihistamine pretreatment in the prevention of adverse reactions to Hymenoptera venom immunotherapy: a prospective randomized placebo-controlled trial. J Allergy Clin Immunol 1997;100:458–463.
5 Capurro N, Levi R: The heart as target organ in systemic allergic reactions. Circ Res 1975;36:520–528.
6 Dale HH, Laidlaw PP: The physiological action of β-imidazolethylamine. J Physiol 1910;41:318–344.
7 Delage C, Irey HC: Anaphylactic deaths: a clinico-pathologic study of 43 cases. J Forens Sci 1972;17:525.
8 De Soto H, Turk P: Cimetidine in anaphylactic shock refractory to standard therapy. Anesth Analg 1989;69:264–265.
9 De Weck AL: Immunochemical particularities of anaphylactic reactions to compounds used in anesthesia. Ann Fr Anesth Réanim 1993;12:126–130.
10 Dukor P, Kallos P, Schlumberger HD, West GB (eds): Pseudo-Allergic Reactions. Basel, Karger, 1980, vol 1–3.
11 Endrich B, Ring J, Intaglietta M: Effects of radiopaque contrast media on the microcirculation of the rabbit omentum. Radiology 1979;132:331–339.

12 Fisher MMD: Clinical observations on the pathophysiology and treatment of anaphylactic cardiovascular collapse. Anesth Intensive Care 1986;17:17–21.
13 Galli S (ed): Anaphylaxis. Novartis Foundation Symposium 157. Chichester, Wiley, 2004.
14 Gronemeyer W: Noradrenalin statt Adrenalin beim anaphylaktischen Schock. Dtsch Med Wochenschr 1980;102:101.
15 Hannaway PJ, Hoppler GDK: Severe anaphylaxis and drug induced β-blockage. N Engl J Med 1983;308:1536.
16 Hermann K, Ring J: The renin-angiotensin system in patients with repeated anaphylactic reactions during Hymenoptera venom hyposensitization and sting challenge. Int Arch Allergy Immunol 1997;11:251–256.
17 Idsoe O, Guthe T, Willcox RR, de Weck AL: Nature and extent of penicillin side-reactions, with particular reference to fatalities from anaphylactic shock. Bull World Health Organ 1968;38:159–188.
18 Johansson SGO, Bieber T, Dahl R, Friedmann PS, Lanier BQ, Lockey RF, Motala C, Martell JAO, Platts-Mills TAE, Ring J, Thien F, Cauwenberge PV, Williams HC: Revised nomenclature for allergy for global use: report of the nomenclature review committee of the World Allergy Organization. J Allergy Clin Immunol 2004;113:832–836.
19 Kleinhans D: Anstrengungs-induzierte Urtikaria und Anaphylaxie. Med Klin 1987;82:103–104.
20 Laubenthal H: Dextrananaphylaxie, Pathomechanismus und Prophylaxe. Ergebnisse einer multizentrischen Studie. Berlin, Springer, 1986.

21 Lockey RF, Benedict LM, Turkeltaub TB, Bukantz SC: Fatalities from immunotherapy and skin testing. J Allergy Clin Immunol 1987;79:666–677.

22 Lorenz W, Doenicke A, Dittmann I, Hug P, Schwarz B: Anaphylaktoide Reaktionen nach Applikation von Blutersatzmitteln beim Menschen. Verhinderung dieser Nebenwirkung von Haemacccel durch Praemedikation mit H_1- und H_2-Antagonisten. Anaesthesist 1977;26:644.

23 Magendie F: Lectures on the blood and on the changes it undergoes during disease. Philadelphia, Harrington, Barungton & Haswell, 1839.

24 Marone G, Patelle V, de Crescanzo A, et al: Human heart mast cells in anaphylaxis and cardiovascular disease. Int Arch Allergy Immunol 1995;107:72–75.

25 Maulitz RM, Pratt DS, Schocket AL: Exercise-induced anaphylactic reaction to shellfish. J Allergy Clin Immunol 1979;63:433.

26 Mueller HL: Diagnosis and treatment of insect sensitivity. J Asthma Res 1966;3:331–333.

27 Müller U: Geschichte der Insektenstichallergie. Allergo J 2009;18:342–352.

28 Neugut AL, Ghatak AT, Miller RL Anaphylaxis in the United States: an investigation into the epidemiology. Arch Intern Med 2001;161:15–21.

29 Von Pirquet C: Allergie. Münch Med Wschr 1906; 30:1457.

30 Pavek K, Wegmann A, Nordström L, Schwander D: Cardiovascular and respiratory mechanisms in anaphylactic and anaphylactoid shock reactions. Klin Wochenschr 1982;60:941–947.

31 Pumphrey RS: Lessons for management of anaphylaxis from a study of fatal reactions. Clin Exp Allergy 2000;30:1144–1150.

32 Ludolph-Hauser D, Ruëff F, Przybilla B: Diagnose und Differentialdiagnose der Anaphylaxie; in Schultze-Werninghaus G, Fuchs T, Bachert C, Wahn U (eds): Manuale allergologicum, 3. Aufl., München, Dustri, 2008, pp 669–685.

33 Richet C: De l'anaphylaxie ou sensibilité croissante des organismes à des doses successives de poison. Arch Fisiol 1904;1:129.

34 Richter W, Hedin H, Ring J, Kraft D, Messmer K: Anaphylaktoide Reaktionen nach Dextran I. Immunologische Grundlagen und klinische Befunde. Allergologie 1980;3:9.

35 Ring J, Messmer K: Incidence and severity of anaphylactoid reactions to colloid volume substitutes. Lancet 1977;i:466–468.

36 Ring J: Allergy in Practice. Berlin, Springer, 2005.

37 Ring J, Galosi A, Przybilla B: Contact anaphylaxis from emulgade F. Contact Derm 1986;15:49–40.

38 Ring J, Behrendt H: Anaphylaxis and anaphylactoid reactions. Classification and pathophysiology. Clin Rev Allergy Immunol 1999;17:387–399.

39 Schadewaldt H: Geschichte der Allergie, vol 1–4. München, Dustri, 1979–1982.

40 Sheffer AL, Austen KF: Exercise-induced anaphylaxis. J Allergy Clin Immunol 1980;66:106.

41 Simons FER (ed): Ancestors of Allergy. New York, Global Medical Communications, 1994.

42 Smedegard G, Revenäs B, Arfors KE: Anaphylaxis in the monkey: hemodynamics and blood flow distribution. Acta Physiol Scand 1979;106:191.

43 Smith PL, Kagey-Sobotka A, Blecker ER, Traystman R, Kaplan AP, Gralink H, Valentine MD, Permut S, Lichtenstein LM: Physiologic manifestations of human anaphylaxis. J Clin Invest 1980;60:1072.

44 Stark BJ, Sullivan TJ: Biphasic and protracted anaphylaxis. J Allergy Clin Immunol 1986;78:76–83.

45 Sullivan TJ: Cardiac disorders in penicillin-induced anaphylaxis: association with intravenous epinephrine therapy. JAMA 1982;248:2161.

46 Tryba M, Ahnefeld FW, Barth J, Dick W, Doenicke A, Fuchs T, Gervais H, Laubenthal H, Löllgen H, Lorenz W, Mehrkens HH, Meuret GH, Möllmann H, Piepenbrock S, Przybilla B, Ring J, Schmutzler W, Schultze-Werninghaus G, Schüttler J, Schuster JP, Sefrin P, Zander J, Zenz M: Akuttherapie anaphylaktoider Reaktionen. Ergebnisse einer interdisziplinären Konsensuskonferenz. Allergo J 1994;3:211–222.

47 Wadell LA: Egyptian Civilization. London, Luzac, 1930.

48 Webb LM, Lieberman P: Anaphylaxis: a review of 601 cases. Ann Allergy Asthma Immunol 2006;97:39–43.

49 Wegmann A, Reuker H, Pavek K, Schwander D: Katecholamintherapie und Herzrhythmusstörungen im anaphylaktischen und anaphylaktoiden Schock. Anaesthesist 1983;32(suppl):320.

50 Wiggins CA, Dykowicz MS, Patterson R: Idiopathic anaphylaxis. Classification, evaluation and treatment of 123 patients. J Allergy Clin Immunol 1988; 82:849–855.

Univ.-Prof. Dr. med. Dr. phil. Johannes Ring
Klinik und Poliklinik für Dermatologie und Allergologie am Biederstein
Klinikum rechts der Isar der Technischen Universität München
Biedersteiner Strasse 29, DE–80802 Munich (Germany)
Tel. +49 89 4140 3170/3217, Fax +49 89 4140 3171, E-Mail johannes.ring@lrz.tum.de

Ring J (ed): Anaphylaxis. Chem Immunol Allergy. Basel, Karger, 2010, vol 95, pp 12–21

Epidemiology of Anaphylaxis

Margitta Worm

Allergie-Centrum-Charité, Klinik für Dermatologie und Allergologie, Berlin, Germany

Abstract

Anaphylaxis is the most severe manifestation of a mast cell-dependent reaction. It is a rare disease and most recent data indicates a continuous increase of affected individuals. Limitations regarding the incidence of anaphylaxis are the lack of a unique definition and the fact that patients are often seen by different medical specialties (e.g. emergency doctors, allergists or other clinicians). However, based on the published data it can be summarized that the most frequent causes of anaphylaxis are food, venom and drugs, and their frequency as an elicitator depend on age. Risk factors for anaphylaxis include age, the presence of other allergic or cardiovascular comorbidities – and gender. More data throughout different countries are needed to monitor the eliciting factors and identify patients at risk.

Published data on the epidemiology of anaphylaxis has been continuously increasing worldwide within the last 2 years. One reason is that anaphylaxis has been more recognized by allergists but also the common community due to the onset of deaths even in small children.

In principal, data on the epidemiology of anaphylaxis will help to identify causes, risk factors and circumstances of the reaction. It will support the medical community to develop measures for the protection of affected patients. A true incidence of anaphylaxis has not been established, reasons are diverse study designs and the fact that there has been no universal consensus as to the definition of anaphylaxis [1].

Sources of Information on the Epidemiology of Anaphylaxis

Whenever data on the epidemiology of anaphylaxis is published it will need to be considered how the data was obtained (table 1). This might affect for example the ranking of eliciting factors. Until now, data has been published including the analysis of hospital and emergency department admissions [1–6], emergency medical services data [7], visits to allergists offices [8], surveys of databases and patient populations [9, 10], and analysis of epinephrine autoinjector prescriptions [11].

Table 1. Data regarding the epidemiology of anaphylaxis [according to 47–51]

Author	Year	Country	Frequency
Emergency department-based data			
Brown et al.	2001	Australia	0.09%
Bellou et al.	2003	France	0.037%
Pastorello et al.	2001	Italy	0.03%
Helbig et al.	2004	Switzerland	0.02%
Population-based data			
Sheikh et al. [51]	2008	England	7.9 per 100,000 persons/year
Decker et al. [48]	2008	USA	49.8 per 100,000 persons/year

Limitations

The data on the epidemiology of anaphylaxis are widely varying estimates on the frequency of this condition. The findings are based on diverse study designs and are often not comparable. A clear conclusion from the data published so far is difficult. One major reason is that there is no universal consensus regarding the definition of anaphylaxis. The International Classification Codes (ICD) recording anaphylaxis are imprecise and do not properly reflect the epidemiological needs.

Causes of Anaphylaxis

The most frequent causes of anaphylaxis are food, insect venom and drugs [1–13]. The exact frequency of the causes depends on age, geographical regions and exposure, but is also highly dependent on the source of the data, e.g. emergency rooms vs. allergists. In a recent study among practicing doctors in Germany, venom was for example referred to as a common cause of anaphylaxis if the data was obtained from general practitioners and dermatologists, whereas drugs were the most common cause if radiologists and oncologists were asked [14].

Food

Food allergy is common in the general population and depending on the study its prevalence varies between 2 and 4% [15]. The rates are much higher if self-reported symptoms are accounted. Food allergy is more frequent in children than in adults

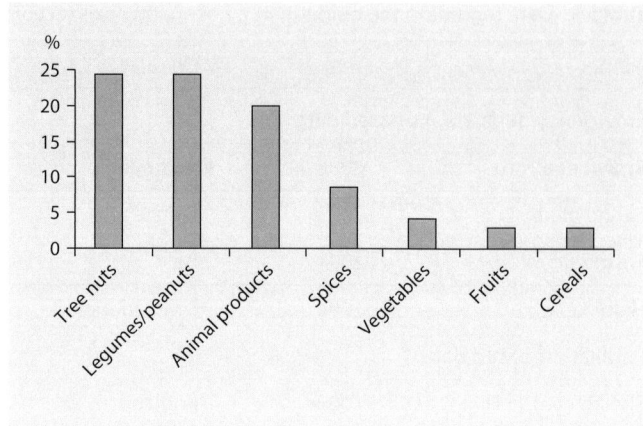

Fig. 1. Food allergens are the most frequent causes of anaphylaxis in children. Data from the anaphylaxis registry of German-speaking countries (ANA-Net), n = 70.

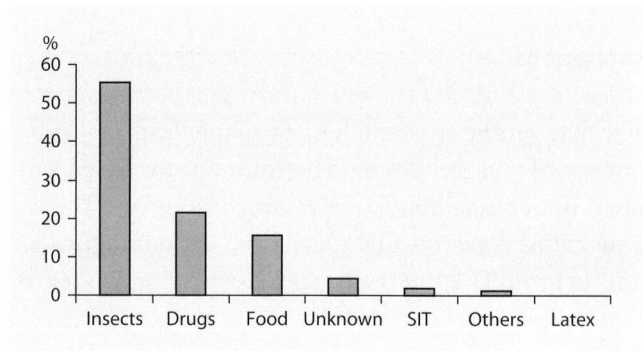

Fig. 2. Venom is the most frequent causes of anaphylaxis in adults. Data from the anaphylaxis registry of German-speaking countries (ANA-Net), n = 734.

[16]. The most frequent elicitators of food allergy in children are peanuts and tree nuts [17]. In France the prevalence of food allergy has been estimated to be 3.2% [18]. Furthermore, in this study, food was identified as the most common cause of anaphylaxis. Here the major identified food allergens besides peanuts and tree nuts were shellfish, wheat and lupine flour [18].

Data from the recently established anaphylaxis registry in German-speaking countries (ANA-Net) is in line with these previously reported data [13]. Here food allergens were among the most frequent causes of anaphylaxis in children (fig. 1), again with peanuts and tree nuts being the most common causes. Among adults, food allergy is the third most frequent cause of anaphylaxis (fig. 2). In addition, food allergens may account as a cofactor in the context of anaphylaxis. In exercised-induced anaphylaxis, food allergens are the most frequent elicitators. Among many possible food allergens which may account for exercise-induced anaphylaxis, it has been shown recently that the allergenic component ω–5 gliadin from wheat is a frequent cause [19]. As this sensitization can now be measured by determination of specific IgE, the diagnostic workup for this clinical entity has been significantly improved [20].

These data suggest that due to an increase of food allergy and in particular tree nut and peanut sensitization, the risk for anaphylaxis has been increased at the same time.

In population-based studies from the USA, self-reported peanut allergy in children rose from 0.4% in 1997 to 0.8% in 2002 [21]. In the UK, prevalence rates for peanut allergy are in excess of 1%. Data from England points in the same direction with a twofold increase in reported peanut allergy.

Recent data from Australia underlines the role of food allergens in causing fatal anaphylaxis in young individuals [22]. 112 fatalities were recognized between 1997 and 2005, and among these, 7 were attributed to food anaphylaxis in the age group of 5–35 years. Five individuals had severe reactions previously and all of these had active asthma. Peanut was the offending allergen in 3 cases. Six had eaten food prepared outside the usual residence. Overall a total of 5,007 food-induced anaphylaxis hospital admissions between 1994 and 2005 with two age peaks – one in 0- to 4-year and the other one in the 15- to 29-year age group. An age-dependent role of gender was identified: in the age group of <15 years male subjects outnumbered female subjects (1.5:1), whereas female subjects outnumbered male subjects (1.4:1) >15 years. Again, this study also describes peanut as the most common allergen (23%), followed by fish (18%), crustaceans (16%), tree nuts (16%), eggs (9%) and milk (8%).

Drugs

Drug allergies rival food allergies in respect to frequency. Among the most frequent causes, antibiotics, NSAIDs, but also radiocontrasts and various other agents administered during the perioperative period are the most common causes [1].

The Australian study identified drugs as the most common cause of anaphylaxis fatalities [22]. Of 105 non-food-induced anaphylaxis cases, 64 were drug-induced. Most deaths occurred in adults 55 to >85 years of age with similar numbers of male and female subjects [22].

Subgroup analysis showed that all penicillin-induced deaths occurred between 60 and 74 years, whereas cephalosporin-induced deaths occurred between 35 and 74 years of age. Significant comorbidities included ischemic heart disease or dysarrhythmia, obstructive airway disease, mastocytosis and hypogammaglobulinemia.

There were a total of 3,019 drug-induced anaphylaxis hospital admissions between 1998 and 2005 reported from Australia [22]. Again, in prepuberty cases, males were more frequently affected and females outnumbered male subjects in the age groups >15 years. The age-specific hospitalization rates were highest for the 55- to 84-year age group (3.8/100,000). In an evaluation of severe anaphylactic episodes, all with circulatory symptoms, performed in Switzerland, the frequency of drug reactions almost doubled that of reactions due to food. Approximately half of the drugs were NSAIDs and antibiotics were the second most frequent drug offender [23].

The data from the anaphylaxis registry in German-speaking countries also indicate that drugs are frequent elicitators of anaphylaxis in adults [13]. They account for the second most frequent cause if patients are registered who consult an allergist (fig. 2). Within this group, antibiotics but also NSAIDs are the most common causes. However, a high underreporting rate must be taken into consideration. In a recent questionnaire study, we were able to identify that not only radiologists but also oncologists frequently see patients experiencing anaphylactic reactions to contrast media and/or chemotherapeuticals [14].

Insect Venom Anaphylaxis

Depending on the country's climate, 50–90% of the interviewees remember being stung by a Hymenoptera insect at least once in their lives [24]. The prevalence of sensitization is estimated between 10 and 30% in the adult population [25]. The prevalence of Hymenoptera sting-induced anaphylaxis varies worldwide. European epidemiological studies report a prevalence of systemic reactions between 0.5 and 7.5% [25]. In the USA the prevalence rate of systemic reactions among adults has been reported to range from 0.5 to 3.3% [26]. The frequency of anaphylactic shock has been reported in 0.6–42% of cases and is generally lower in children. In analyses of the latest population-based studies of anaphylaxis due to any cause [27–33], insect sting-induced anaphylaxis is responsible for 7.3–59% of the total number of cases reported. Emergency department studies indicate lower numbers with percentages ranging from 1.5 to 34%. These broad variations are due to the fact that the exposure of individuals to e.g. bees or wasps depends on the climate and outdoor activity behavior of a population. In Germany approximately 20 persons die from an anaphylactic reaction every year due to an insect sting.

The risk of systemic reactions is determined by previous reaction severity: the more serious the initial reaction, the greater the risk of recurrence. The estimated risk of a systemic reaction with a recent history of anaphylaxis is 40–60% reacting to a future sting. Bee venom-allergic patients are at a greater risk of a systemic reaction on their next sting than those with wasp venom allergy. The relative risk for life-threatening sting reactions in the Mediterranean area is about three times higher for hornet stings than for honeybee or wasp stings [25]. Preexisting cardiovascular diseases are in particular risk factors for severe and fatal sting reactions. Frequently prescribed drugs in these patients are β-blockers and ACE inhibitors, which may account for an increased severity of such reactions.

16

Table 2. Predisposing factors of anaphylaxis

A	Risk factors for food-induced anaphylaxis:
	Children and young adults
	Active allergic asthma
	Peanut allergy
	Ingestion of food prepared outside of the subjects residence
	Delayed administration of adrenaline
B	Risk factors for drug-induced anaphylaxis:
	Age of 55-85 years
	Presence of respiratory and cardiovascular comorbidities
	Antibiotics and anesthetic agents
C	Risk factors for insect sting-induced anaphylaxis:
	Age of 35–84 years
	Male sex

Finally, patients suffering from mastocytosis have a higher risk of developing severe anaphylaxis after an insect sting [34]. In venom-allergic patients with mastocytosis, elevated baseline serum tryptase levels were found to be associated with severe anaphylactic reactions to stings [35].

Biphasic Anaphylactic Reaction

Anaphylactic reactions may exhibit a biphasic pattern. Different studies indicated a wide variation regarding the incidence of biphasic reactions. These range from 3 to 20% regarding the incidence of biphasic reactions. The time from the initial symptoms to the onset of the secondary reaction varied from >1 up to 47 h [36].

Age

As mentioned above, age may account as a risk factor for anaphylaxis (table 2). Whereas food allergy and fatal anaphylaxis occur more frequently in younger age groups, drugs as causes for anaphylaxis increase continuously throughout life [22]. A recent study analyzing the population-based deaths from anaphylaxis in Florida indicated that among 89 registered deaths, 28 were related to drugs [37]. The annual death rate for anaphylaxis in Florida was 5.02/10 million. The relative risk of death from anaphylaxis was 14.09 for individuals >65 years old and 6.38 for individuals 35–64 years old.

Atopy

The role of atopy in anaphylaxis has not completely been resolved. On the one hand there is for example no evidence of a higher risk of severe reactions in venom-allergic patients. A recent study by Sturm et al. [38] indicated that patients with high total IgE levels predominantly developed mild to moderate reactions. By contrast, atopy may increase the risk and severity of systemic reactions in beekeepers and their family numbers [39]. On the other hand, atopy and in particular allergic asthma are risk factors for food allergy and therefore are also important risk factors for food-induced anaphylaxis. This is most likely also true for exercise-induced anaphylaxis, but also non-IgE-dependent anaphylaxis induced by NSAIDs or contrast media.

The role of atopy among drug-induced anaphylaxis depends probably on the elicitating drug; here clearly more data are needed.

Geography

A distinct effect of geographical location on the incidence of anaphylaxis was suggested by two studies, one from England [40] and one from the USA [11]. The US study assessed epinephrine autoinjector prescriptions and found a north (Massachusetts) – south gradient for anaphylactic episodes. In the northern part of the USA, 11.81 prescriptions per 1,000 persons and in the southern part, 3 prescriptions per 1,000 persons were found. Interestingly, the rate of prescriptions was inversely related to sunlight exposure and it was postulated that relative vitamin D deficiency may play a role in increasing the incidence of anaphylaxis. The study from England analyzed the emergency admissions and they determined up to 25 emergency admissions per 100,000 in the south whereas in the north the rate was less than 15 per 100,000 emergency admissions. These results are somewhat contradictory and indicate that factors which are associated with geography will need to be identified.

Gender

The impact of gender on the onset of anaphylaxis is age-dependent. In children, boys predominate whereas after puberty this relationship reverses (fig. 3). Similar observations have been described for allergic asthma but not atopic eczema previously [41].

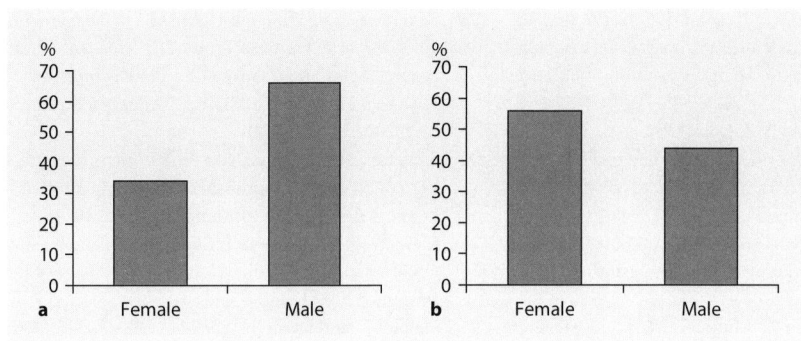

Fig. 3. Onset at anaphylaxis related to gender: (**a**) children and adolescents (n = 135) and (**b**) adults (n = 734).

The incidence of anaphylaxis is significantly higher in adult women and this attributes for the overall increased incidence of anaphylaxis in women. The exact contribution of biological and sociological factors for these observations is not completely delineated so far. Estrogens have been shown to promote the mediator release of mast cells and basophils [reviewed in 42]. In addition, it has been shown that sex hormones can affect the sensitization and elicitation of allergic reactions. In general, estrogens can enhance humoral immunity and antibody synthesis, while androgens and progesterone seem to suppress immunity and inflammation [reviewed in 42]. Recent data from epidemiological studies indicate that sex is a risk factor for food allergy, which plays an important role as a trigger factor for anaphylaxis [43].

Socioeconomic Status

Areas with a higher socioeconomic status seem to be related to an increased number of anaphylactic reactions [44–46]. Data from Canada and Wales indicate that prescriptions for epinephrine autoinjectors were higher in populations of relative wealth, whereas these findings could not be explained by access to medical care or other factors.

References

1 Lieberman P: Epidemiology of anaphylaxis. Curr Opin Allergy Clin Immunol 2008;8:316–320.
2 Anthony F, Brown T, McKinnon D, Chu K: Emergency department anaphylaxis: a review of 142 patients in a single year. J Allergy Clin Immunol 2001;108:861–866.
3 Kane KE, Cone DC: Anaphylaxis in the prehospital setting. J Emerg Med 2004;27:371–377.
4 Smit DV, Cameron PA, Rainer TH: Anaphylaxis presentation in a emergency department in Hong Kong: incidence and predictors of biphasic reactions. J Emerg Med 2005;28:381–388.
5 Kiratiseavee S, Ranesg S: Evaluation of pediatric patients admitted with adverse food reactions to an inner-city pediatric ED. J Allergy Clin Immunol 2007;119:S114.

6 Mulla ZD, Simon MR: Hospitalizations for anaphylaxis in Florida: epidemiologic analysis of a population-based dataset. J Allergy Clin Immunol 2007; 119:S32.

7 Poulos LM, Waters AM, Correl PK, et al: Trends in hospitalizations for anaphylaxis, angioedema, and urticaria in Australia, 1993–1994 to 2004–2005. J Allergy Clin Immunol 2007;120:878–884.

8 Webb LM, Lieberman P: Anaphylaxis: a review of 601 cases. Ann Allergy Asthma Immunol 2006;97: 39–43.

9 Furlong T, Stivers T, Munoz-Furlong A, Sicherer SH: A registry of self-reported seafood allergy: demographic and allergic characteristic of the first 1,000 registrants. J Allergy Clin Immunol 2005;115: S62.

10 Bohlke K, Davis RL, DeStefano F, et al: Epidemiology of anaphylaxis among children and adolescents enrolled in a health maintenance organization. J Allergy Clin Immunol 2004;113:536–542.

11 Camargo CA, Clark S, Kaplan MS, et al: Regional differences in EpiPen prescriptions in the United States. J Allergy Clin Immunol 2007;120:131–136.

12 Clark S, Camargo CA Jr: Epidemiology of anaphylaxis. Immunol Allergy Clin North Am 2007;27:145–163.

13 Hompes S, Kirschbaum J, Scherer K, Treudler R, Przybilla B, Henzgen M, Worm M: Erste Daten der Pilotphase des Anaphylaxie-Registers im deutschsprachigen Raum. Allergo J 2008;7:550–555.

14 Worm M, Hompes S, Vogel N, Kirschbaum J, Zuberbier T: Care of anaphylaxis among practising doctors. Allergy 2008;63:1562–1563.

15 Zuberbier T, Edenharter G, Worm M, Ehlers I, Reimann S, Hantke T, Roehr CC, Bergmann KE, Niggemann B: Prevalence of adverse reactions to food in Germany – a population study. Allergy 2004;59:338–345.

16 Roehr CC, Edenharter G, Reimann S, Ehlers I, Worm M, Zuberbier T, Niggemann B: Food allergy and non-allergic food hypersensitivity in children and adolescents. Clin Exp Allergy 2004;34:1534–1541.

17 Sicherer SH, Muñoz-Furlong A, Sampson HA: Prevalence of peanut and tree nut allergy. Clin Immunol 2003;112:1203–1207.

18 Kanny G, Moneret-Vautrin DA, Flabbee J, Beaudouin E, Morisset M, Thevenin F: Population study of food allergy in France. J Allergy Clin Immunol 2001;108:133–140.

19 Jacquenet S, Morisset M, Battais F, Denery-Papini S, Croizier A, Baudouin E, Bihain B, Moneret-Vautrin DA: Interest of ImmunoCAP system to recombinant omega–5 gliadin for the diagnosis of exercise-induced wheat allergy. Int Arch Allergy Immunol 2008;149:74–80.

20 Beyer K, Chung D, Schulz G, Mishoe M, Niggemann B, Wahn U, Sampson HA: The role of wheat omega–5 gliadin IgE antibodies as a diagnostic tool for wheat allergy in childhood. J Allergy Clin Immunol 2008;122:419–421.

21 Sicherer SH, Sampson HA: Peanut allergy: emerging concepts and approaches for an apparent epidemic. J Allergy Clin Immunol 2007;120:491–505.

22 Liew WK, Williamson E, Tang ML: Anaphylaxis fatalities and admissions in Australia. J Allergy Clin Immunol 2009;123:434–442.

23 Helbling A, Hurni T, Mueller UR, Pichler WJ: Incidence of anaphylaxis with circulatory symptoms: a study over a 3-year period comprising 940,000 inhabitants of the Swiss Canton Bern. Clin Exp Allergy 2004;34:285–290.

24 Antonicelli L, Bilò MB, Bonifazi F: Epidemiology of Hymenoptera allergy. Curr Opin Allergy Clin Immunol 2002;2:341–346.

25 Bonifazi F, Jutel M, Biló BM, Birnbaum J, Muller U; EAACI Interest Group on Insect Venom Hypersensitivity: Prevention and treatment of Hymenoptera venom allergy: guidelines for clinical practice. Allergy 2005;60:1459–1470.

26 Golden DB: Patterns of anaphylaxis: acute and late phase features of allergic reactions; in Bock G, Goode J (eds): Anaphylaxis. Novartis Found Symp 257. Chichester, Wiley, 2004, pp 1–101.

27 Mullins RJ: Anaphylaxis: risk factors for recurrence. Clin Exp Allergy 2003;33:1033–1040.

28 Peng MM, Jick H: A population-based study of the incidence, cause, and severity of anaphylaxis in the United Kingdom. Arch Intern Med 2004;164:317–319.

29 Bohlke K, Davis RL, DeStefano F, et al: Vaccine Safety Datalink Team. Epidemiology of anaphylaxis among children and adolescents enrolled in a health maintenance organization. J Allergy Clin Immunol 2004;113:536–542.

30 Thong BY, Cheng YK, Leong KP, et al: Anaphylaxis in adults referred to a clinical immunology/allergy centre in Singapore. Singapore Med J 2005;46:529–534.

31 Mehl A, Wahn U, Niggemann B: Anaphylactic reactions in children – a questionnaire-based survey in Germany. Allergy 2005;60:1440–1445.

32 Yang MS, Lee SH, Kim TW, et al: Epidemiologic and clinical features of anaphylaxis in Korea. Ann Allergy Asthma Immunol 2008;100:31–36.

33 De Swert LF, Bullens D, Raes M, Dermaux AM: Anaphylaxis in referred pediatric patients: demographic and clinical features, triggers, and therapeutic approach. Eur J Pediatr 2008;167:1251–1261.

34 Brockow K, Jofer C, Behrendt H, Ring J: Anaphylaxis in patients with mastocytosis: a study on history, clinical features and risk factors in 120 patients. Allergy 2008;63:226–232.

35 Ruëff F, Placzek M, Przybilla B: Mastocytosis and Hymenoptera venom allergy. Curr Opin Allergy Clin Immunol 2006;6:284–288.

36 Smit DV, Cameron PA, Rainer TH: Anaphylaxis presentations to an emergency department in Hong Kong: incidence and predictors of biphasic reactions. J Emerg Med 2005;28:381–388.

37 Simon MR, Mulla ZD: A population-based epidemiologic analysis of deaths from anaphylaxis in Florida. Allergy 2008;63:1077–1083.

38 Sturm GJ, Heinemann A, Schuster C, et al: Influence of total IgE levels on the severity of sting reactions in Hymenoptera venom allergy. Allergy 2007;62:884–889.

39 Müller UR: Bee venom allergy in beekeepers and their family members. Curr Opin Allergy Clin Immunol 2005;5:343–347.

40 Sheikh A, Alves B: Age, sex, geographical and socioeconomic variations in admissions for anaphylaxis: analysis of four years of English hospital data. Clin Exp Allergy 2001;31:1571–1576.

41 Siroux V, Curt F, Oryszczyn MP, Maccario J, Kauffmann F: Role of gender and hormone-related events on IgE, atopy, and eosinophils in the Epidemiological Study on the Genetics and Environment of Asthma, bronchial hyperresponsiveness and atopy. J Allergy Clin Immunol 2004;114:491–498.

42 Chen W, Mempel M, Schober W, Behrendt H, Ring J: Gender difference, sex hormones, and immediate type hypersensitivity reactions. Allergy 2008;63:1418–1427.

43 Soost S, Leynaert B, Almquist C, Edenharter G, Zuberbier T, Worm M: Risk factor of adverse reactions to food in German adults. Clin Exp Allergy 2009;39:1036–1044.

44 Simons FE, Peterson S, Black CD: Epinephrine dispensing patterns for an out-of-hospital population: a novel approach to studying the epidemiology of anaphylaxis. J Allergy Clin Immunol 2002;110:647–651.

45 Simons FE, Peterson S, Black CD: Epinephrine dispensing for the out-of-hospital treatment of anaphylaxis in infants and children: a population-based study. Ann Allergy Asthma Immunol 2001;86:622–626.

46 Rangaraj S, Tuthill D, Burr M, Alfaham M: Childhood epidemiology of anaphylaxis and epinephrine in Wales: 1994–1999. J Allergy Clin Immunol 2000;109:S75.

47 Moneret-Vautrin DA, Morisset M, Flabbee J, Beaudouin E, Kanny G: Epidemiology of life-threatening and lethal anaphylaxis: a review. Allergy 2005;60:443–451.

48 Decker WW, Campbell RL, Manivannan V, Luke A, St Sauver JL, Weaver A, Bellolio MF, Bergstralh EJ, Stead LG, Li JT: Etiology and incidence of anaphylaxis in Rochester, Minnesota: a report from the Rochester Epidemiology Project. J Allergy Clin Immunol 2008;122:1161–1165.

49 Simons FE, Sampson HA: Anaphylaxis epidemic: fact or fiction? J Allergy Clin Immunol 2008;122:1166–1168.

50 Pumphrey RS: Fatal anaphylaxis in the UK, 1992–2001; in Bock G, Goode J (eds): Anaphylaxis. Novartis Found Symp 257. Chichester, Wiley, 2004, pp 116–128.

51 Sheikh A, Hippisley-Cox J, Newton J, Fenty J: Trends in national incidence, lifetime prevalence and adrenaline prescribing for anaphylaxis in England. J R Soc Med 2008;101:139–143.

Prof. Dr. Margitta Worm
Allergie-Centrum-Charité, Klinik für Dermatologie und Allergologie
Charité Platz 1, DE–10117 Berlin (Germany)
Tel. +49 30 450 518 105, Fax +49 30 450 518 919
E-Mail margitta.worm@charite.de

Ring J (ed): Anaphylaxis. Chem Immunol Allergy. Basel, Karger, 2010, vol 95, pp 22–44

T-Cell Response to Allergens

Cevdet Ozdemir[a] · Mübeccel Akdis[b] · Cezmi A. Akdis[b]

[a]Marmara University, Division of Pediatric Allergy and Immunology, Istanbul, Turkey, and [b]Swiss Institute of Allergy and Asthma Research (SIAF), Davos, Switzerland

Abstract

Anaphylaxis is a life-threatening IgE-dependent type 1 hypersensitivity reaction in which multiple organ systems are involved. The existence of allergen exposure and specific IgE are the major contributors to this systemic reaction. The decision of the immune system to respond to allergens is highly dependent on factors including the type and load of allergen, behavior and type of antigen-presenting cells, innate immune response stimulating substances in the same micromilieu, the tissue of exposure, interactions between T and B lymphocytes, costimulators, and genetic propensity known as atopy. Antigen-presenting cells introduce processed allergens to T-helper lymphocytes, where a decision of developing different types of T-cell immunity is given under the influence of several cytokines, chemokines, costimulatory signals and regulatory T cells. Among Th2-type cytokines, interleukin (IL)-4 and IL-13 are responsible for class switching in B cells, which results in production of allergen-specific IgE antibodies that bind to specific receptors on mast cells and basophils. After re-exposure to the sensitized allergen, this phase is followed by activation of IgE Fc receptors on mast cells and basophils resulting in biogenic mediator releases responsible for the symptoms and signs of anaphylaxis. Since the discovery of regulatory T cells, the concepts of immune regulation have substantially changed during the last decade. Peripheral T-cell tolerance is a key immunologic mechanism in healthy immune response to self antigens and non-infectious non-self antigens. Both naturally occurring CD4+CD25+ regulatory T (Treg) cells and inducible populations of allergen-specific, IL-10-secreting Treg type 1 cells inhibit allergen-specific effector cells and have been shown to play a central role in the maintenance of peripheral homeostasis and the establishment of controlled immune responses. On the other hand, Th17 cells are characterized by their IL-17 (or IL-17A), IL-17F, IL-6, tumor necrosis factor-α, and IL-22 expressions, which coordinate local tissue inflammation through upregulation of proinflammatory cytokines and chemokines. This chapter is mainly focused on antigen presentation pathways and allergen-specific T-cell responses.

The terms 'allergy' and 'atopy' are in close proximity of our lives in the new millennium since our lifestyles have enormously changed. Encounters with various new molecules in air, water and diet, living in a more polluted world with less exposure to infections, and infectious agents are supposed to be the major causative factors added to the genetic propensity of developing IgE antibodies responsible for symptoms and signs of allergic disorders [1]. Clinical manifestations are allergic rhinitis, allergic asthma, food allergy, allergic skin inflammation, ocular allergy as a single or combined disease and anaphylaxis [2].

Allergens are almost always proteins, but not all proteins are allergens. Understanding what makes a protein an allergen is essential to develop strategies for immune intervention [2]. For a protein antigen to display allergenic activity, it must induce IgE production, which must lead to a type 1 hypersensitivity response upon subsequent exposure to the same protein [3]. Biochemical properties of the allergen, stimulating factors of the innate immune response around the allergen substances at the time of exposure, stability of the allergen in the tissues, digestive system, skin or mucosa, and the dose and time of stay in lymphatic organs during the interaction with the immune system are all possible confounding factors causing an antigen to become an allergen [2]. Foods (especially peanuts and tree nuts), medications (also allergen immunotherapy injections), insect venoms and latex constitute the major allergens causing anaphylaxis [4, 5]. Early detection of the responsible allergen is a requisite and an important prognostic factor in controlling allergic diseases and anaphylaxis [6].

Dendritic cells (DCs) are complex cell populations that differ in their anatomic location, antigen recognition, processing machinery, and migratory capacity. DCs stay as sentinels that take up exogenous antigens and transmit the information into immune system by migrating to draining lymph nodes, and presenting the processed antigens to T cells resulting in T-cell differentiation and activation [7, 8]. Content of micromilieu and several cytokines and other cofactors released from DCs are essential for the differentiation of naive T cells into T-helper (Th)1, Th2, Th9, Th17 effector T-cell subsets [9]. Expansion of allergen-specific Th2 cells results in production of interleukin (IL)-4 and IL-13, which induce immunoglobulin class switching to IgE and clonal expansion of naive and IgE+ memory B-cell populations. In the presence of IL-4 also differentiation of naive T cells into Th2 takes place (fig. 1). When IgE bound to FcεRI (high-affinity receptor for IgE) on mast cells and basophils crosslinks with the specific allergen, release of vasoactive amines (such as histamine), lipid mediators (such as prostaglandin D, platelet-activating factor, leukotriene C_4 (LTC_4), LTD_4 and LTE_4), chemokines (CXC-chemokine ligand 8 (CXCL8), CXCL10, CC-chemokine ligand 2 (CCL2), CCL4 and CCL5) and other cytokines (such as IL-4, IL-5 and IL-13) occur, which are responsible for the signs and symptoms of immediate phase of the allergic reactions [3].

Allergen Recognition by the Immune System

Pathogen-Associated Molecular Patterns and Pattern Recognition Receptors
Recent investigations have greatly increased our understanding of immunological mechanisms involved in the pathogenesis of allergic disease [10–12]. Presentation

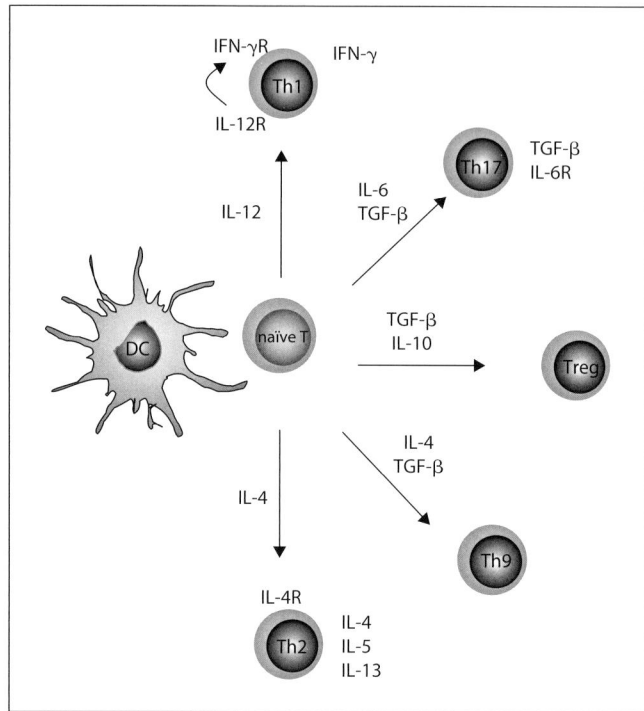

Fig. 1. Differentiation of T cells: content of micromilieu and several cytokines and other cofactors released from DCs are essential for the differentiation of naive T cells into T-helper (Th)1, Th2, Th9, Th17 effector T-cell subsets.

of allergens by antigen-presenting cells (APCs) or by other means and initiation of allergen-specific immune response represents the first step in sensitization to allergens. New allergens and their cross-reactivities are continuously being identified and types of immune response to them are demonstrated [13, 14]. Allergic inflammation results from the activation of tissue migrating hematopoietic and resident non-hematopoietic cells. This coordinated activation leads to increased production of a variety of soluble factors including chemokines and cytokines. Direct or indirect effects of the innate immune response are decisive in the development of adoptive immunity to allergens [15]. In principle, it is not only the protein allergen, but the adjuvants in the surrounding of the allergens are decisive for the type of the immune response [16, 17].

Mammals execute host defense against pathogens through two different types of immunity: innate and adaptive immune responses [18]. APCs and lymphocytes act as important contributors in the imminent relationship between these two systems. Innate immunity is designed to recognize small molecular motifs that are unique and essential for the survival of pathogens, which do not exist in mammalians termed as pathogen-associated molecular patterns (PAMPs) [19–21]. PAMPs are recognized by pattern recognition receptors (PRRs) that are expressed by DCs. Among the well-known PRRs, TLRs are the best-characterized group that recognize bacteria or viruses [22, 23]. TLR3, TLR7, TLR8, and TLR9 recognize viral RNAs and bacterial

DNA [24]. TLR3 is expressed on the surface of airway epithelial cells [25]. Moreover, TLR engagement on DCs polarizes T-cell response and while TLR2 and TLR4 may favor both Th1 and Th2 responses, and TLR9 induces the development of regulatory T cells [26]. Toll is a type I transmembrane receptor containing extracellular leucine-rich repeat (LRR) motifs and cytoplasmic Toll/IL-1 receptor homology domain (TIR) [27]. TLRs activate nuclear factor (NF)-κB and other signaling pathways such as mitogen-associated protein (MAP) kinases, signal transducer and activator of transcription (STAT)-1 through the adapter protein MyD88, TIR containing adaptor protein (TIRAP), TIR containing adaptor inducing interferon (IFN)-β (TRIF) and TRIF-related adaptor molecule (TRAM) [26, 28–30].

PAMPs and various tissue factors can prime DCs to produce T-cell-polarizing factors [21]. IL-12 is a pro-inflammatory cytokine that induces IFN-γ and promotes the development of Th1-cell differentiation [31]. Other Th1-polarizing factors are IFN-α and IFN-β [32] and cell-surface expressed intracellular adhesion molecule (ICAM)-1 [33]. On the other hand, it has been shown that NF-κB inducing kinase (NIK), which is known to regulate B-cell maturation and lymphoid organogenesis, is important for the induction of Th17 cells [34].

TLR signals in DCs increase expression of major histocompatibility complex (MHC) proteins and T-cell coreceptors, resulting in greater T-cell activation with Th1 bias [35, 36]. TLR signals in mast cells increase their release of IL-5 and in airway epithelial cells enhance airway generation of proallergic cytokines [36, 37]. Multiple bacterial TLR ligands such as unmethylated CpG motif-containing DNA and lipopolysaccharides have also been shown to stimulate production of IL-12 in host cells and consequently downregulate Th2 responses in animal models of allergy [38–40]. Nevertheless, at the slowly developing adaptive immunity site, antigen specificity in an evolved response of both T and B lymphocytes takes part. T lymphocytes are responsible for cell-mediated immune responses, where B lymphocytes are for humoral immune responses [41]. Exosomes are vesicles of 30–100 nm produced by inward budding of endosomal compartments and are released by a range of different cell types. Exosomes from APCs carry immunorelevant molecules like MHC class I and II and costimulatory molecules and thus are suggested to have a role in immune modulation. Recently, exosomes were isolated from supernatants of B-cell lines derived from patients with birch pollen allergy [42]. They showed expression of MHC, costimulatory molecules like CD86, tetraspanin proteins such as CD81, and CD19. Furthermore, B-cell-derived exosomes bound Bet v 1-derived peptides and subsequently induced a dose-dependent T-cell proliferation, and IL-5 and IL-13 production. These results demonstrate that exosomes from B lymphocytes are an immunostimulatory factor in allergic immune responses. Overall, antigenic recognition has major contributions in directing immune response into either innate or adaptive responses. This is the most important step and is essential for an intact immune response in addition to a true discrimination of self and non-self, which is essential for a healthy immune response.

Dendritic Cell Subsets

The immune response to foreign proteins strongly depends on the efficiency and selectivity of antigen uptake by DCs. DCs play roles in the induction of protective T-cell immunity, as well as in tolerance induction. After contact with antigens, DCs mature and migrate from peripheral tissues to the T-cell areas of secondary lymphoid organs, where they produce regulatory cytokines and prime naive T lymphocytes [43]. The two distinct DC subsets that have been recognized in humans are myeloid DCs (mDCs) and plasmacytoid DCs (pDCs) [44]. mDCs express TLR2–TLR6 and TLR8 and can produce IL-12 in response to the bacterial and viral stimuli, whereas pDCs express TLR7 and TLR9 and have the ability to produce large amounts of type 1 IFNs in antiviral immune responses [43, 45–47] It has been suggested that pDCs directly suppress the potential of mDCs to generate effector T cells [48]. It was reported that pDCs could stimulate the formation of Treg cells, possibly in an inducible costimulator (ICOS)-L-dependent way [46, 48]. Depletion of pDCs from the lungs has abolished tolerance to inhaled antigens [48, 49]. On the other hand, the two distinct DC populations that have been identified in inflamed epidermis of atopic dermatitis are the classical Langerhans' cells and the inflammatory dendritic epidermal cells (IDEC) [50]. The IDEC population clearly induces a Th1 profile, while the Langerhans' cell population rather induces a Th2 type of T-cell response [51]. Concerning DCs and LCs, the expression of IgE FcεRI and its increase on the surface of these cells is strongly related to distinct type of inflammatory status [52].

C-kit (CD117) is a receptor tyrosine kinase, which has role in maintenance and survival of hematopoietic stem cells and mast cells. Stem cell factor (SCF) is the ligand for c-kit. The effect of c-kit on DCs is through the expression of IL-6 and Jagged-2, the ligand of Notch, which is known to regulate Th-cell differentiation, promotes Th2 and Th17 responses but not Th1 response [53]. Engagement of Notch at the surface of T cells with jagged on DCs and T cell receptor (TCR) with MHC-II-coupled antigen induces priming of Th cells [54].

Dendritic Cell/T-Cell Interaction

As the T lymphocytes cannot directly recognize antigens, a need for the specialized introduction of antigenic materials is essential, mostly for the peptide fragments (epitopes) that are generated by proteolytic degradation of antigens via highly specialized APCs [55]. DCs, monocytes, macrophages and B cells act as professional APCs, whereas fibroblasts, thymic epithelial cells, thyroid epithelial cells, glial cells, pancreatic β cells and vascular endothelial cells present the antigens non-professionally [56]. Antigenic peptide presentation to T cells is coupled to MHC molecules on the cell surface (fig. 2). Out of three classes, the two MHC molecules, class I and II, are important contributors in this recognition [57, 58]. When an intracellular pathogen like a virus invades a host cell, intracellular antigens are produced by viral replication. The host is capable of digestion of these viral associated proteins into small peptides via specialized enzyme complexes termed as proteasomes [55]. Sometimes endogenous

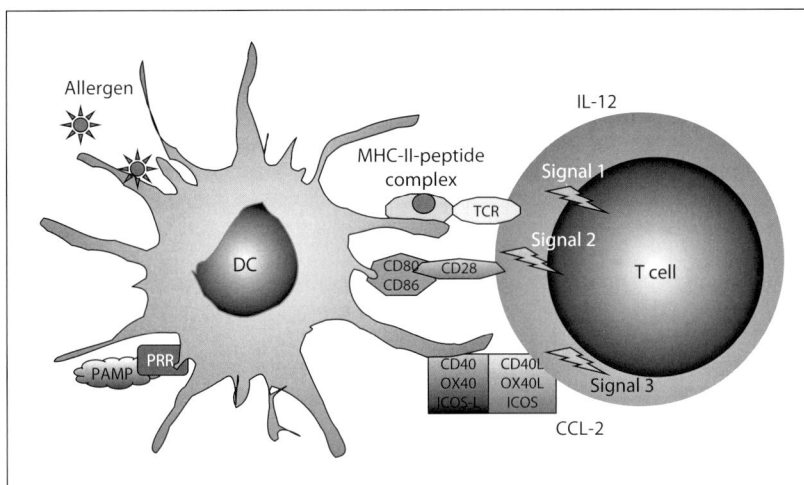

Fig. 2. Antigens (allergen) captured by the DCs, which reside as sentinels in the skin and mucosal surfaces, are processed and presented to T cells. PRRs recognize PAMPs and direct the immune differentiation on either the innate or adaptive side. Presentation to T-helper cells occurs via MHC-II-coupled peptide complexes along with costimulatory signals known as CD80/CD86-CD28 and CD40-CD40L, OX40-OX40L and ICOSL-ICOS interactions.

self proteins and tumor-associated antigens can also be digested in the same manner. Then peptides were moved to endoplasmic reticulum where MHC class I molecules are coupled to be presented on the cell surface. The role of MHC class I is to present antigens to CD8+ cytotoxic T cells. Almost all host cells can express MHC class I. MHC class I coupled antigenic material expression means a signal for destruction of the host cells is given, which leads to clearance of intracellular antigens due to infected, cancerous, damaged or dysfunctional cells [59, 60]. Modular antigen translocation (MAT) molecules have been engineered by protein transduction domain technology. MAT vaccines are composed of three modules: (i) a protein translocation domain to deliver cargo molecules to immune cells, (ii) a truncated invariant chain addressing the delivered cargo molecule to the MHC class II compartment, and (iii) an antigen of interest. MHC class II molecules are targeted to endocytic compartments by the invariant chain (li) that is degraded upon arrival in these compartments. MHC II acquires antigenic fragments from endocytosed proteins for presentation at the cell surface, and the strength of the immune response directly depends from the efficacy of the presentation. Direct targeting of the MHC class II pathway results in an increased antigen presentation and as a consequence thereof in robust protective humoral immune responses. MAT vaccines induced a strong proliferation of PBMCs at a low concentration and induced a Th2/Treg cell shift in the cytokine profile. Also in allergic mouse models, MAT vaccines are highly efficient in desensitizing mice and protect them from anaphylactic shock [61].

DCs have a significant impact on the development of allergic response because they play a role in differentiation of naive T cells. DCs are generated in the bone marrow and migrate as precursor cells into peripheral tissues, particularly to antigen entry sites like skin and mucosa in an immature form, where they stay as sentinels ready to capture antigens [62]. Understanding the importance of DCs in Th-cell activation and polarization is pivotal to ascertain developmental mechanisms of allergic disorders. Antigens and several tissue factors can activate DCs, which induce the maturation process. Expression of CC-chemokine receptor 7 (CCR-7) is increased which is an important homing molecule controlling the lymph node entry of naive T cells and of activated mature DCs [21, 63, 64]. This step is followed by migration of DCs to local draining lymph nodes where naive T cells are primed in an antigen-specific manner.

T-Cell Activation Signals

The immune system behaves in a different way to extracellular pathogens than bacteria and parasites. Initially, capture of exogenous pathogens by dendritic cells results in phagocytosis, which is then followed by migration to local lymph nodes through chemotactic signals where DCs mature and lose their phagocytic capacity and improve the antigen presentation capacity of T cells. In T-cell activation, several signals are essential for the differentiation of naive T cells to cytokine-producing effector Th cells.

Signal 1 is the interaction of MHC-II-coupled peptides with TCR [65]. TCR is a heterodimer consisting mainly of $\alpha\beta$ chains and also $\delta\gamma$ chains, which are the members of the immunoglobulin superfamily [66]. Each chain has complementarity determining regions (CDRs) that are amino acid sequences found in the variable domains of antigen receptor. CDRs recognize processed antigens and MHC [66]. However, signal 1 itself is not sufficient for the entire activation. Signaling through the TCR must be accompanied by costimulatory signals. In the absence of costimulation, T-cell activation results in T-cell anergy [67].

Signal 2 is mediated by triggering of CD28 by CD80 (B7.1) and CD86 (B7.2) that are expressed by DCs after ligation of PRRs [21, 67]. This costimulatory signal through CD28 is required for T-cell activation resulting in increased IL-2 production, which is the T-cell growth factor [68]. This also induces upregulation of CD40 ligands on T cells, which bind to CD40 on the DCs. CD28 costimulation upregulates ICOS for a costimulation by DC expressed ICOS ligand [69]. Aims to modulate antigen presentation through intracellular targeting of the MHC II presentation pathway is a recent issue in allergy vaccine development [61].

CD28 is critical for initiating T-cell responses, whereas CD40 ligand (CD40L) is required for sustained Th1 responses. The importance of CD28 and CD40L in T-cell activation and tolerance induction were evaluated in TCR transgenic T cells lacking either CD28 or CD40L. It has been reported that the absence of CD28 resulted in defective Th2 responses, whereas CD40L–/– T cells are defective in Th1 development

[70]. The importance of CD28 came out when the phase I clinical trial with the humanized monoclonal superagonist of the CD28, TGN1412, resulted in an unexpected cytokine storm with multiorgan failure in 2006 in the UK [71].

Effector T-Cell Subsets

Th1 and Th2 Cells

Activated effector T cells play an essential role in allergy and asthma. Formerly, subsets of CD4+ Th lymphocytes were categorized as Th1 and Th2 based on their distinct cellular functions and cytokine secretion capacities [72]. Although originally interpreted within the framework of a binary Th1/Th2 paradigm, our knowledge of the pathogenesis of atopic diseases has broadened to incorporate the contribution of Treg cells and the newly described proinflammatory Th17 cell lineage. The commitment of peripheral T-cell clones to undergo differentiation into one of those lineages is shaped by self-reinforcing transcriptional circuitries that center on key transcriptional regulators: T-box expressed in T cells (T-bet), (Th1), GATA-3 (Th2), forkhead box p3 (FOXP3, Treg cells), and retinoid-related orphan receptor γt/retinoid-related orphan receptor α (Th17). Counter-regulation between the three effector subsets has been continuously proposed [11, 73–75]. The activation of T-bet as a key transcription factor of Th1 cells inhibits both Th2 cell-mediated eosinophil recruitment and Th17 cell-mediated neutrophil recruitment into the airways [76]. An association between a specific T-bet haplotype and allergic asthma in children is demonstrated [77].

A predominant Th2 profile in atopic diseases might be the result of an increased tendency to activation and apoptosis of high IFN-γ-producing Th1 cells [78]. Th1 cells, particularly their high IFN-γ-producing fraction, and CXCR3+ T cells showed significantly increased apoptosis in atopic individuals. During their in vitro differentiation, significantly high apoptosis in Th1 cells was observed in atopic individuals compared to non-atopic individuals [78]. Th1 cells are implicated in cell-mediated defense against intracellular microorganisms and in promotion of memory IgG responses, and are characterized by IL-2, IFN-γ and tumor necrosis factor-β cytokine profiles. Th1-cell differentiation occurs in the presence of IL-12, IL-18 and IL-17. These cells can efficiently contribute to the effector phases in allergic diseases by exerting their roles in apoptosis of the epithelium in asthma and atopic dermatitis [79, 80].

The proinflammatory cytokines IL-4, IL-5, and IL-13 are clustered on chromosome 5q with GM-CSF in close proximity, and each of these cytokines has been implicated in the pathogenesis of IgE and eosinophilia-associated inflammations. Th2 cells engage in immunity to parasites, secrete IL-4, IL-5 and IL-13, and predominantly mediate IgE responses and allergic inflammation [3, 81] (fig. 3). Monocytic chemotactic protein 1 (MCP-1) and OX40 ligand are the Th2-polarizing factors that have been defined [82]. During priming, Th2 polarization is critically dependent on the presence of IL-4. It has been shown that OX40 ligation upregulates IL-4 production which promotes Th2

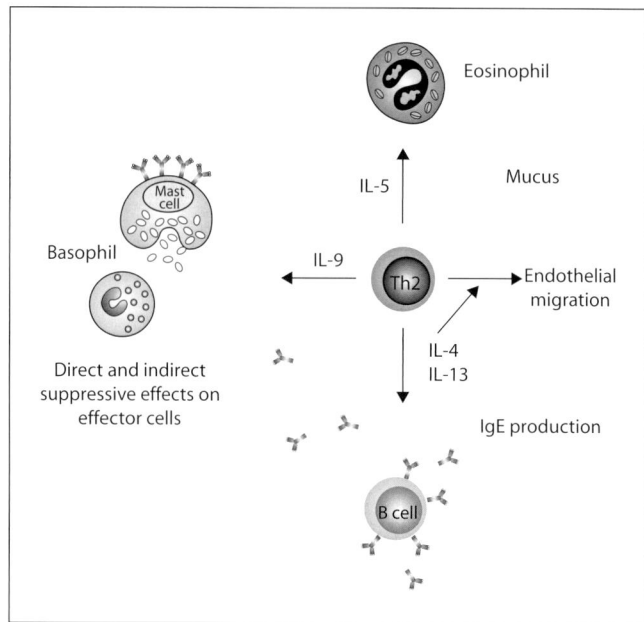

Fig. 3. Th2 cells provide cytokines such as IL-4, IL-5, IL-9 and IL-13, which are essential for differentiation, survival and activity of basophils, mast cells and eosinophils. IL-4 and IL-13 induce IgE production from B cells. IL-5 induces eosinophils, increases eosinophil survival and reduces apoptosis. IL-9 stimulates mast cells.

polarization with the resultant IL-4, IL-5 and IL-13 production [82]. Thymic stromal lymphopoietin (TSLP) as a novel growth factor, found to promote the proliferation and differentiation of committed B-cell progenitors and can replace the activity of IL-7, which is essential in supporting B-cell development. TSLP is produced by epithelial cells and has master roles at the epithelial cell and DC interface of allergic inflammation [83]. TSLP has been suggested to activate human mDCs to induce inflammatory Th2 responses [84]. TSLP is also elevated in asthma and triggers DC-mediated activation of Th2 inflammatory responses [85]. TSLP-induced DCs mature and migrate into the draining lymph nodes to initiate the adaptive phase of allergic immune response. TSLP-induced DCs express OX40L, which triggers the differentiation of allergen-specific naive CD4+ T cells to inflammatory Th2 cells [86]. It has also been reported that apoptosis-resistant DCs have the capability to generate antigen-specific Th2 cells in vitro and in vivo and induce IgE responses in vivo compared to freshly isolated DCs, independently of the sensitization status of the host [87]. IL-25 (IL-17E), a member of the IL-17 family of immunoregulatory cytokines, has been implicated in the regulation of Th2-type immunity. Blocking IL-25 in an experimental model of allergic asthma prevented AHR and reduced IL-5 and IL-13 production, eosinophil infiltration, goblet cell hyperplasia, and serum IgE secretion [88].

T-Helper-17 Cells

In 2006, another subset of Th cells was recognized, known as Th17 cells [89]. These cells have been described to exert major functions in induction of tissue inflammation and host protection against extracellular pathogens [74, 90]. Th17 cells are distinct from Th1 and Th2 cells with IL-17-producing capacity and mediate a variety of autoimmune diseases [91]. IL-17 family cytokines (IL-17A to F) induce various signaling molecules and have crucial functions in immune regulation. Most notably, IL-17 coordinates local tissue inflammation through upregulation of proinflammatory cytokines and chemokines [89, 92]. Differentiation of Th17 (IL-17A- and IL-17F-producing) cells is induced by IL-6, IL-21, IL-23, and transforming growth factor (TGF)-β [9]. The reciprocal interaction present between Treg cells and Th17 cells has suggested that induction of Treg cells can suppress autoimmunity or induction of Th17 cells can start tissue inflammation [93]. IL-17 act as a recruitment and survival factor for macrophages and coordinate granulocyte influx in allergic airway inflammation models [94, 95]. The role of Th17 cells in tissue inflammation has been shown by improvement in joint destruction that has been observed in an experimental arthritis model after neutralization of IL-17 with IL-17 receptor IgG1 Fc fusion protein [96]. Among IL-17 family members, IL-17F (IL-25) has specific functions in promoting a Th2-type response [97]. IL-25 induces eosinophilia, increases serum IgE and IgG1 and also upregulates tissue expression of IL-4, IL-5, and IL-13 [98, 99], so it can be classified in the Th2 group.

T-Helper-9 Cells
A distinct population of effector T cells that promote tissue inflammation has been described without suppressive functions [9]. This population is termed as Th9 cells and exerts IL-9 and IL-10 secretion capacities. IL-4 and TGF-β promotes an IL-9-producing subset, Th9 cells, which have roles in mucus production and tissue inflammation [100, 101].

Regulatory T Cells
Although pathogenesis of both autoimmune and allergic disorders had initially been committed to a dysbalance between Th1 and Th2, in 1995 a new population of T cells with suppressive roles which are termed as regulatory T cells was described [102] (fig. 4). These cells are characterized by their IL-10 and TGF-β secretion capacities. The Treg cells cause an abolished allergen-induced specific T-cell proliferation and suppressed Th1- and Th2-type cytokine secretion. In addition, Treg cells directly or indirectly suppress effector cells of allergic inflammation such as mast cells, basophils and eosinophils [103, 104]. Moreover, Treg cells can potently suppress IgE production while simultaneously increasing production of non-inflammatory isotypes IgG4 and IgA, respectively [103]. Subsets of Treg cells with distinct phenotypes and mechanisms of action include the naturally occurring thymus-selected CD4+CD25+ FOXP3+ Treg cells and the inducible type 1 IL-10-secreting Treg cells (TR1 cells) [105]. Additionally, subsets of CD8+ T cells, γδ T cells, DCs, IL-10-producing B cells, natural killer (NK) cells and resident tissue cells, which might promote the generation of Treg cells, could contribute to suppressive and regulatory events [106]. Both naturally occurring and inducible Treg cells have been extensively studied to understand

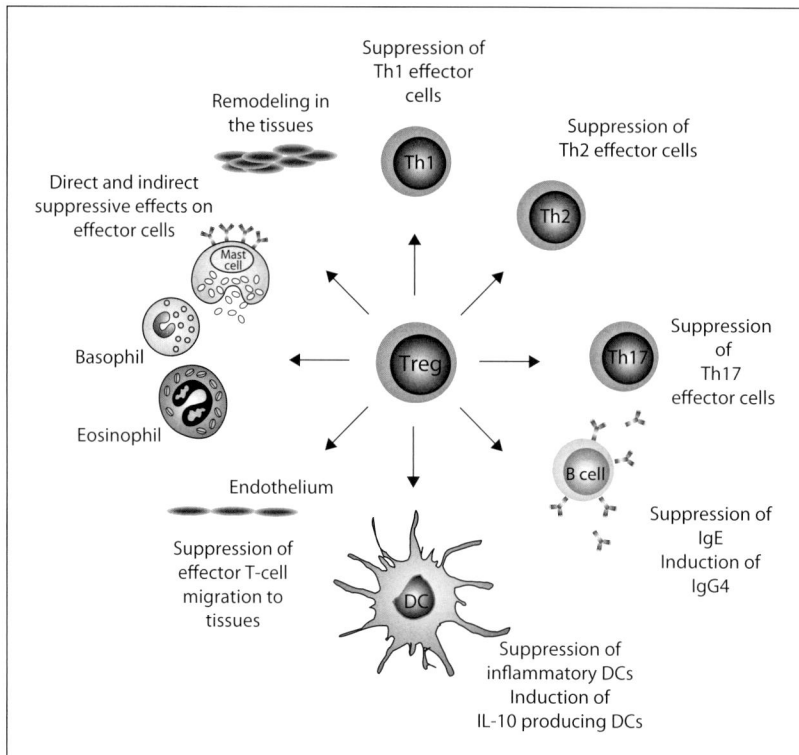

Fig. 4. Regulatory T-cell functions: suppression of DCs that support the generation of effector T cells; suppression of T_H1, T_H2, and T_H17 cells; suppression of allergen-specific IgE and induction of IgG4, IgA, or both; suppression of mast cells, basophils, and eosinophils; interaction with resident tissue cells and remodeling, and suppression of effector T-cell migration to tissues.

the mechanisms of peripheral tolerance development and induction of either Th1 or Th2 immunity [107].

Treg cells have both direct and indirect impacts on effector cells of allergic inflammation and potently suppress IgE production [104, 108, 109]. It is essential to delineate interaction between Treg cells and DCs to understand the mechanisms of peripheral tolerance to allergens. It has recently been reported that Treg cells compete with naive T cells in a physical manner by creating aggregates around DCs in vitro and inhibit their maturation [110]. It was also shown that Treg cells downregulate the expression of CD80/CD86 on DCs [110]. Naturally occurring Treg cells highly express cytotoxic T-lymphocyte antigen-4 (CTLA-4). CD28 and CTLA-4 signaling are required for T-cell priming leading to IL-4 cytokine production, B-cell activation, and IgE secretion during both immune responses [111]. CTLA-4 is a CD28 family member that binds CD80/CD86 as CD28 but with a higher affinity. In contrast to stimulatory effects of CD28, CTLA-4 inhibits T-cell activation [112, 113]. The polarizing signals that are mediated by various soluble or membrane-bound factors, such as IL-12 that promote the development of Th1 and CC-chemokine ligand 2 (CCL2) for Th2 cells, are regarded as signal 3 [21].

The immune regulatory role of T-cell-derived IL-10 in allergic disease has been extensively studied. In this context, functionally different properties of other cells that produce IL-10 are being investigated. It was suggested that controlling alternatively activated macrophages in Th2-driven inflammatory processes might be a novel target for immune intervention. Compared with healthy control subjects, the percentage of IL-10-producing monocytes was significantly increased in atopic patients [114]. IL-10-secreting monocytes were isolated by using an IL-10 secretion assay, and analysis of these sorted cells revealed that IL-10-secreting monocytes preferentially differentiate into suppressor of cytokine signalling 3 (SOCS3) expressing alternatively activated macrophages, which perpetuate Th2 immune response [114]. Whether IL-10-released from macrophages directly plays a role in lung inflammation or is released to keep the level of the inflammation in low levels remains to be investigated. IL-10-treated DCs are potent suppressors of the development of AHR, inflammation, and Th2 cytokine production; these regulatory functions are at least in part through the induction of endogenous production of IL-10 [115]. In human cells and mouse models, IL-10 has been repeatedly shown to suppress not only allergic inflammation, but also to play a role in transplantation tolerance, tumor cell tolerance, and suppression of autoimmunity. IL-10 inhibits CD28 and ICOS costimulations of T cells via Src homology 2 domain-containing protein tyrosine phosphatase (SHP)-1 [116]. IL-10 receptor-associated tyrosine kinase Tyk-2 acts as a constitutive reservoir for SHP-1 in resting T cells, and then tyrosine phosphorylates SHP-1 on IL-10 binding. SHP-1 rapidly binds to CD28 and ICOS costimulatory receptors and dephosphorylates them within minutes. In consequence, the binding of phosphatidylinositol 3-kinase to either costimulatory receptor no longer occurs, and downstream signaling is inhibited. Accordingly, spleen cells from SHP-1-deficient mice showed increased proliferation with CD28 and ICOS stimulation in comparison with wild-type mice, which was not suppressed by IL-10. Generation of dominant-negative SHP-1-overexpressing T cells or silencing of the SHP-1 gene by small inhibitory RNA both altered SHP-1 functions and abolished the T-cell-suppressive effect of IL-10. In conclusion, the rapid inhibition of the CD28 or ICOS costimulatory pathways by SHP-1 represents a novel mechanism for direct T-cell suppression by IL-10 [116]. Supporting these findings, Src homology 2 domain-containing inositol 5-phosphatase 1 inhibits allergic responses as a negative regulator of cytokine and immune receptor signaling. Its deficiency leads to a spontaneous development of allergic-like inflammation in the murine lung [117].

In addition to IL-10, TGF-β is a key cytokine in immune tolerance. It was investigated whether orally administered TGF-β, such as TGF-β in human milk, retains and exerts its activity in the intestinal mucosa and can induce immune tolerance to dietary antigens. In a relevant mice model the oral administration of TGF-β increased activation and response in TGF-β-related responsive elements and increased serum TGF-β levels [118]. BALB/c mice treated orally with OVA and TGF-β showed augmented reduction of OVA-specific IgE and IgG1 antibodies, T-cell reactivity, and immediate-type skin reactions when compared with the mice treated orally with OVA alone [118]. The data suggest that oral administration of TGF-β might become a potential strategy to prevent allergic diseases, such as food allergy.

T Cells in Allergen-Specific Immunotherapy

Allergen-specific immunotherapy (allergen-SIT) is the only curative treatment modality for the treatment of allergic disorders targeting to induce a tolerant state, which is essential for a healthy immune response. Development of peripheral T-cell tolerance is characterized mainly by the generation of allergen-specific Treg cells, which suppress proliferative and cytokine responses against the major allergens [104, 119–121]. In allergen-SIT, peripheral T-cell tolerance is initiated by the autocrine action of increasing levels of the anti-inflammatory cytokines IL-10 and TGF-β, produced by antigen-specific Treg cells [103, 122, 123]. Although earlier studies emphasized a switch from Th2 cells to Th1 cells in the course of allergen-SIT, recently, it was shown that allergen-SIT increased the expression of mucosal and peripheral T-cell IL-10 and TGF-β levels [124–127]. The role of Treg cells in the induction of allergen-specific tolerance was supported by the demonstration of local FOXP3+CD25+ T cells in the nasal mucosa and their increased numbers after immunotherapy [128]. A gradual decrease in IgE levels can be observed over months or years in allergen-SIT [129]. On the other hand, analysis of the IgG subtypes induced by allergen-SIT has shown increases in allergen-specific IgG4 and IgG1, with 10- to 100-fold increases in their serum levels [130, 131]. IL-10 is a potent suppressor of both total and allergen-specific IgE, while it simultaneously increases IgG4 production. Thus, IL-10 not only generates tolerance in T cells; it also regulates specific isotype formation and skews the specific response from an IgE- to an IgG4-dominated phenotype [104].

Treg Cells in Suppression of Effector Cells

The effector cells of allergic inflammation are directly or indirectly under the influence of Treg cells [7]. Even in early phases of allergen-SIT, responsiveness and thresholds for activation of mast cells and basophils are increased [132, 133]. Following bee venom allergen immunotherapy, histamine release was decreased in response to stimulation even after the first days of injections [124]. Treg cells directly inhibited the FcεRI-dependent mast cell degranulation through cell-cell contact involving OX40-OX40 ligand interactions between Treg cells and mast cells, respectively. Mast cells showed increased cyclic adenosine monophosphate levels and reduced Ca^{2+} influx when activated in the presence of Treg cells [134]. On the other hand, it has been reported that in vivo depletion or inactivation of Treg cells caused enhancement of the anaphylactic response [9, 134]. IL-10 plays a role in homeostatic mechanisms of mast cell numbers and functions in peripheral tissues by regulating mast cell maintenance and proliferation [135]. IL-10 was shown to reduce proinflammatory cytokine release from mast cells [136]. In addition, IL-10 downregulates eosinophil function and activity, and suppresses IL-5 production by human resting Th0 and Th2 cells [137].

T-Cell/B-Cell Interaction, IgE Production

Priming of Th2 cells results in the production of Th2 cytokines (such as IL-4 and IL-13) that are responsible for the somatic recombination process by which the class of immunoglobulin is switched from IgM to IgE in B cells [3]. In Th-cell/B-cell inter-action costimulatory signals between CD40L and CD40 as well as CD28 and CD80/CD86 are also necessary. Interaction of IgE with its receptors, known as FcεR on mast cells and basophils, is the key process in allergic immune response. Based on affinities, Fcε receptors are classified as FcεRI and FcεRII. The high-affinity recep-tor, FcεRI, is previously thought to be present on only mast cells and basophils of humans and rodents. However, demonstration of FcεRI on Langerhans' cells, eosino-phils and epidermal cells highlighted the role of IgE-mediated antigen presentation of this receptor [138–140]. Low-affinity receptor, FcεRII (also known as CD23), has a widespread cellular distribution and is expressed on B cells, some T cells, eosinophils, macrophages, monocytes and platelets of humans [141–145]. Both types of IgE Fc receptors are thought to play a role in IgE-mediated antigen presentation [146–149]. IgE-facilitated antigen presentation enhances especially very low doses of allergen to CD4+ T cells [148–150]. Binding of allergen with its specific IgE antibody bound on FcεRI of the mast cells and basophils causes release of preformed mediators from secretory granules that include histamine, tryptase and proteases. Also, release of newly generated lipid-derived mediators such as leukotrienes and platelet-activating factor as well as cytokines and chemokines responsible for the symptoms and signs of allergic disorders as well as anaphylaxis takes place [151], as described elsewhere in other chapters.

B cells also have impact on T-cell differentiation. B-cell antigen presentation plays an important role at promoting Th2 responses and pathophysiology during allergic disorders. It has been shown that B-cell –/– mice and in mice selectively deficient in MHC II on B cells had decreased Th2 cytokines IL-4 and IL-5 [152]. Also in another study it has been reported that B-cell-derived exosomes can present allergen peptides and activate allergen-specific T cells to proliferate and produce Th2 cytokines IL-5 and IL-13 [42].

In addition to binding of FcεRII at the surface of B cells, IgE also binds FcεRI at the surface of DCs and monocytes. This process increases the uptake of allergen by DCs and the subsequent presentation to specific Th cells, which drive the late phase of the allergic inflammation [3, 144].

IgE can be an important target for the treatment of allergic diseases. One of the promising developments in the area of allergy treatment is monoclonal antibody ther-apy against different molecular targets [153]. Omalizumab is a humanized monoclo-nal anti-IgE antibody acting by reducing serum levels of free IgE and downregulating of IgE receptors on circulating basophils and DCs [154]. Until today, three Cochrane analyses about omalizumab have been performed [155–157]. These analyses have determined the efficacy of omalizumab compared with placebo in patients with allergic asthma [155–157]. Omalizumab was also reported to be effective in patients with moderate-to-severe allergic asthma and in patients with allergic rhinitis [158]. Its impacts on effector cells, such as nasal and bronchial eosinophils, bronchial mast cells, T and B cells, have promising results opening an area of extensive research. Although recommendations have been released by task forces for some omalizumab-associated anaphylaxis cases [159], its usage in the treatment of unprovoked anaphylaxis in mastocytosis patients and pretreatment before rush immunotherapies has revealed hopeful results [160, 161].

IL-10 and Treg Cells in Suppression of IgE
IL-10 is a potent suppressor of allergen-specific IgE, whereas it induces IgG4 production [103]. It has been shown that IL-10 decreases ε transcript expression, thus down-regulating IgE production, while enhancing γ4 transcript expression and increasing IgG4 production [162]. This alteration in the isotypes of immunoglobins is marked especially in allergen-SIT trials [103]. Also, supporting evidence has been released on Treg cell subset/B-cell interaction experiments through GITR/GITR-L interaction, IL-10 and TGF-β [163]. On the other hand, demonstrating the induction of IgG4 and suppression of IgE in healthy individuals has recently showed the direct influence of Treg cells on B cells [108]. Moreover, neither IL-10-secreting Tr1 cells nor CD4+CD25+FOXP3+ Treg cells have been shown to exert any influence on IgA production.

T Cells in Late-Phase Reactions
Type 1 hypersensitivity reaction is followed by a late-phase allergic reaction, which appears 6–12 h after allergen exposure in which allergen-specific T cells migrate and are reactivated and clonally expand under the influence of chemokines and other cytokines at the site of allergen exposure. Eosinophils constitute the major percentage of the cellular infiltrate, where Th1 cells, mast cells and basophils also contribute to this phase of reaction [3]. This phase is also a cellular-driven process with migration and infiltration of eosinophils, basophils, macrophages and T cells. These effector cells release additional inflammatory mediators and cytokines that elicit continuance of the inflammatory response. A chronic late-phase response due to continuous allergen exposure is thought to be responsible for the persistent, chronic signs and symptoms [164]. After a successful allergen-SIT course, hyperreactivity levels to non-specific stimuli, which seem to reflect underlying mucosal inflammation decreases in correlation with clinical improvements [165]. DC recruitment and activation are also important contributors of late-phase reactions which have been shown to be augmented by TSLP [166]. Platelets also have an impact on late-phase reactions. It has recently been suggested that platelets play important roles through chemokines

that attract leukocytes to the skin and by forming platelet-leukocyte complexes via P-selectin [167].

Conclusion

Understanding the mechanisms enrolled in the development of anaphylaxis, the systemic life-threatening IgE-mediated type 1 hypersensitivity reaction is essential for developing strategies for treatment and prevention from the reaction. Capture and recognition of antigens need specialized APCs with highly distinctive features acting for introduction to the immune effector cells, especially to T lymphocytes. Recent developments in T-cell subsets, particularly the extension of the knowledge on reciprocal regulation and counterbalance between Th1 and Th2 cells to Th17 and Treg cells, has increased our knowledge in mechanisms of immunoregulation. Allergen-specific strategies for targeting immune responses have significantly evolved and new insights into the mechanism of immunoregulation are leading to novel approaches for allergen-SIT vaccine development. Many different elements behave synergistically in directing the immune system into the Th2 profile in atopic individuals, whereas IL-4 and IL-13 exert an important role in class switching in B lymphocytes with the resultant IgE production. Allergen-specific IgE molecules bind to mast cells and basophils via specialized receptors where they stay ready for a subsequent exposure. Upon challenge, a specific allergen release of mediators as well as cytokines happens which causes symptoms and signs of anaphylaxis. All APCs, T and B lymphocytes, mast cells and basophils as well as several cellular elements play a synchronized active role in this sequential process of allergy.

Acknowledgements

The authors' laboratories are funded by the Swiss National Science Foundation (grants SNF-32-112306/1 and 32-118226) and Global Allergy and Asthma European Network (GA²LEN).

References

1 Yazdanbakhsh M, Kremsner PG, van Ree R: Allergy, parasites, and the hygiene hypothesis. Science 2002; 296:490–494.

2 Akdis CA: Allergy and hypersensitivity: mechanisms of allergic disease. Curr Opin Immunol 2006; 18:718–726.

3 Larche M, Akdis CA, Valenta R: Immunological mechanisms of allergen-specific immunotherapy. Nat Rev Immunol 2006;6:761–771.

4 De Silva IL, Mehr SS, Tey D, Tang ML: Paediatric anaphylaxis: a 5-year retrospective review. Allergy 2008;63:1071–1076.

5 Sampson HA, Mendelson L, Rosen JP: Fatal and near-fatal anaphylactic reactions to food in children and adolescents. N Engl J Med 1992;327:380–384.

6 De Bilderling G, Mathot M, Agustsson S, Tuerlinckx D, Jamart J, Bodart E: Early skin sensitization to aeroallergens. Clin Exp Allergy 2008;38:643–648.

7 Ozdemir C, Akdis M, Akdis CA: T regulatory cells and their counterparts: masters of immune regulation. Clin Exp Allergy 2009;39:626–639.

8 Romani N, Koide S, Crowley M, Witmer-Pack M, Livingstone AM, Fathman CG, Inaba K, Steinman RM: Presentation of exogenous protein antigens by dendritic cells to T cell clones. Intact protein is presented best by immature, epidermal Langerhans' cells. J Exp Med 1989;169:1169–1178.

9 Akdis CA, Akdis M: Mechanisms and treatment of allergic disease in the big picture of regulatory T cells. J Allergy Clin Immunol 2009;123:735–748.

10 Akdis CA, Akdis M, Bieber T, Bindslev-Jensen C, Boguniewicz M, Eigenmann P, Hamid Q, Kapp A, Leung DY, Lipozencic J, Luger TA, Muraro A, Novak N, Platts-Mills TA, Rosenwasser L, Scheynius A, Simons FE, Spergel J, Turjanmaa K, Wahn U, Weidinger S, Werfel T, Zuberbier T: Diagnosis and treatment of atopic dermatitis in children and adults. European Academy of Allergology and Clinical Immunology/American Academy of Allergy, Asthma and Immunology/PRACTALL Consensus Report. J Allergy Clin Immunol 2006;118:152–169.

11 Romagnani S: Coming back to a missing immune deviation as the main explanatory mechanism for the hygiene hypothesis. J Allergy Clin Immunol 2007;119:1511–1513.

12 Munitz A, Levi-Schaffer F: Inhibitory receptors on eosinophils: a direct hit to a possible Achilles heel? J Allergy Clin Immunol 2007;119:1382–1387.

13 Adedoyin J, Gronlund H, Oman H, Johansson SG, van Hage M: Cat IgA, representative of new carbohydrate cross-reactive allergens. J Allergy Clin Immunol 2007;119:640–645.

14 Soeria-Atmadja D, Onell A, Kober A, Matsson P, Gustafsson MG, Hammerling U: Multivariate statistical analysis of large-scale IgE antibody measurements reveals allergen extract relationships in sensitized individuals. J Allergy Clin Immunol 2007; 120:1433–1440.

15 Kiss A, Montes M, Susarla S, Jaensson EA, Drouin SM, Wetsel RA, Yao Z, Martin R, Hamzeh N, Adelagun R, Amar S, Kheradmand F, Corry DB: A new mechanism regulating the initiation of allergic airway inflammation. J Allergy Clin Immunol 2007; 120:334–342.

16 Hsu SC, Tsai TH, Kawasaki H, Chen CH, Plunkett B, Lee RT, Lee YC, Huang SK: Antigen coupled with Lewis-x trisaccharides elicits potent immune responses in mice. J Allergy Clin Immunol 2007;119: 1522–1528.

17 Liotta F, Frosali F, Querci V, Mantei A, Fili L, Maggi L, Mazzinghi B, Angeli R, Ronconi E, Santarlasci V, Biagioli T, Lasagni L, Ballerini C, Parronchi P, Scheffold A, Cosmi L, Maggi E, Romagnani S, Annunziato F: Human immature myeloid dendritic cells trigger a T_H2-polarizing program via Jagged-1/Notch interaction. J Allergy Clin Immunol 2008;121: 1000–1005 e1008.

18 Kaisho T, Akira S: Toll-like receptor function and signaling. J Allergy Clin Immunol 2006;117:979–988.

19 Janeway CA Jr: Approaching the asymptote? Evolution and revolution in immunology. Cold Spring Harb Symp Quant Biol 1989;54:1–13.

20 Janeway CA Jr, Medzhitov R: Innate immune recognition. Annu Rev Immunol 2002;20:197–216.

21 Kapsenberg ML: Dendritic-cell control of pathogen-driven T-cell polarization. Nat Rev Immunol 2003;3: 984–993.

22 Kopp EB, Medzhitov R: The Toll-receptor family and control of innate immunity. Curr Opin Immunol 1999;11:13–18.

23 Van Vliet SJ, den Dunnen J, Gringhuis SI, Geijtenbeek TB, van Kooyk Y: Innate signaling and regulation of dendritic cell immunity. Curr Opin Immunol 2007;19:435–440.

24 Gon Y: Toll-like receptors and airway inflammation. Allergol Int 2008;57:33–37.

25 Hewson CA, Jardine A, Edwards MR, Laza-Stanca V, Johnston SL: Toll-like receptor 3 is induced by and mediates antiviral activity against rhinovirus infection of human bronchial epithelial cells. J Virol 2005;79:12273–12279.

26 Duez C, Gosset P, Tonnel AB: Dendritic cells and toll-like receptors in allergy and asthma. Eur J Dermatol 2006;16:12–16.

27 Takeuchi O, Akira S: Toll-like receptors; their physiological role and signal transduction system. Int Immunopharmacol 2001;1:625–635.

28 Fitzgerald KA, Rowe DC, Barnes BJ, Caffrey DR, Visintin A, Latz E, Monks B, Pitha PM, Golenbock DT: LPS-TLR4 signaling to IRF-3/7 and NF-κB involves the toll adapters TRAM and TRIF. J Exp Med 2003;198:1043–1055.

29 Horng T, Barton GM, Medzhitov R: TIRAP: an adapter molecule in the Toll signaling pathway. Nat Immunol 2001;2:835–841.

30 Yamamoto M, Sato S, Hemmi H, Hoshino K, Kaisho T, Sanjo H, Takeuchi O, Sugiyama M, Okabe M, Takeda K, Akira S: Role of adaptor TRIF in the MyD88-independent toll-like receptor signaling pathway. Science 2003;301:640–643.

31 Trinchieri G: Interleukin-12 and the regulation of innate resistance and adaptive immunity. Nat Rev Immunol 2003;3:133–146.

32 Kadowaki N, Antonenko S, Lau JY, Liu YJ: Natural interferon α/β-producing cells link innate and adaptive immunity. J Exp Med 2000;192:219–226.

33 Salomon B, Bluestone JA: LFA-1 interaction with ICAM-1 and ICAM-2 regulates Th2 cytokine production. J Immunol 1998;161:5138–5142.

34 Jin W, Zhou XF, Yu J, Cheng X, Sun SC: Regulation of Th17 cell differentiation and EAE induction by the MAP3K NIK. Blood 2009;113:6603–6610.

35 Cella M, Engering A, Pinet V, Pieters J, Lanzavecchia A: Inflammatory stimuli induce accumulation of MHC class II complexes on dendritic cells. Nature 1997;388:782–787.

36 Inaba K, Turley S, Iyoda T, Yamaide F, Shimoyama S, Reis e Sousa C, Germain RN, Mellman I, Steinman RM: The formation of immunogenic major histocompatibility complex class II-peptide ligands in lysosomal compartments of dendritic cells is regulated by inflammatory stimuli. J Exp Med 2000;191:927–936.

37 Varadaradjalou S, Feger F, Thieblemont N, Hamouda NB, Pleau JM, Dy M, Arock M: Toll-like receptor 2 (TLR2) and TLR4 differentially activate human mast cells. Eur J Immunol 2003;33:899–906.

38 Hemmi H, Takeuchi O, Kawai T, Kaisho T, Sato S, Sanjo H, Matsumoto M, Hoshino K, Wagner H, Takeda K, Akira S: A Toll-like receptor recognizes bacterial DNA. Nature 2000;408:740–745.

39 Mizel SB, Snipes JA: Gram-negative flagellin-induced self-tolerance is associated with a block in interleukin-1 receptor-associated kinase release from toll-like receptor 5. J Biol Chem 2002;277:22414–22420.

40 Sel S, Wegmann M, Bauer S, Garn H, Alber G, Renz H: Immunomodulatory effects of viral TLR ligands on experimental asthma depend on the additive effects of IL-12 and IL-10. J Immunol 2007;178:7805–7813.

41 Tosi MF: Innate immune responses to infection. J Allergy Clin Immunol 2005;116:241–240.

42 Admyre C, Bohle B, Johansson SM, Focke-Tejkl M, Valenta R, Scheynius A, Gabrielsson S: B-cell-derived exosomes can present allergen peptides and activate allergen-specific T cells to proliferate and produce T$_H$2-like cytokines. J Allergy Clin Immunol 2007;120:1418–1424.

43 Jarrossay D, Napolitani G, Colonna M, Sallusto F, Lanzavecchia A: Specialization and complementarity in microbial molecule recognition by human myeloid and plasmacytoid dendritic cells. Eur J Immunol 2001;31:3388–3393.

44 Rissoan MC, Soumelis V, Kadowaki N, Grouard G, Briere F, de Waal Malefyt R, Liu YJ: Reciprocal control of T-helper cell and dendritic cell differentiation. Science 1999;283:1183–1186.

45 Ito T, Kanzler H, Duramad O, Cao W, Liu YJ: Specialization, kinetics, and repertoire of type 1 interferon responses by human plasmacytoid pre-dendritic cells. Blood 2006;107:2423–2431.

46 Ito T, Yang M, Wang YH, Lande R, Gregorio J, Perng OA, Qin XF, Liu YJ, Gilliet M: Plasmacytoid dendritic cells prime IL-10-producing T regulatory cells by inducible costimulator ligand. J Exp Med 2007;204:105–115.

47 Kadowaki N, Ho S, Antonenko S, Malefyt RW, Kastelein RA, Bazan F, Liu YJ: Subsets of human dendritic cell precursors express different toll-like receptors and respond to different microbial antigens. J Exp Med 2001;194:863–869.

48 De Heer HJ, Hammad H, Soullie T, Hijdra D, Vos N, Willart MA, Hoogsteden HC, Lambrecht BN: Essential role of lung plasmacytoid dendritic cells in preventing asthmatic reactions to harmless inhaled antigen. J Exp Med 2004;200:89–98.

49 Kool M, Lambrecht BN: Dendritic cells in asthma and COPD: opportunities for drug development. Curr Opin Immunol 2007;19:701–710.

50 Wollenberg A, Kraft S, Hanau D, Bieber T: Immuno-morphological and ultrastructural characterization of Langerhans' cells and a novel, inflammatory dendritic epidermal cell population in lesional skin of atopic eczema. J Invest Dermatol 1996;106:446–453.

51 Novak N, Bieber T: The role of dendritic cell subtypes in the pathophysiology of atopic dermatitis. J Am Acad Dermatol 2005;53:S171–S176.

52 Bieber T, Braun-Falco O: IgE-bearing Langerhans' cells are not specific to atopic eczema but are found in inflammatory skin diseases. J Am Acad Dermatol 1991;24:658–659.

53 Ray P, Krishnamoorthy N, Ray A: Emerging functions of c-kit and its ligand stem cell factor in dendritic cells: regulators of T cell differentiation. Cell Cycle 2008;7:2826–2832.

54 Galli SJ, Tsai M, Piliponsky AM: The development of allergic inflammation. Nature 2008;454:445–454.

55 Goldberg AL, Rock KL: Proteolysis, proteasomes and antigen presentation. Nature 1992;357:375–379.

56 Nickoloff BJ, Turka LA: Immunological functions of non-professional antigen-presenting cells: new insights from studies of T-cell interactions with keratinocytes. Immunol Today 1994;15:464–469.

57 Belov K, Deakin JE, Papenfuss AT, Baker ML, Melman SD, Siddle HV, Gouin N, Goode DL, Sargeant TJ, Robinson MD, Wakefield MJ, Mahony S, Cross JG, Benos PV, Samollow PB, Speed TP, Graves JA, Miller RD: Reconstructing an ancestral mammalian immune supercomplex from a marsupial major histocompatibility complex. PLoS Biol 2006;4:e46.

58 Kumanovics A, Takada T, Lindahl KF: Genomic organization of the mammalian MHC. Annu Rev Immunol 2003;21:629–657.

59 Kloetzel PM: Antigen processing by the proteasome. Nat Rev Mol Cell Biol 2001;2:179–187.

60 York IA, Goldberg AL, Mo XY, Rock KL: Proteolysis and class I major histocompatibility complex antigen presentation. Immunol Rev 1999;172:49–66.

61 Rhyner C, Kundig T, Akdis CA, Crameri R: Targeting the MHC II presentation pathway in allergy vaccine development. Biochem Soc Trans 2007;35: 833–834.

62 Bancereau J, Briere F, Caux C, Davoust J, Lebecque S, Liu YJ, Pulendran B, Palucka K: Immunobiology of dendritic cells. Annu Rev Immunol 2000;18:767–811.

63 Worbs T, Forster R: A key role for CCR7 in establishing central and peripheral tolerance. Trends Immunol 2007;28:274–280.

64 Yoshida R, Imai T, Hieshima K, Kusuda J, Baba M, Kitaura M, Nishimura M, Kakizaki M, Nomiyama H, Yoshie O: Molecular cloning of a novel human CC chemokine EBI1-ligand chemokine that is a specific functional ligand for EBI1, CCR7. J Biol Chem 1997;272:13803–13809.

65 Frauwirth KA, Thompson CB: Activation and inhibition of lymphocytes by costimulation. J Clin Invest 2002;109:295–299.

66 Janeway CA Jr: The T cell receptor as a multicomponent signalling machine: CD4/CD8 coreceptors and CD45 in T cell activation. Annu Rev Immunol 1992;10:645–674.

67 Freeman GJ, Gribben JG, Boussiotis VA, Ng JW, Restivo VA Jr, Lombard LA, Gray GS, Nadler LM: Cloning of B7-2: a CTLA-4 counter-receptor that costimulates human T cell proliferation. Science 1993;262:909–911.

68 Gillis S, Ferm MM, Ou W, Smith KA: T cell growth factor: parameters of production and a quantitative microassay for activity. J Immunol 1978;120:2027–2032.

69 Yoshinaga SK, Whoriskey JS, Khare SD, Sarmiento U, Guo J, Horan T, Shih G, Zhang M, Coccia MA, Kohno T, Tafuri-Bladt A, Brankow D, Campbell P, Chang D, Chiu L, Dai T, Duncan G, Elliott GS, Hui A, McCabe SM, Scully S, Shahinian A, Shaklee CL, Van G, Mak TW, Senaldi G: T-cell co-stimulation through B7RP-1 and ICOS. Nature 1999;402:827–832.

70 Howland KC, Ausubel LJ, London CA, Abbas AK: The roles of CD28 and CD40 ligand in T cell activation and tolerance. J Immunol 2000;164:4465–4470.

71 Wadman M: London's disastrous drug trial has serious side effects for research. Nature 2006;440:388–389.

72 Mosmann TR, Cherwinski H, Bond MW, Giedlin MA, Coffman RL: Two types of murine helper T cell clone. I. Definition according to profiles of lymphokine activities and secreted proteins. J Immunol 1986;136:2348–2357.

73 Wells JW, Cowled CJ, Giorgini A, Kemeny DM, Noble A: Regulation of allergic airway inflammation by class I-restricted allergen presentation and CD8 T-cell infiltration. J Allergy Clin Immunol 2007;119:226–234.

74 Schmidt-Weber CB, Akdis M, Akdis CA: T_H17 cells in the big picture of immunology. J Allergy Clin Immunol 2007;120:247–254.

75 Chatila TA, Li N, Garcia-Lloret M, Kim HJ, Nel AE: T-cell effector pathways in allergic diseases: transcriptional mechanisms and therapeutic targets. J Allergy Clin Immunol 2008;121:812–823; quiz 824–815.

76 Fujiwara M, Hirose K, Kagami S, Takatori H, Wakashin H, Tamachi T, Watanabe N, Saito Y, Iwamoto I, Nakajima H: T-bet inhibits both T_H2 cell-mediated eosinophil recruitment and T_H17 cell-mediated neutrophil recruitment into the airways. J Allergy Clin Immunol 2007;119:662–670.

77 Munthe-Kaas MC, Carlsen KH, Haland G, Devulapalli CS, Gervin K, Egeland T, Carlsen KL, Undlien D: T cell-specific T-box transcription factor haplotype is associated with allergic asthma in children. J Allergy Clin Immunol 2008;121:51–56.

78 Akkoc T, de Koning PJ, Ruckert B, Barlan I, Akdis M, Akdis CA: Increased activation-induced cell death of high IFN-γ-producing T_H1 cells as a mechanism of T_H2 predominance in atopic diseases. J Allergy Clin Immunol 2008;121:652–658 e651.

79 Trautmann A, Akdis M, Kleemann D, Altznauer F, Simon HU, Graeve T, Noll M, Brocker EB, Blaser K, Akdis CA: T cell-mediated Fas-induced keratinocyte apoptosis plays a key pathogenetic role in eczematous dermatitis. J Clin Invest 2000;106:25–35.

80 Trautmann A, Schmid-Grendelmeier P, Kruger K, Crameri R, Akdis M, Akkaya A, Brocker EB, Blaser K, Akdis CA: T cells and eosinophils cooperate in the induction of bronchial epithelial cell apoptosis in asthma. J Allergy Clin Immunol 2002;109:329–337.

81 Romagnani S: Regulation of the T cell response. Clin Exp Allergy 2006;36:1357–1366.

82 Ohshima Y, Yang LP, Uchiyama T, Tanaka Y, Baum P, Sergerie M, Hermann P, Delespesse G: OX40 costimulation enhances interleukin-4 (IL-4) expression at priming and promotes the differentiation of naive human CD4+ T cells into high IL-4-producing effectors. Blood 1998;92:3338–3345.

83 Liu YJ: Thymic stromal lymphopoietin and OX40 ligand pathway in the initiation of dendritic cell-mediated allergic inflammation. J Allergy Clin Immunol 2007;120:238–246.

84 Ray RJ, Furlonger C, Williams DE, Paige CJ: Characterization of thymic stromal-derived lymphopoietin in murine B-cell development in vitro. Eur J Immunol 1996;26:10–16.

85 Kato A, Favoreto S Jr, Avila PC, Schleimer RP: TLR3- and Th2 cytokine-dependent production of thymic stromal lymphopoietin in human airway epithelial cells. J Immunol 2007;179:1080–1087.

86 Ito T, Wang YH, Duramad O, Hori T, Delespesse GJ, Watanabe N, Qin FX, Yao Z, Cao W, Liu YJ: TSLP-activated dendritic cells induce an inflammatory T-helper type 2 cell response through OX40 ligand. J Exp Med 2005;202:1213–1223.

87 Arques JL, Regoli M, Bertelli E, Nicoletti C: Persistence of apoptosis-resistant T cell-activating dendritic cells promotes T-helper type-2 response and IgE antibody production. Mol Immunol 2008;45:2177–2186.

88 Ballantyne SJ, Barlow JL, Jolin HE, Nath P, Williams AS, Chung KF, Sturton G, Wong SH, McKenzie AN: Blocking IL-25 prevents airway hyperresponsiveness in allergic asthma. J Allergy Clin Immunol 2007;120:1324–1331.

89 Bettelli E, Carrier Y, Gao W, Korn T, Strom TB, Oukka M, Weiner HL, Kuchroo VK: Reciprocal developmental pathways for the generation of pathogenic effector T_H17 and regulatory T cells. Nature 2006;441:235–238.

90 Weaver CT, Harrington LE, Mangan PR, Gavrieli M, Murphy KM: Th17: an effector CD4 T cell lineage with regulatory T cell ties. Immunity 2006;24:677–688.

91 Harrington LE, Hatton RD, Mangan PR, Turner H, Murphy TL, Murphy KM, Weaver CT: Interleukin-17-producing CD4+ effector T cells develop via a lineage distinct from the T-helper type 1 and 2 lineages. Nat Immunol 2005;6:1123–1132.

92 Mangan PR, Harrington LE, O'Quinn DB, Helms WS, Bullard DC, Elson CO, Hatton RD, Wahl SM, Schoeb TR, Weaver CT: Transforming growth factor-β induces development of the T_H17 lineage. Nature 2006;441:231–234.

93 Bettelli E, Korn T, Oukka M, Kuchroo VK: Induction and effector functions of T_H17 cells. Nature 2008;453:1051–1057.

94 Hellings PW, Kasran A, Liu Z, Vandekerckhove P, Wuyts A, Overbergh L, Mathieu C, Ceuppens JL: Interleukin-17 orchestrates the granulocyte influx into airways after allergen inhalation in a mouse model of allergic asthma. Am J Respir Cell Mol Biol 2003;28:42–50.

95 Sergejeva S, Ivanov S, Lotvall J, Linden A: Interleukin-17 as a recruitment and survival factor for airway macrophages in allergic airway inflammation. Am J Respir Cell Mol Biol 2005;33:248–253.

96 Bush KA, Farmer KM, Walker JS, Kirkham BW: Reduction of joint inflammation and bone erosion in rat adjuvant arthritis by treatment with interleukin-17 receptor IgG1 Fc fusion protein. Arthritis Rheum 2002;46:802–805.

97 Dong C: Regulation and pro-inflammatory function of interleukin-17 family cytokines. Immunol Rev 2008;226:80–86.

98 Fort MM, Cheung J, Yen D, Li J, Zurawski SM, Lo S, Menon S, Clifford T, Hunte B, Lesley R, Muchamuel T, Hurst SD, Zurawski G, Leach MW, Gorman DM, Rennick DM: IL-25 induces IL-4, IL-5, and IL-13 and Th2-associated pathologies in vivo. Immunity 2001;15:985–995.

99 Hurst SD, Muchamuel T, Gorman DM, Gilbert JM, Clifford T, Kwan S, Menon S, Seymour B, Jackson C, Kung TT, Brieland JK, Zurawski SM, Chapman RW, Zurawski G, Coffman RL: New IL-17 family members promote Th1 or Th2 responses in the lung: in vivo function of the novel cytokine IL-25. J Immunol 2002;169:443–453.

100 Veldhoen M, Uyttenhove C, van Snick J, Helmby H, Westendorf A, Buer J, Martin B, Wilhelm C, Stockinger B: Transforming growth factor-β 'reprograms' the differentiation of T-helper-2 cells and promotes an interleukin-9-producing subset. Nat Immunol 2008;9:1341–1346.

101 Dardalhon V, Awasthi A, Kwon H, Galileos G, Gao W, Sobel RA, Mitsdoerffer M, Strom TB, Elyaman W, Ho IC, Khoury S, Oukka M, Kuchroo VK: IL-4 inhibits TGF-β-induced Foxp3+ T cells and, together with TGF-β, generates IL-9+ IL-10+ Foxp3– effector T cells. Nat Immunol 2008;9:1347–1355.

102 Chen Y, Kuchroo VK, Inobe J, Hafler DA, Weiner HL: Regulatory T cell clones induced by oral tolerance: suppression of autoimmune encephalomyelitis. Science 1994;265:1237–1240.

103 Akdis CA, Blesken T, Akdis M, Wuthrich B, Blaser K: Role of interleukin-10 in specific immunotherapy. J Clin Invest 1998;102:98–106.

104 Jutel M, Akdis CA: T-cell regulatory mechanisms in specific immunotherapy. Chem Immunol Allergy 2008;94:158–177.

105 Cottrez F, Hurst SD, Coffman RL, Groux H: T regulatory cells 1 inhibit a Th2-specific response in vivo. J Immunol 2000;165:4848–4853.

106 Bellinghausen I, Konig B, Bottcher I, Knop J, Saloga J: Inhibition of human allergic T-helper type 2 immune responses by induced regulatory T cells requires the combination of interleukin-10-treated dendritic cells and transforming growth factor-β for their induction. Clin Exp Allergy 2006;36:1546–1555.

107 Akdis M, Blaser K, Akdis CA: T regulatory cells in allergy: novel concepts in the pathogenesis, prevention, and treatment of allergic diseases. J Allergy Clin Immunol 2005;116:961–969.

108 Meiler F, Klunker S, Zimmermann M, Akdis CA, Akdis M: Distinct regulation of IgE, IgG4 and IgA by T regulatory cells and toll-like receptors. Allergy 2008;63:1455–1463.

109 Verhagen J, Blaser K, Akdis CA, Akdis M: Mechanisms of allergen-specific immunotherapy: T-regulatory cells and more. Immunol Allergy Clin North Am 2006;26:207–231.

110 Onishi Y, Fehervari Z, Yamaguchi T, Sakaguchi S: Foxp3+ natural regulatory T cells preferentially form aggregates on dendritic cells in vitro and actively inhibit their maturation. Proc Natl Acad Sci USA 2008;105:10113–10118.

111 Gause WC, Urban JF, Linsley P, Lu P: Role of B7 signaling in the differentiation of naive CD4+ T cells to effector interleukin-4-producing T-helper cells. Immunol Res 1995;14:176–188.

112 Read S, Malmstrom V, Powrie F: Cytotoxic T lymphocyte-associated antigen 4 plays an essential role in the function of CD25+CD4+ regulatory cells that control intestinal inflammation. J Exp Med 2000; 192:295–302.

113 Salomon B, Lenschow DJ, Rhee L, Ashourian N, Singh B, Sharpe A, Bluestone JA: B7/CD28 costimulation is essential for the homeostasis of the CD4+CD25+ immunoregulatory T cells that control autoimmune diabetes. Immunity 2000;12:431–440.

114 Prasse A, Germann M, Pechkovsky DV, Markert A, Verres T, Stahl M, Melchers I, Luttmann W, Muller-Quernheim J, Zissel G: IL-10-producing monocytes differentiate to alternatively activated macrophages and are increased in atopic patients. J Allergy Clin Immunol 2007;119:464–471.

115 Koya T, Matsuda H, Takeda K, Matsubara S, Miyahara N, Balhorn A, Dakhama A, Gelfand EW: IL-10-treated dendritic cells decrease airway hyperresponsiveness and airway inflammation in mice. J Allergy Clin Immunol 2007;119:1241–1250.

116 Taylor A, Akdis M, Joss A, Akkoc T, Wenig R, Colonna M, Daigle I, Flory E, Blaser K, Akdis CA: IL-10 inhibits CD28 and ICOS costimulations of T cells via Src homology 2 domain-containing protein tyrosine phosphatase 1. J Allergy Clin Immunol 2007;120:76–83.

117 Oh SY, Zheng T, Bailey ML, Barber DL, Schroeder JT, Kim YK, Zhu Z: Src homology 2 domain-containing inositol 5-phosphatase 1 deficiency leads to a spontaneous allergic inflammation in the murine lung. J Allergy Clin Immunol 2007;119:123–131.

118 Ando T, Hatsushika K, Wako M, Ohba T, Koyama K, Ohnuma Y, Katoh R, Ogawa H, Okumura K, Luo J, Wyss-Coray T, Nakao A: Orally administered TGF-β is biologically active in the intestinal mucosa and enhances oral tolerance. J Allergy Clin Immunol 2007;120:916–923.

119 Akdis M: Healthy immune response to allergens: T regulatory cells and more. Curr Opin Immunol 2006;18:738–744.

120 Ling EM, Smith T, Nguyen XD, Pridgeon C, Dallman M, Arbery J, Carr VA, Robinson DS: Relation of CD4+CD25+ regulatory T-cell suppression of allergen-driven T-cell activation to atopic status and expression of allergic disease. Lancet 2004;363:608–615.

121 Sakaguchi S, Yamaguchi T, Nomura T, Ono M: Regulatory T cells and immune tolerance. Cell 2008; 133:775–787.

122 Francis JN, Till SJ, Durham SR: Induction of IL-10+CD4+CD25+ T cells by grass pollen immunotherapy. J Allergy Clin Immunol 2003;111:1255–1261.

123 Jutel M, Akdis M, Budak F, Aebischer-Casaulta C, Wrzyszcz M, Blaser K, Akdis CA: IL-10 and TGF-β cooperate in the regulatory T cell response to mucosal allergens in normal immunity and specific immunotherapy. Eur J Immunol 2003;33:1205–1214.

124 Jutel M, Pichler WJ, Skrbic D, Urwyler A, Dahinden C, Muller UR: Bee venom immunotherapy results in decrease of IL-4 and IL-5 and increase of IFN-γ secretion in specific allergen-stimulated T cell cultures. J Immunol 1995;154:4187–4194.

125 Nouri-Aria KT, Wachholz PA, Francis JN, Jacobson MR, Walker SM, Wilcock LK, Staple SQ, Aalberse RC, Till SJ, Durham SR: Grass pollen immunotherapy induces mucosal and peripheral IL-10 responses and blocking IgG activity. J Immunol 2004;172:3252–3259.

126 Pilette C, Nouri-Aria KT, Jacobson MR, Wilcock LK, Detry B, Walker SM, Francis JN, Durham SR: Grass pollen immunotherapy induces an allergen-specific IgA2 antibody response associated with mucosal TGF-β expression. J Immunol 2007;178:4658–4666.

127 Varney VA, Hamid QA, Gaga M, Ying S, Jacobson M, Frew AJ, Kay AB, Durham SR: Influence of grass pollen immunotherapy on cellular infiltration and cytokine mRNA expression during allergen-induced late-phase cutaneous responses. J Clin Invest 1993; 92:644–651.

128 Radulovic S, Jacobson MR, Durham SR, Nouri-Aria KT: Grass pollen immunotherapy induces Foxp3-expressing CD4+ CD25+ cells in the nasal mucosa. J Allergy Clin Immunol 2008;121:1467–1472, 1472 e1461.

129 Muller U, Helbling A, Bischof M: Predictive value of venom-specific IgE, IgG and IgG subclass antibodies in patients on immunotherapy with honey bee venom. Allergy 1989;44:412–418.

130 Jutel M, Jaeger L, Suck R, Meyer H, Fiebig H, Cromwell O: Allergen-specific immunotherapy with recombinant grass pollen allergens. J Allergy Clin Immunol 2005;116:608–613.

131 Van der Giessen M, Homan WL, van Kernbeek G, Aalberse RC, Dieges PH: Subclass typing of IgG antibodies formed by grass pollen-allergic patients during immunotherapy. Int Arch Allergy Appl Immunol 1976;50:625–640.

132 Shim JY, Kim BS, Cho SH, Min KU, Hong SJ: Allergen-specific conventional immunotherapy decreases immunoglobulin E-mediated basophil histamine releasability. Clin Exp Allergy 2003;33: 52–57.

133 Treter S, Luqman M: Antigen-specific T cell tolerance down-regulates mast cell responses in vivo. Cell Immunol 2000;206:116–124.

134 Gri G, Piconese S, Frossi B, Manfroi V, Merluzzi S, Tripodo C, Viola A, Odom S, Rivera J, Colombo MP, Pucillo CE: CD4+CD25+ regulatory T cells suppress mast cell degranulation and allergic responses through OX40-OX40L interaction. Immunity 2008;29:771–781.

135 Thompson-Snipes L, Dhar V, Bond MW, Mosmann TR, Moore KW, Rennick DM: Interleukin-10: a novel stimulatory factor for mast cells and their progenitors. J Exp Med 1991;173:507–510.

136 Marshall JS, Leal-Berumen I, Nielsen L, Glibetic M, Jordana M: Interleukin (IL)-10 inhibits long-term IL-6 production but not preformed mediator release from rat peritoneal mast cells. J Clin Invest 1996; 97:1122–1128.

137 Schandene L, Alonso-Vega C, Willems F, Gerard C, Delvaux A, Velu T, Devos R, de Boer M, Goldman M: B7/CD28-dependent IL-5 production by human resting T cells is inhibited by IL-10. J Immunol 1994;152:4368–4374.

138 Kinet JP: Atopic allergy and other hypersensitivities. Curr Opin Immunol 1999;11:603–605.

139 Natter S, Seiberler S, Hufnagl P, Binder BR, Hirschl AM, Ring J, Abeck D, Schmidt T, Valent P, Valenta R: Isolation of cDNA clones coding for IgE autoantigens with serum IgE from atopic dermatitis patients. FASEB J 1998;12:1559–1569.

140 Stingl G, Maurer D: IgE-mediated allergen presentation via FcεRI on antigen-presenting cells. Int Arch Allergy Immunol 1997;113:24–29.

141 Finbloom DS, Metzger H: Binding of immunoglobulin E to the receptor on rat peritoneal macrophages. J Immunol 1982;129:2004–2008.

142 Larche M: Immunoregulation by targeting T cells in the treatment of allergy and asthma. Curr Opin Immunol 2006;18:745–750.

143 Melewicz FM, Plummer JM, Spiegelberg HL: Comparison of the Fc receptors for IgE on human lymphocytes and monocytes. J Immunol 1982;129: 563–569.

144 Mudde GC, Hansel TT, von Reijsen FC, Osterhoff BF, Bruijnzeel-Koomen CA: IgE: an immunoglobulin specialized in antigen capture? Immunol Today 1990;11:440–443.

145 Tunon de Lara JM: Immunoglobulins E and inflammatory cells (in French). Rev Mal Respir 1996;13:27–36.

146 Maurer D, Ebner C, Reininger B, Fiebiger E, Kraft D, Kinet JP, Stingl G: The high affinity IgE receptor (FcεRI) mediates IgE-dependent allergen presentation. J Immunol 1995;154:6285–6290.

147 Pirron U, Schlunck T, Prinz JC, Rieber EP: IgE-dependent antigen focusing by human B lymphocytes is mediated by the low-affinity receptor for IgE. Eur J Immunol 1990;20:1547–1551.

148 Santamaria LF, Bheekha R, van Reijsen FC, Perez Soler MT, Suter M, Bruijnzeel-Koomen CA, Mudde GC: Antigen focusing by specific monomeric immunoglobulin E bound to CD23 on Epstein-Barr virus-transformed B cells. Hum Immunol 1993;37: 23–30.

149 Van der Heijden FL, Joost van Neerven RJ, van Katwijk M, Bos JD, Kapsenberg ML: Serum-IgE-facilitated allergen presentation in atopic disease. J Immunol 1993;150:3643–3650.

150 Van Neerven RJ, Wikborg T, Lund G, Jacobsen B, Brinch-Nielsen A, Arnved J, Ipsen H: Blocking antibodies induced by specific allergy vaccination prevent the activation of CD4+ T cells by inhibiting serum-IgE-facilitated allergen presentation. J Immunol 1999;163:2944–2952.

151 Peavy RD, Metcalfe DD: Understanding the mechanisms of anaphylaxis. Curr Opin Allergy Clin Immunol 2008;8:310–315.

152 Lindell DM, Berlin AA, Schaller MA, Lukacs NW: B-cell antigen presentation promotes Th2 responses and immunopathology during chronic allergic lung disease. PLoS ONE 2008;3:e3129.

153 Ozdemir C, Akdis CA: Discontinued drugs in 2006: pulmonary-allergy, dermatological, gastrointestinal and arthritis drugs. Expert Opin Investig Drugs 2007;16:1327–1344.

154 Holgate S, Casale T, Wenzel S, Bousquet J, Deniz Y, Reisner C: The anti-inflammatory effects of omalizumab confirm the central role of IgE in allergic inflammation. J Allergy Clin Immunol 2005;115: 459–465.

155 Walker S, Monteil M, Phelan K, Lasserson TJ, Walters EH: Anti-IgE for chronic asthma. Cochrane Database Syst Rev 2003:CD003559.

156 Walker S, Monteil M, Phelan K, Lasserson TJ, Walters EH: Anti-IgE for chronic asthma in adults and children. Cochrane Database Syst Rev 2004:CD003559.

157 Walker S, Monteil M, Phelan K, Lasserson TJ, Walters EH: Anti-IgE for chronic asthma in adults and children. Cochrane Database Syst Rev 2006:CD003559.

158 Holgate ST, Chuchalin AG, Hebert J, Lotvall J, Persson GB, Chung KF, Bousquet J, Kerstjens HA, Fox H, Thirlwell J, Cioppa GD: Efficacy and safety of a recombinant anti-immunoglobulin E antibody (omalizumab) in severe allergic asthma. Clin Exp Allergy 2004;34:632–638.

159 Cox L, Platts-Mills TA, Finegold I, Schwartz LB, Simons FE, Wallace DV: American Academy of Allergy, Asthma & Immunology/American College of Allergy, Asthma and Immunology Joint Task Force Report on omalizumab-associated anaphylaxis. J Allergy Clin Immunol 2007;120:1373–1377.

160 Carter MC, Robyn JA, Bressler PB, Walker JC, Shapiro GG, Metcalfe DD: Omalizumab for the treatment of unprovoked anaphylaxis in patients with systemic mastocytosis. J Allergy Clin Immunol 2007;119:1550–1551.

161 Casale TB, Busse WW, Kline JN, Ballas ZK, Moss MH, Townley RG, Mokhtarani M, Seyfert-Margolis V, Asare A, Bateman K, Deniz Y: Omalizumab pretreatment decreases acute reactions after rush immunotherapy for ragweed-induced seasonal allergic rhinitis. J Allergy Clin Immunol 2006;117:134–140.

162 Jeannin P, Lecoanet S, Delneste Y, Gauchat JF, Bonnefoy JY: IgE versus IgG4 production can be differentially regulated by IL-10. J Immunol 1998; 160:3555–3561.

163 Satoguina JS, Adjobimey T, Arndts K, Hoch J, Oldenburg J, Layland LE, Hoerauf A: Tr1 and naturally occurring regulatory T cells induce IgG4 in B cells through GITR/GITR-L interaction, IL-10 and TGF-β. Eur J Immunol 2008;38:3101–3113.

164 Kay AB: Asthma and inflammation. J Allergy Clin Immunol 1991;87:893–910.

165 Rak S, Lowhagen O, Venge P: The effect of immunotherapy on bronchial hyperresponsiveness and eosinophil cationic protein in pollen-allergic patients. J Allergy Clin Immunol 1988;82:470–480.

166 Corrigan CJ, Jayaratnam A, Wang Y, Liu Y, de Waal Malefyt R, Meng Q, Kay AB, Phipps S, Lee TH, Ying S: Early production of thymic stromal lymphopoietin precedes infiltration of dendritic cells expressing its receptor in allergen-induced late phase cutaneous responses in atopic subjects. Allergy 2009;64: 1014–1022.

167 Tamagawa-Mineoka R, Katoh N, Kishimoto S: Platelets play important roles in the late phase of the immediate hypersensitivity reaction. J Allergy Clin Immunol 2009;123:581–587, 587.e1-9.

Dr. Cezmi A. Akdis
Swiss Institute of Allergy and Asthma Research (SIAF)
Obere Strasse 22, CH–7270 Davos (Switzerland)
Tel. +41 81 410 0848, Fax +41 81 410 0840
E-Mail akdisac@siaf.unizh.ch

Ring J (ed): Anaphylaxis. Chem Immunol Allergy. Basel, Karger, 2010, vol 95, pp 45–66

Anaphylaxis: Mechanisms of Mast Cell Activation

Janet Kalesnikoff · Stephen J. Galli

Department of Pathology, Stanford University School of Medicine, Stanford, Calif., USA

Abstract

Anaphylaxis is a severe systemic allergic response that is rapid in onset and potentially lethal, and that typically is induced by an otherwise innocuous substance. In IgE-dependent and other examples of anaphylaxis, tissue mast cells and circulating basophilic granulocytes (basophils) are thought to represent major (if not the major) sources of the biologically active mediators that contribute to the pathology and, in unfortunate individuals, fatal outcome, of anaphylaxis. In this chapter, we will describe the mechanisms of mast cell (and basophil) activation in anaphylaxis, with a focus on IgE-dependent activation, which is thought to be responsible for most examples of antigen-induced anaphylaxis in humans. We will also discuss the use of mouse models to investigate the mechanisms that can contribute to anaphylaxis in that species in vivo, and the relevance of such mouse studies to human anaphylaxis.

Anaphylaxis is a catastrophic, rapid in onset, and sometimes fatal acute allergic reaction to what typically is an otherwise innocuous substance; no one who has witnessed (or survived) an episode of anaphylaxis is likely soon to forget it. In humans and other mammals, anaphylaxis can be induced when certain unfortunate subjects previously sensitized to an allergen (i.e., an antigen that can induce an allergic reaction) are later exposed to even very small amounts of that allergen. The most common allergens include foods (e.g., peanuts), drugs (e.g., β-lactam antibiotics), natural rubber latex or components of insect venoms [1, 2]. Because anaphylaxis can be induced by allergens derived from intrinsically innocuous substances, such as components of peanuts or other foods, it represents arguably the most grotesque example of a pathological imbalance between the cost and benefit of an acquired immune response.

Our understanding of anaphylaxis has advanced substantially since the original description of this phenomenon in the scientific literature over 100 years ago. There is now little reasonable doubt that the IgE-dependent activation of mast cells and basophils is the key event underlying most examples of allergen-induced anaphylaxis in humans [3–5]. IgE binds to the high-affinity IgE receptor, FcεRI, expressed on the surface of mast cells and basophils. Aggregation of FcεRI by binding of FcεRI-bound IgE to bivalent or multivalent allergen activates downstream events that lead to the secretion of three classes of mediators: (1) the extracellular release of preformed mediators stored in the cells' cytoplasmic granules, including vasoactive amines (in humans, histamine), neutral proteases, proteoglycans and some cytokines and growth factors, by a process called degranulation; (2) the de novo synthesis of pro-inflammatory lipid mediators, such as prostaglandins and leukotrienes; and (3) the synthesis and secretion of many growth factors, cytokines and chemokines [6]. Thus, FcεRI aggregation induces the rapid and sustained release of mast cell and basophil mediators, which in turn induces the pathophysiologic consequences of anaphylaxis.

This chapter highlights the mechanisms responsible for mast cell activation during anaphylactic responses to environmental substances. In addition to discussing in detail the activation of mast cells and basophils by IgE and antigen, we also will describe how mouse models have been used to analyze the importance of various proteins, cells, mediators and activation mechanisms in the expression of anaphylaxis in that species.

Use of Mouse Models to Study Anaphylaxis

Laboratory mice represent a powerful model organism for studying the pathogenesis of anaphylaxis; it is now possible rather easily to manipulate the mouse genome and study the influence of specific genetic pathways on biological processes and diseases. Moreover, despite the obvious anatomical and physiological differences between mice and humans, it has been argued that the mouse and human immune systems are sufficiently similar that many basic observations made about models of anaphylaxis in mice are likely to apply to humans [4]. However, as summarized in table 1, there are some differences (as well as many similarities) between mice and humans that must be kept in mind when considering the relevance of mouse models to human anaphylaxis. For example, FcεRI complexes are expressed on more cell types in human beings compared to mice [4, 7–9], and both IgE and IgG1 antibodies can make major contributions to anaphylaxis in mice whereas it has been more difficult to implicate antibody isotypes other than IgE in the pathogenesis of allergen-induced anaphylaxis in humans [1, 4, 5, 10].

The in vivo relevance and biological importance of in vitro observations about mast cell function, as well as the contributions of mast cells towards the expression of particular biological responses (such as various models of anaphylaxis) in vivo, can be assessed using c-*kit* mutant mice (e.g., WBB6F$_1$-*Kit*$^{W/W-v}$ or C57BL/6-*Kit*$^{W-sh/W-sh}$ mice) that virtually lack mast cell populations. Mice with mutations of c-*kit* [6, 11] or mutations that affect KIT expression [12–14] have other abnormalities of phenotype besides a mast cell deficiency. However, the mast cell deficiency of these mice can be selectively repaired by the adoptive transfer of genetically compatible, in vitro-derived

Table 1. Key concepts about the roles of mast cells in systemic anaphylaxis in mice and humans

–   It is generally accepted (based on clinical and in vitro studies) that mast cells (and basophils), IgE and FcεRI are involved in most cases of allergen-induced anaphylaxis in humans. However, it is difficult to define the exact roles and relative importance of mast cells, basophils, and other potential effector cells (e.g., monocytes/macrophages, dendritic cells) in either IgE-dependent or IgE-independent human anaphylaxis. Unlike in mice, we neither have access to mast cell- or basophil-deficient humans nor can we genetically manipulate human subjects to produce such phenotypes.

–   In mice, in vivo studies with mutant mice, in vitro studies with mutant cells, and in vitro and in vivo studies with pharmacological agents show that anaphylaxis can occur through an IgE/FcεRI-dependent or IgG/FcγRIII-dependent pathway, or can result from the activation of both pathways. The IgE/FcεRI-dependent pathway critically involves mast cells, whereas the IgG/FcγRIII-dependent pathways can involve basophils and/or macrophages (probably reflecting the details of the models being investigated). While mast cells are not required for mice to express IgG/FcγRIII-dependent anaphylaxis, mast cells can influence certain pathophysiological features of such responses.

–   While it had been thought that, in mice, only mast cells and basophils expressed FcεRI, it has been shown that FcεRI can be expressed by certain dendritic cells as well. In rats, it has been reported that certain rat nerve cells may express FcεRI. In humans, FcεRI is also expressed on monocytes/macrophages, Langerhans' cells, dendritic cells, eosinophils (although typically in very low numbers on the cell surface), and on other cell types (e.g., some FcεRI expression has been reported on neutrophils, platelets, and on bronchial smooth muscle cells, although the clinical significance of such findings is not yet clear). It is possible that other cell types may also be found to express FcεRI.

–   In mice and humans, it is possible that mast cells and basophils contribute to the pathophysiology of anaphylaxis both via direct effects on end organ targets and also by indirect effects, including the ability of mast cells and basophils to influence the responsiveness of such target cells to mediators generated in subjects with anaphylaxis.

–   It remains to be determined whether, and, if so under what circumstances, IgG-mediated anaphylaxis exists in humans.

–   The roles of potential effector cells other than mast cells and basophils (e.g. monocytes/macrophages, dendritic cells) in IgE-dependent and IgE-independent anaphylaxis in mice and humans remain to be determined.

–   There may be substantial variation both within and among species (e.g., in mice vs. humans) in the expression of various proteins, receptors and/or ligands that influence the activation of mast cells (or basophils or other potential effector cell types), or that can regulate the responsiveness of end organ target cells (e.g., bronchial or gastrointestinal smooth muscle cells, vascular endothelial cells) to potential mediators of anaphylaxis derived from mast cells.

–   In humans, it is not known why some patients develop anaphylactic reactivity to certain antigens whereas others, including those who bear IgE antibodies reactive with the same antigens, do not.

mast cells from congenic wild-type mice or various transgenic or mutant mice, or from mouse embryonic stem cells, or by using mast cells that have been transduced with short hairpin (sh)RNA to reduce expression of proteins of interest [12, 14, 15]. These 'mast cell knockin mice' are now widely used to assess the contributions of mast cells or specific mast cell products in diverse biological responses in vivo, and they have proven extremely beneficial for dissecting the mechanisms of anaphylaxis. Two groups recently reported the generation of mast cell-specific 'Cre' mice [16, 17]. Given that mutation of c-*kit* affects a variety of cell lineages and c-*kit* mutant mice have a number of other phenotypic abnormalities (in addition to lacking mast cells), it is likely that mice with confirmed mast cell-specific Cre expression and mice with inducible mast cell-specific Cre expression will also become powerful genetic models for investigating the contributions of mast cells or mast cell-specific products to health and disease.

Anaphylaxis is a systemic reaction involving multiple organ systems in humans [10]. In mice, models of systemic anaphylaxis also can induce rapid and potentially reversible hypotension, hypothermia, and decreased mobility [4]. Although it is not clear to what extent antibody isotypes other than IgE contribute to the expression of anaphylaxis in humans [1, 4, 5, 10], it is well known that either IgE or IgG antibodies acting via FcεRI or FcγRIII, respectively, can induce potentially fatal systemic anaphylactic reactions in mice [4]. The elicitation of antigen-specific fatal anaphylaxis in mice that virtually lack mast cells [18], IgE [19], or the IgE-binding α chain of FcεRI [20], provided evidence for the existence of IgE-independent, but IgG-dependent, anaphylaxis in mice. The IgE-dependent mechanism, which is mediated mainly by mast cells, histamine, and, to a lesser extent, platelet-activating factor (PAF), requires smaller amounts of antibody and antigen than the IgG-dependent mechanism [4]. Although clinical observations indicate that most cases of allergen-induced anaphylaxis in humans likely reflect activation of the IgE-dependent pathway (in that the disorder can be induced by small amounts of allergen and, at least in the case of peanut allergy, the threshold of sensitivity to the allergen can be ameliorated significantly in subjects treated with anti-IgE), it is possible that the IgG-dependent pathway may account for disease in some subjects repeatedly exposed to large quantities of allergen (which, in rare instances, may even be anti-IgE antibody itself) [1, 4, 5] or in subjects in which little or no allergen-specific IgE can be detected by skin testing or based on measurements in vitro [1].

The relatively large amount of antigen required to initiate IgG-dependent anaphylaxis in mice is consistent with the much lower affinity of FcγRIII for IgG than FcεRI for IgE. Moreover, whereas antigen binds directly to FcεRI-bound IgE on mast cells, antigen/IgG immune complexes must form in the blood and lymph prior to binding FcγRIII [4]. For years, the macrophage was thought to be the main source of PAF and perhaps other mediators that are responsible for IgG-dependent systemic anaphylaxis in mice [4]. However, recent lines of evidence strongly implicate basophils as an important source of PAF, and as the cell type most responsible for a fatal outcome in some models of IgG-mediated anaphylaxis in mice [21]. It is important to remember that the conclusions of all studies of models of anaphylaxis in mice (or other species) are based on the characteristics of the anaphylaxis models investigated. While there is very strong evidence that basophils play a critical role in models of active anaphylaxis to Penicillin V or 2,4,6-trinitrophenol (TNP)-BSA in C57BL/6 mice [21], it is possible that macrophages (as well as additional cell types that can produce PAF or other bioactive mediators) contribute to the pathology observed in other models of anaphylaxis, such as those studied by Finkelman and colleagues [reviewed in 4], and/or in models of anaphylaxis induced in other strains of mice. Moreover, mast cells can also contribute to some of the pathological feature of IgG-immune complex-dependent anaphylaxis in mice [22].

The route of antigen administration can alter the speed of antigen access to the circulation and, thus, the systemic symptoms in anaphylaxis models. For example, allergen ingestion typically induces anaphylaxis that includes gastrointestinal symptoms, such as diarrhea [4]. These 'intestinal anaphylaxis' models in mice are dependent on IgE-induced mast cell activation, and the release of PAF and serotonin (rather than histamine) [1, 4].

Although human anaphylaxis is a systemic reaction, the mouse model of passive cutaneous anaphylaxis (PCA) has been used extensively to enhance our understanding of mechanisms which also may contribute to systemic anaphylaxis. Unlike systemic anaphylaxis in the mouse, PCA appears to be entirely dependent on mast cells [4, 6]. While IgE appears to be the primary antibody isotype that mediates PCA reactions in actively immunized mice, activation of FcγRIII by a fraction of IgG1 antibodies (called anaphylactic IgG1) can also mediate PCA reactions in mice [4].

IgE-Dependent Anaphylaxis: FcεRI Signaling

In both humans and rodents, FcεRI is expressed on the surface of mast cells (and basophils) as a heterotetrameric receptor ($\alpha\beta\gamma_2$) composed of an α subunit, a four transmembrane-spanning β subunit, and two identical disulphide-linked γ subunits [7–9, 23]. Murine FcεRI expression once was thought to be restricted to the surface of mast cells and basophils [7, 8], however viral infection (Sendai virus) induces expression of trimeric ($\alpha\gamma_2$) FcεRI complexes on lung dendritic cells in mice [24]. In humans, trimeric ($\alpha\gamma_2$) FcεRI complexes can be expressed on eosinophils (although typically at very low numbers), monocytes and macrophages, Langerhans' cells, and dendritic cells (myeloid and plasmacytoid) [7, 8]. FcεRI has also been detected on human platelets and neutrophils, but the subunit composition on these cell types remains to be defined [7]. Finally, a few reports have described evidence that certain non-hematopoietic cells, including bronchial smooth muscle cells in humans and some nerve cells in rats, may express FcεRI [9]. The clinical significance of such findings remains to be determined.

The two extracellular immunoglobulin-related domains of the FcεRI α subunit bind to the Fc portion of a single IgE molecule [7, 8]. Monomeric IgE binds to FcεRI at a very high affinity (1×10^{10} M^{-1}), and this interaction has a low dissociation rate [7], thus FcεRI binds IgE and retains it for long periods, setting the stage for an immediate response upon subsequent exposure to antigen. The FcεRI β and γ chains each contain an immunoreceptor tyrosine-based activation motif (ITAM) that becomes tyrosine phosphorylated after receptor aggregation (fig. 1). While the β chain is an important amplifier of IgE and antigen-induced signaling events and FcεRI cell surface expression, the γ subunits are indispensible for initiating signaling events downstream of FcεRI [7].

Critical to understanding the mechanisms of anaphylaxis is defining the intracellular signaling pathways that regulate mast cell mediator release. Many researchers deserve credit for elucidating important components of this pathogenetic pathway and a number of excellent reviews on mast cell signaling via FcεRI have been published recently [2, 7, 25, 26]. This section focuses on some new developments that employ genetically-altered mice and/or in vivo models of anaphylaxis to elucidate aspects of the positive or negative regulation of signaling initiated by FcεRI.

Proximal Signaling Events

Like all immunoreceptor family members, FcεRI lacks intrinsic tyrosine kinase activity. IgE and antigen-induced crosslinking of FcεRI initiates a complex series of phosphate transfer events via the activation of non-receptor Src, Syk and Tec family protein tyrosine kinases (fig. 1). The Src family kinase Lyn, which associates with the FcεRI β subunit in mast cells, transphosphorylates neighboring FcεRI ITAMs after receptor aggregation [7, 26]. Once phosphorylated, the β chain ITAM binds to the SH2 domain of additional Lyn molecules, while the phosphorylated γ chain ITAM recruits Syk to the receptor complex, where it is activated by both autophosphorylation and phosphorylation by Lyn [2, 7, 15, 26].

Lyn and Syk then phosphorylate several enzymes (e.g., phospholipase Cγ [PLCγ]) and adaptor molecules (e.g., linker for activation of T cells [LAT] 1 and LAT2 [also known as NTAL or LAB]). Phosphorylated adaptor molecules coordinate the assembly of membrane-localized signaling networks containing additional adaptor molecules including Grb2, Gads, Shc, SLP-76 and Vav, the guanine nucleotide exchange factor SOS, and signaling enzymes, including PLCγ, to regulate mast cell activation (fig. 1). For example, recruitment and activation of SLP-76, Vav, Shc, Grb2 and SOS culminate in the activation of the small GTPase, Ras, which activates the MAPK cascade, leading to the activation of transcription factors important for cytokine production and for the activation of PLA$_2$, which then initiates the generation of arachidonic acid metabolites.

In addition to Lyn, a second Src family kinase, Fyn, associates with the FcεRI β chain and is activated after FcεRI aggregation [26]. Fyn phosphorylates the adaptor Gab2 to activate the phosphatidylinositol-3-OH kinase (PI3K) pathway; the SH2 domain-

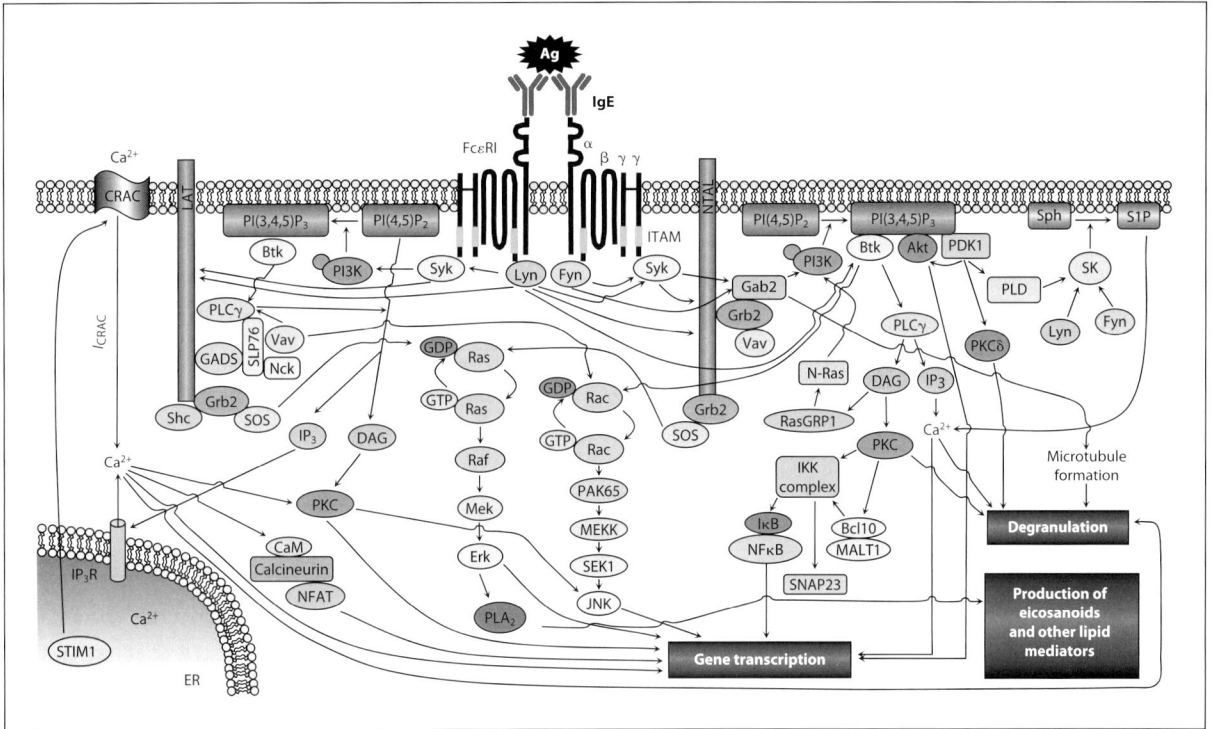

Fig. 1. Simplified scheme of early FcεRI-mediated signaling events. Antigen- (Ag-) induced crosslinking of FcεRI induces activation of Lyn and Fyn; Lyn phosphorylates FcεRI ITAMs (grey) and activates Syk following ITAM binding of Syk, and Fyn phosphorylates the adaptor Gab2 to activate the PI3K pathway. Lyn and Syk phosphorylate many adaptor molecules (e.g., LAT and NTAL) and enzymes, which regulate activation of the Ras, PLCγ, PI3K and other pathways. Grb2 and SOS activate the Ras/Erk pathway, which regulates transcription factor activation and arachidonic acid metabolism (through PLA$_2$ activation). PLCγ can either be activated through the coordinated function of LAT/Gads/SLP-76/Vav and Btk (left side of figure) or independently of LAT through a PI3K/Btk-dependent pathway (right side of figure). PLCγ activation regulates classical PKC activation (through DAG generation) and calcium responses (through the generation of IP$_3$). IP$_3$ binding to the IP$_3$R triggers Ca^{2+} release from the ER; STIM1 couples ER Ca^{2+} store depletion with the activation of CRAC channels, leading to the influx of extracellular Ca^{2+} and activation of the Ca^{2+} release activated current (I_{CRAC}). The PI3K product, PI(3,4,5)P$_3$, is an important lipid mediator that regulates the activity of various enzymes, e.g., Btk, Akt, and PDK1 and (via PDK1) PLD and SK, and the formation of other lipid mediators, e.g., DAG and S1P (which regulates extracellular Ca^{2+} influx). The IKK complex consists of two catalytic subunits, IKKα/IKK1 and IKKβ/IKK2, and a regulatory subunit, NEMO/IKKγ; this complex phosphorylates IκB to activate the transcription factor NFκB. IKKβ/IKK2 also phosphorylates SNAP23 to facilitate SNARE complex formation (not shown). Arrows indicate the contributions of these signaling pathways toward mast cell degranulation, arachidonic acid metabolism, and cytokine/chemokine/growth factor production. Note: some arrows do not indicate direct interactions or targets. Bcl10 = B cell lymphoma 10; Btk = Bruton's tyrosine kinase; Ca^{2+} = calcium; CaM = calmodulin; CRAC = Ca^{2+} release activated calcium channel; DAG = diacylglycerol; Gab2 = Grb2-associated binding protein 2; GADS = Grb2-related adaptor downstream of Shc; ER = endoplasmic reticulum; Erk = extracellular signal-regulated kinase; I_{CRAC} = Ca^{2+} release activated current; IκB = inhibitor of κB; IKK = IκB kinase; IP$_3$ = inositol 1,4,5-trisphosphate; IP$_3$R = IP$_3$ receptor; ITAM = immunoreceptor tyrosine-based activation motif; LAT = linker for activation of T cells; MALT1 = mucosa-associated lymphoid tissue lymphoma translocation protein 1; NEMO = NFκB essential modulator; NFAT = nuclear factor of activated T cells; NFκB = nuclear factor κB; NTAL = non-T-cell activation linker; PI3K = phosphoinositide 3-kinase; PI(3,4,5)P$_3$ = phosphatidylinositol 3,4,5-trisphosphate; PKC = protein kinase C; PL = phospholipase; RasGRP = Ras guanyl nucleotide-releasing protein; S1P = sphingosine 1 phosphate; SK = sphingosine kinase; SLP-76 = SH2-domain containing leukocyte protein of 76 kDa; SOS = son of sevenless homolog; Sph = sphingosine; STIM1 = stromal interaction molecule 1.

containing p85 regulatory subunit of PI3K binds to phosphorylated Gab2, which allows the associated p110 catalytic subunit to phosphorylate phosphatidylinositol 4,5-bisphosphate [PI(4,5)P$_2$] to generate the important second messenger, PI(3,4,5)P$_3$ (PIP$_3$) (fig. 1). Thus, Fyn functions as a positive regulator of FcεRI-mediated mast cell activation because PIP$_3$ is essential for many aspects of mast cell responsiveness. In addition to Fyn and Gab2, RasGRP1 was recently identified as a positive regulator of FcεRI-mediated PI3K activation [27]. PI3K activation was diminished in RasGRP1 knockout mouse bone marrow-derived cultured mast cells (BMCMCs), and these cells exhibited decreased IgE and antigen-induced degranulation, as well as impaired release of the cytokines TNF, IL-3, and IL-4 (but not IL-6). Moreover, RasGRP1-deficient mice failed to mount a passive systemic anaphylactic response upon systemic administration of DNP-HSA 24 h after injection of a monoclonal anti-DNP IgE antibody. It has been proposed that RasGRP1 activates PI3K through N-Ras following membrane recruitment of p85 by Gab2 (fig. 1) [27].

In addition to its signal-initiating activity described above, Lyn can also negatively regulate FcεRI-induced signaling events, including Fyn activation [26]. A third Src family kinase, Hck, plays a positive regulatory role in FcεRI-induced mast cell degranulation and cytokine release via Lyn-dependent and Lyn-independent mechanisms (both of which are dependent, at least in part, on phosphorylation of the FcεRI β chain) [28]. The Lyn-dependent mechanism involves Hck-mediated suppression of Lyn's negative regulatory kinase activity (i.e., Lyn activity and the phosphorylation of various Lyn targets, for example, the phosphatase SHIP, were increased in $Hck^{-/-}$ BMCMCs) [28]. Based on these findings, the authors proposed a hierarchical relationship among the Src family kinases downstream of FcεRI; Hck negatively regulates Lyn, which negatively regulates Fyn [28]. However, additional studies are required to understand more fully the interplay among Src family kinases downstream of FcεRI.

Calcium Regulation

Calcium influx plays a central role in mast cell activation events, such as IgE and antigen-induced degranulation. Several proteins and channels that regulate calcium entry in mast cells have been identified to date. One of the key enzymes that positively regulates FcεRI-induced calcium entry in mast cells is PLC-γ, which hydrolyzes PI(4,5)P$_2$ to form soluble inositol-1,4,5-trisphosphate (IP$_3$) and membrane-bound diacylglycerol (DAG) [6, 7, 15, 25, 26]. IP$_3$ binding to its receptor in the endoplasmic reticulum (ER) rapidly induces the first stage of calcium (Ca^{2+}) mobilization, the transient release of Ca^{2+} from ER stores, which in turn induces prolonged influx of Ca^{2+} through store-operated calcium release-activated calcium (CRAC) channels in the plasma membrane (fig. 1).

The recent identification of STIM1, a sensor of ER Ca^{2+} concentrations that couples depletion of ER Ca^{2+} stores with activation of CRAC channels, and CRACM1 (also known as Orai1), the pore-forming subunit of the CRAC channel, has increased our understanding of CRAC currents at the molecular level [7, 15]. Investigators using STIM1-deficient mice showed that STIM1 is required for FcεRI-induced Ca^{2+} influx, degranulation, NF-κB and NFAT transcription factor activation in mast cells and IgE-dependent anaphylaxis in vivo [29]. Others used CRACM1-deficient mice to show that CRACM1 is required for FcεRI-induced degranulation, lipid mediator synthesis and cytokine release in mast cells and IgE-dependent allergic responses in vivo [30]. These studies demonstrate conclusively that the second stage of FcεRI-induced Ca^{2+} mobilization, the influx of Ca^{2+} mediated by STIM1 and CRACM1, is essential for mast cell activation in vitro and in vivo [29, 30].

The rate of Ca^{2+} influx through store-operated channels is also dependent on the membrane potential, which is regulated by calcium-activated non-selective cation channels, such as TRPM4 (transient receptor potential cation channel, subfamily M, member 4). TRPM4 activates a cation current that depolarizes membrane potential and limits the driving force for Ca^{2+} entry through CRAC channels in mouse BMCMCs [31]. FcεRI-induced degranulation, leukotriene release and TNF production (but not that of IL-6), is increased in TRPM4-deficient BMCMCs and TRPM4-deficient mice exhibited more severe acute (but not late-phase) inflammation during IgE-mediated PCA responses [31]. This work indicates that TRPM4 is a negative regulator of FcεRI-induced calcium influx in mast cells in vitro and in vivo.

The tyrosine kinases Lyn, Fyn and Syk positively regulate IgE and antigen-induced calcium influx in mast cells [26]. The exact mechanism(s) by which Fyn contributes to calcium influx remain(s) undefined, however the Fyn-mediated generation of sphingosine 1-phosphate (S1P), a recently recognized mediator of anaphylaxis, likely represents one such mechanism [2, 26]. The sphingosine kinases (SK) SK1 and SK2 convert sphingosine to S1P in a PIP$_3$-dependent manner downstream of activated FcεRI (fig. 1). S1P acts both intracellularly and extracellularly to regulate mast cell degranulation. Intracellular S1P positively regulates IgE and antigen-induced Ca^{2+} influx (and degranulation) independently of PLCγ and IP$_3$. Following secretion from the cell, extracellular S1P mediates its functional effect on mast cells by binding to the S1P1 or S1P2 surface receptor, thereby inducing cytoskeletal rearrangement or enhancing degranulation, respectively. In mouse models of anaphylaxis, increased circulating S1P is associated with increased in vivo mast cell responsiveness (i.e., there is a close correlation between the levels of S1P and histamine in the plasma following anaphylactic challenge) [2, 26]. Although S1P can act in an autocrine manner to activate mast cells, the generation of S1P from other sources (such as endothelial cells or platelets) likely represents an important source of S1P following anaphylactic challenge [2, 26].

Membrane Fusion Events

Downstream of early FcεRI-induced signaling events (such as Ca^{2+} influx), the final stages of mast cell degranulation require membrane fusion events. The exocytosis of mast cell granules, also called secretory granules, is regulated by Rab GTPases and membrane fusion proteins called SNAREs (soluble N-ethyl-maleimide-sensitive factor [NSF] attachment protein receptors) [32, 33]. SNARES are divided into t-SNAREs, localized on the target membrane (e.g., syntaxins and soluble NSF attachment proteins [SNAPs]) and v-SNAREs, localized on the vesicle membrane (e.g., vesicle-associated membrane proteins [VAMPs]). Murine rodent and human mast cells express VAMP-2, -3, -7 and -8. Two groups recently showed that FcεRI-induced exocytosis is reduced in VAMP-8-deficient mouse mast cells [34, 35]. One group reported that this defect is limited to a distinct subset of secretory granules that contain serotonin and cathepsin D [34]. However, in this study, VAMP-8-deficient mast cells did not display any defects in the regulated exocytosis of granules containing histamine [34]. By contrast, the other group showed that FcεRI-induced β-hexosaminidase and histamine release in vitro was reduced by approximately 50% in the absence of VAMP-8 [35]. Moreover, they showed that VAMP-8-deficient mice had reduced concentrations of blood histamine during passive systemic anaphylaxis [35]. Although these groups used different VAMP-8-deficient mice, the reason for the discrepancies in their findings remains to be determined. Another study reported that inhibition of syntaxin 4, SNAP-23, VAMP-7 or VAMP-8, but not VAMP-2 or VAMP-3, blocked FcεRI-induced histamine release in primary human mast cells [36].

The t-SNAREs syntaxin 4 and SNAP23 regulate FcεRI-induced exocytosis from mast cells [15, 32, 33], and the phosphorylation of SNAP23 (on Ser120 and Ser95) has been shown to modulate exocytic events [15]. IκB kinase β (IKKβ, also termed IKK2), one of two catalytically active subunits of the IKK complex, phosphorylates SNAP23 on Ser120 and Ser95 [37]. Although the IKK complex is best known for its role in activating the transcription factor NFκB, the IKKβ-mediated phosphorylation of SNAP23 upregulates FcεRI-induced degranulation in vitro in an NFκB-independent manner [37]. Moreover, in mouse mast cells, IKKβ plays a critical role in enhancing IgE-mediated acute local or systemic anaphylaxis reactions in vivo independently of NFκB [37]. Conversely, the IKKβ-mediated enhancement of cutaneous late phase reactions in vivo (which are promoted by the release of pro-inflammatory cytokines) occurs in an NFκB-dependent manner [37]. These results suggest that IKKβ may have additional substrates that allow this kinase to regulate NFκB-independent mast cell activation events, such as SNARE complex formation.

Negative Regulation of FcεRI-Dependent Mast Cell Activation

Several intracellular regulators can diminish FcεRI-induced signaling events. These negative regulators include the tyrosine phosphatase SHP-1 (SH2-containing protein tyrosine phosphatase-1) and the lipid phosphatases SHIP (SH2-containing inositol 5′ phosphatase), SHIP2 and PTEN [2, 7, 26] (fig. 2). Some signaling molecules initiate

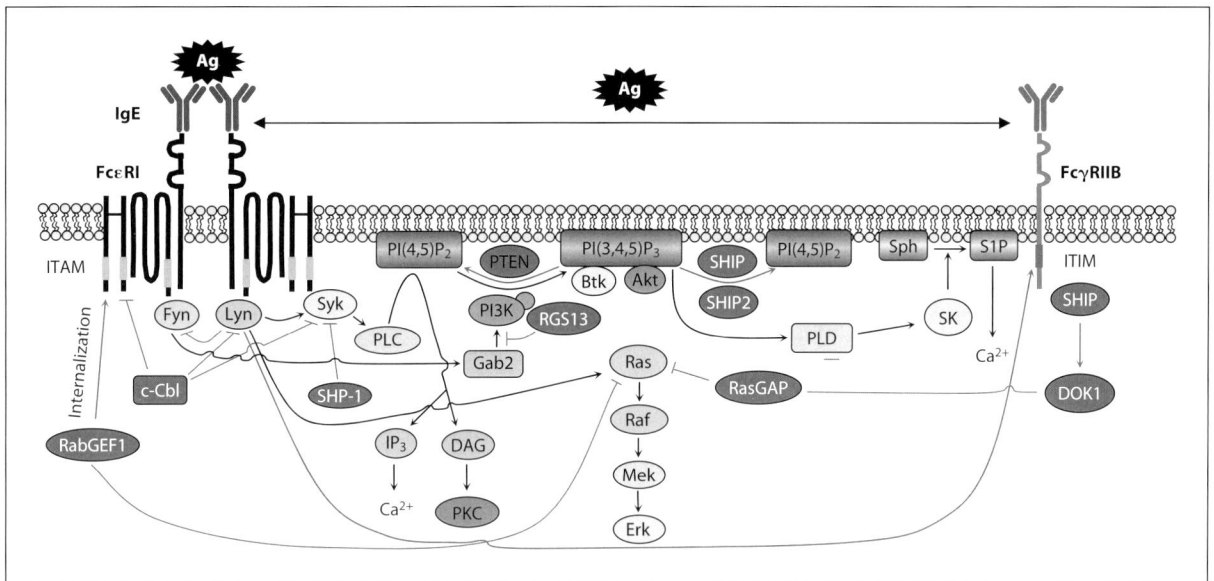

Fig. 2. Negative regulation of FcεRI-mediated signaling events. FcεRI aggregation activates a number of proteins that can negatively regulate the positive signaling pathways activated downstream of this receptor. For example, Lyn, which initiates both activating and inhibitory signals, negatively regulates Fyn activity (by phosphorylating Csk-binding protein, which allows Csk to negatively regulate Fyn activity) and, thus, Gab2 phosphorylation. Other negative regulators include c-Cbl (which facilitates the ubiquitination of FcεRI, Lyn and Syk), the tyrosine phosphatase SHP-1 (which dephosphorylates Syk), the lipid phosphatases SHIP and (not shown) SHIP2 (which catalyze the hydrolysis of $PI(3,4,5)P_3$ to $PI(3,4)P_2$) as well as PTEN (which catalyzes the hydrolysis of $PI(3,4,5)P_3$ to $PI(4,5)P_2$), RasGAP (which enhances the intrinsic GTPase activity of Ras), RabGEF1 (which enhances FcεRI internalization and can bind to GTP-bound Ras), and RGS13 (which binds to the p85α subunit of PI3K and disrupts its association with Gab2 and Grb2 in mice). Antigen- (Ag-) induced coaggregation of FcεRI with FcγRIIB inhibits FcεRI-induced signaling events and mast cell activation via Lyn-mediated phosphorylation of the FcγRIIB ITIM (grey) and the subsequent recruitment of SHIP (which binds to the phosphorylated ITIM) and DOK1 (which is activated by SHIP). Csk = C-terminal Src kinase; DOK1 = docking protein 1; Gab2 = Grb2-associated binding protein 2; ITAM = immunoreceptor tyrosine-based activation motif; ITIM = immunoreceptor tyrosine-based inhibitory motif; NFκB = nuclear factor κB; PI3K = phosphoinositide 3-kinase; PKC = protein kinase C; PLD = phospholipase D; PTEN = phosphatase and tensin homolog; RabGEF = Rab5 guanine nucleotide exchange factor; RasGAP = Ras GTPase-activating protein; RGS = regulator of G protein signaling; SHIP = Src homology 2 (SH2) domain-containing inositol 5′-phosphatase; SHP-1 = SH2 domain-containing tyrosine phosphatase-1; SK = sphingosine kinase.

both activating and inhibitory signals; for example, Lyn phosphorylates FcεRI ITAMs (an activating signal) as well as inhibitory receptor immunoreceptor tyrosine-based inhibitory motifs (ITIMs), the latter of which leads to recruitment of inhibitory signaling molecules, such as SHIP. Other signaling molecules can negatively regulate FcεRI-induced mast cell activation events by altering the rate of FcεRI internalization (e.g., one function of RabGEF1 is to enhance FcεRI internalization [38]) or the levels of FcεRI expressed on the mast cell surface (e.g., Rabaptin-5 deficiency markedly diminished expression of FcεRI on the mast cell surface by diminishing receptor surface stability [39]).

The number of lipid phosphatases that can negatively regulate PIP_3 levels highlights the importance of the PI3K pathway and intracellular PIP_3 levels in regulating mast cell activation events. Both SHIP and SHIP2 dephosphorylate PIP_3 at the 5′ position to generate $PI(3,4)P_2$, whereas PTEN directly opposes PI3K function by dephosphorylating PIP_3 at the 3′ position to generate $PI(4,5)P_2$ (fig. 2). Mast cells derived from SHIP knockout mice demonstrate increased FcεRI-induced PIP_3 levels, degranulation and cytokine production [6]. Similarly, the downregulation of SHIP2 or PTEN by silencing RNA strategies in mouse or human mast cells, respectively, resulted in enhanced FcεRI-mediated degranulation and cytokine release [26]. While calcium influx was increased in the absence of SHIP or PTEN, it was normal in SHIP2-deficient mast cells; the authors propose that the enhanced responsiveness in the SHIP2-deficient cells was due to increased activation of Rac and enhanced microtubule polymerization [40]. Interestingly, it was recently shown that small-molecule activators of SHIP can inhibit PI3K-mediated phosphorylation events (including phosphorylation of the serine/threonine kinase Akt on Thr308) in vitro and the administration of these compounds in vivo was protective in a mouse model of acute cutaneous anaphylaxis [41]. These findings suggest that it will be worthwhile to investigate whether the activation of these negative regulatory phosphatases may represent an effective strategy for the treatment of anaphylaxis or other inflammatory disorders.

Intracellular PIP_3 levels can also be modulated by altering PI3K activity. In mice, RGS13 (regulator of G protein signaling [RGS] 13) was identified as a novel negative regulator of FcεRI-induced degranulation (but not production of the cytokines TNF, IL-6 or IL-13) in vitro and IgE-dependent passive cutaneous and systemic anaphylaxis in vivo [42]. RGS proteins typically inhibit G protein-coupled receptor (GPCR) signaling events through GTPase-accelerating protein (GAP) activity on $G_α$ subunits. Although GPCR signaling can amplify FcεRI-mediated responses through activation of PI3Kγ, RGS13-mediated inhibition of FcεRI-induced activation occurs independently of RGS13's GAP activity [42]. Instead, it was proposed that RGS13, which is upregulated following antigen stimulation, binds to the p85α subunit of PI3K and disrupts its association with an FcεRI-activated signaling complex containing Gab2 and Grb2 in mice [42] (fig. 2). The same group recently reported that RGS13 can inhibit a number of GPCR-mediated biological responses in human mast cells; depletion of RGS12 in the human mast cell leukemia line, HMC-1, by RNA interference enhanced adenosine-, S1P-, C5a- and CXCL12-induced signaling events and increased the migration of these cells in response to a CXCL12 gradient [43]. Reduced expression of RGS13 in LAD2 human mast cells lead to enhanced degranulation in response to S1P, but not to the GPCR ligand, C3a. Moreover, in contrast to the results obtained in mouse BMCMCs, FcεRI-induced degranulation was not enhanced following the depletion of RGS13 in LAD2 cells [43]. The authors propose that dysregulated signaling components in the LAD2 cells might mitigate the loss of RGS13 [43]; however, studies in primary mast cells will be required to assess whether RGS13 is also a negative regulator of PI3K activity downstream of FcεRI in normal human mast cells.

In addition to negative intracellular regulators, signaling events initiated by FcεRI and other ITAM-containing immunoreceptors can be negatively regulated by their coaggregation with ITIM-containing receptors. Each of these receptors contains at least one cytoplasmic ITIM (I/VxYxxL) that becomes phosphorylated after coaggregation with FcεRI and attenuates immunoreceptor-induced signaling events through the recruitment of specific SH2-containing phosphatases (i.e., SHP-1, SHP-2, SHIP or SHIP2). Mast cells express several such inhibitory receptors, including FcγRIIB, gp49B1, MAFA and PIR-B [5–7].

The low-affinity IgG receptor, FcγRIIB, was the first identified ITIM-containing receptor. Both IgE- and IgG-dependent anaphylaxis are exacerbated in FcγRIIB-deficient mice [4]. FcγRIIB is an attractive therapeutic target for mast cell activation events because it recruits SHIP following coaggregation with FcεRI in vivo [44] (fig. 2). Indeed, an IgG-IgE fusion protein designed to inhibit FcεRI signaling by coaggregating FcεRI with FcγRIIB blocks mast cell activation in vitro and, when administered in vivo, inhibits PCA and passive systemic anaphylaxis in mice through the activation of SHIP and SHP-1/2 [45].

Factors Modulating (or 'Tuning') FcεRI-Dependent Mast Cell Functional Activation

Effects of IgE on Surface Levels of FcεRI, Survival and Mediator Production

Several lines of evidence indicate that IgE can contribute to the intensity of anaphylaxis by mechanisms beyond simply sensitizing or priming mast cells (and basophils) to undergo activation and to release mediators when the cells encounter the antigen for which that IgE has specificity. IgE also has the ability, independently of its antigen specificity, to enhance significantly the effector function of these cells. The best understood mechanism by which this occurs is via the IgE-dependent enhancement of FcεRI surface expression, which reflects the stabilization of FcεRI on the mast cell surface by occupancy with IgE. It has long been noted that there is a strong positive correlation in humans between levels of circulating IgE and levels of surface expression of FcεRI on blood basophils [46–48]. In 1985, using RBL (rat basophil leukemia) cells, two groups reported that the presence of IgE in the media could cause a modest increase in the number of FcεRI expressed on these cells, by inhibiting the elimination of the receptor from the cell surface [49, 50]. Subsequently, two groups [51, 52] reported that this IgE-dependent enhancement of FcεRI surface expression can be quite striking, quantitatively, in non-neoplastic in vitro-derived [51, 52] or in vivo-derived [52] mouse mast cells, and that this phenomenon has significant functional consequences. These include enhancing the capacity of the mast cells to bind more IgE [51, 52], thereby potentially rendering the cells sensitive to an expanded panel of unrelated antigens, lowering the antigen concentration necessary to activate the cells [52], increasing the amounts of mediators released by the cells at a given concentration of antigen [51, 52], and, at least in mouse mast cells, permitting the cells to release an additional product (i.e., IL-4) that may not be detectably released by cells that express lower amounts of the receptor [52].

It is now clear that the basic findings regarding the IgE-dependent enhancement of FcεRI surface expression, and its functional consequences, which were first identified in the mouse system, also occur in humans [23, 52]. The implications of these findings are that subjects with high levels of IgE, and therefore with high levels of FcεRI expression on the surface of mast cells and basophils, may have key effector cells of anaphylaxis (i.e., mast cells and basophils) that are primed to be more exquisitely sensitive to antigen, and to release larger amounts of mediators in response to allergen challenge, than are those in subjects with lower levels of IgE.

Moreover, it has been reported that IgE, again in the absence of known specific antigen, can enhance the survival of mouse mast cells and, in some cases, induce mouse or human mast cells to release mediators [5, 23, 53]. In such settings, it appears that the IgE antibodies themselves can induce FcεRI aggregation. How they can do this (apart from the trivial explanation that some IgE preparations may contain dimers or aggregates of IgE) is not fully understood. For one of the monoclonal mouse IgE antibodies with this property (SPE-7, produced by Sigma), this may reflect the molecule's ability to assume at least two distinct isomeric conformations in its antigen-binding site, one of which can bind the known antigen and the other of which can bind, albeit with a lower affinity, a structurally and chemically distinct antigen [54]. The extent to which these findings can be generalized to other rodent or human IgE antibodies remains to be determined. The same is true with respect to the clinical implications (if any) of the ability of IgE to enhance mast cell survival and/or secretory function in the absence of the antigen for which that IgE is known to have specificity.

Variation in the Mast Cell's Responsiveness to Activation

Evidence has been presented that mast cells can exhibit variation in their intrinsic responsiveness to various activating stimuli, and in some cases may actually secrete products in the absence of known mast cell stimuli. For example, mast cells derived from mice lacking certain proteins that negatively regulate mast cell activation (e.g., SHIP, RabGEF1, etc.) or mast cells in which certain proteins that negatively regulate mast cell activation (e.g., PTEN) were knocked down by silencing RNA strategies, exhibit increased sensitivity to activating stimuli, and/or release substantially larger amounts of mediators once stimulated; in some cases, such cells exhibit evidence of activation even in the absence of known stimuli [6, 26]. These findings suggest that naturally occurring variations in levels of expression of such proteins (and/or of proteins that positively regulate secretion) within the population, or genetic variations (i.e., polymorphisms, mutations, etc.) that alter the structure and/or function of such proteins, also may contribute to variation in the secretory phenotype of mast cells in different individuals and thereby influence their susceptibility to the development (and/or the severity) of anaphylaxis, allergic inflammation or other mast cell-associated responses. Indeed, deficiencies in a positive signaling molecule downstream of FcεRI (i.e., Syk) have been reported in 'non-releaser' basophils (that do not degranulate in response to FcεRI crosslinking) [55] whereas deficiencies in a negative signaling molecule (i.e., SHIP) have been reported in 'hyper-releasable' basophils derived from highly allergic donors [56].

Further highlighting the effects of genetic background and variability on mast cell degranulation and anaphylactic responses, one recent study comparing FcεRI-induced mast cell activation events in mast cells derived from Lyn knockout mice on two pure genetic backgrounds (C57BL/6 vs. 129/SvJ) showed that Lyn deficiency enhanced degranulation in 129/SvJ BMCMCs but inhibited this response in C57BL/6 cells (perhaps at least in part because these Lyn-deficient BMCMCs also had reduced expression of Fyn) [57]. Prior to this study, it had been reported that Lyn knockout mice or mast cells exhibit increased [58, 59], decreased [60], or normal [61] IgE and antigen-induced responses when compared to wild-type, thus making it difficult to define Lyn's role in FcεRI-induced signaling events; however, these studies used mast cells derived from mice on different genetic backgrounds (C57BL/6 mice or mixed background 129/SvJ × C57BL/6 mice). In human mast cells, the silencing of Lyn expression enhanced FcεRI-induced degranulation [57] indicating that, like in 129/SvJ BMCMCs, Lyn was a negative regulator of FcεRI-induced signaling events in the human mast cells that were examined in that study. Although it seems likely that genetic factors may influence the induction and severity of anaphylaxis, few studies have examined the role of genetic factors in human anaphylaxis.

Endogenous Products that Modulate Responses to Aggregation of FcεRI

Adding another layer of complexity to the regulation of mast cell activation levels in vivo is the observation that activated mast cells can respond to, and in some cases produce, a myriad of mediators that may serve to amplify FcεRI-induced responses. For example, stem cell factor (SCF), the ligand for KIT, both can enhance FcεRI-dependent activation of mouse or human mast cells and, under certain circumstances, can directly induce mast cell degranulation [6, 25, 62]. Thus, elevated SCF levels and/or activating KIT mutations (such as those that occur in mastocytosis) may exacerbate mast cell-driven reactions. Indeed, patients (both adult and children) with extensive skin disease associated with mastocytosis are at increased risk to develop severe anaphylaxis [63]. Moreover, it was recently reported that cases of idiopathic anaphylaxis are often associated with mastocytosis [64], suggesting that the activating KIT mutations in mastocytosis may also exacerbate IgE-independent mast cell-driven reactions.

In addition to KIT, GPCRs expressed by mast cells may contribute to the modulation of mast cell activation, via either autocrine or paracrine mechanisms [2, 25]. Ligand binding induces a conformational change in GPCRs, which in turn promotes the exchange of GDP for GTP on Gα subunits of heterotrimeric G proteins (Gαβγ) and the concurrent dissociation of the now active GTP-Gα subunit and Gβγ complex. These G protein components stimulate downstream effectors, such as PLCβ and PI3Kγ, to mediate GPCR-induced mast cell degranulation or to enhance IgE and antigen-induced mast cell activation [25].

The GPCR ligand adenosine represents a potentially important autocrine signal for the activation of mast cells. IgE and antigen-mediated mast cell activation induces the release of adenosine, which, through the A3 adenosine receptor expressed on mast cells [65], activates PI3Kγ and results in a transient increase in PIP_3 levels that can initiate a sustained calcium influx and mast cell degranulation. Signaling via PI3Kγ also is required for optimal enhancement of cutaneous vascular permeability during IgE-dependent passive systemic anaphylaxis in vivo, although this may reflect the PI3Kγ-dependent signaling from GPCRs that are activated by ligands other than adenosine that also are released during this immune response [65, 66]. Mast cells also express the A2B adenosine receptor. Based on pharmacological studies, this receptor was thought to mediate pro-inflammatory effects of adenosine in HMC-1 cells [67]. However, mice lacking this receptor display increased sensitivity to IgE-mediated PCA and passive systemic anaphylaxis [68], suggesting that the A2B receptor functions as a negative regulator of mast cell degranulation in vivo in the mouse. Interestingly, a recent pharmacological analysis of A2B receptor-deficient mouse BMCMCs proposed that the exaggerated antigen-induced degranulation observed in these cells may be completely unrelated to the adenosine signaling function of A2B receptors [69]. Moreover, these investigators showed that genetic ablation of the A2B receptor abrogated the adenosine-dependent stimulation of IL-13 and VEGF (but not IL-6) secretion following the FcεRI-dependent activation of these cells, offering further support for a pro-inflammatory role of adenosine signaling via A2B receptors in mouse BMCMCs.

While the findings in mice are of interest, it is important to note that there are four known mammalian adenosine receptors and that the pattern of adenosine receptor expression on mast cells (as well as other immune cells and/or structural cells), and the regulation of their expression by such cells (e.g., during inflammatory responses), which can represent major determinants of adenosine responses, vary substantially among species [70–72]. For example, it is thought that adenosine-induced bronchoconstriction is mediated by adenosine A1 and A2B receptors in rats and mice, A3 receptors in rats, guinea-pigs and mice, and A2B receptors in humans [72].

Other GPCRs that positively influence FcεRI-induced mast cell activation events include the receptors for prostaglandin E_2 (the EP3 receptor), S1P (the SIP2 receptor), and the complement component C3a (the C3aR) [2, 26]. For example, it is known that peanut proteins can activate complement to produce the anaphylatoxin C3a, which can synergize with IgE-induced mast cell activation to exacerbate anaphylaxis [4]. Finally, it is likely that signaling via other receptors expressed on the mast cell surface, such as Toll-like receptors (TLRs) [6], may have effects that can alter mast cell responsiveness to signaling via the FcεRI. Of note, many of these ligands, including C3a, S1P and various TLR ligands (LPS, etc.), can also activate mast cells independently of IgE and antigen.

Taken together, these findings indicate that in addition to responding to external factors (such as dose of foreign antigen), FcεRI-induced mast cell activation events can be 'tuned' by a number of genetically-determined or microenvironmental host factors that may importantly influence the responsiveness of mast cells and therefore the features or severity of anaphylaxis. How differences in genetic makeup influence mast cell responsiveness in human anaphylaxis remains to be defined; so does the pathological relevance of the ability of the various factors described above to enhance FcεRI-dependent mast cell activation. A recent review discusses the mechanisms by which the diverse groups of receptors listed above may influence the signaling pathways initiated downstream of FcεRI [25]. Finally, in addition to factors which can directly influence mast cell activation, it is important to recognize that a number of agents, such as IL-4 and IL-13 (produced by T cells and basophils), as well as nitric oxide (produced by endothelial cells and other cell types), can exacerbate anaphylaxis at the target cell level by increasing responsiveness to mast cell mediators such as PAF, histamine, and serotonin [4].

Other Immune and Non-Immune Mechanisms of Anaphylaxis

Although clinical observations indicate that anaphylaxis in humans is usually triggered through a mechanism involving IgE, responses clinically indistinguishable from IgE and allergen-induced anaphylaxis can also be triggered by other immune and/ or non-immune mechanisms [reviewed in 1]. Other potential immunologic mechanisms in anaphylaxis include activation of the complement or coagulation system, immune complexes, and platelet or T-cell activation [1, 10]. However, it is not clear whether any of these mechanisms critically require mast cells or basophils for their expression. For example, the immune complex, complement-mediated activation of anaphylaxis in humans (which can occur, for example, following the administration of blood products) is dependent on the generation of the complement components known as anaphylatoxins (C3a and C5a). These anaphylatoxins can directly increase vascular permeability (causing hypotension or shock) and enhance smooth muscle contraction (causing bronchoconstriction and respiratory impairment), as well as induce mast cell and/or basophil degranulation [73]. Complicating matters further, it is likely that many anaphylactic triggers act through more than one mechanism [1].

Even though current definitions of anaphylaxis characteristically include the term 'allergic reaction', it is clear that responses that are clinically indistinguishable from IgE and allergen-induced anaphylaxis can be induced by non-immunological mechanisms [1, 10]. Non-immunologic mechanisms that trigger such anaphylaxis include exercise, exposure to cold air or water, and certain medications (such as opioids, vancomycin, and COX-1 inhibitors) [1, 73]. The exact mechanisms by which these non-immunologic factors activate mast cells remain to be fully elucidated, e.g., some of them may (e.g., opioids) or may not (e.g., hyperosmolarity) involve the activation of specific receptors. It also is not yet clear to what extent mast cells or basophils contribute to the pathophysiology of anaphylaxis in such settings. Although the clinical diagnosis and acute treatment of anaphylaxis do not depend on which of the many different potential effector mechanisms initially triggered the disorder, a better understanding of the effector mechanisms leading to mast cell (and basophil) activation in anaphylaxis may offer novel targets for therapeutic intervention and may also provide valuable information for long-term risk reduction [1].

Concluding Remarks

Although there has been impressive progress towards understanding the mechanisms of anaphylaxis, a number of important questions remain unanswered. One of the biggest challenges is to understand why only some individuals, among the many who bear IgE antibodies reactive with potential environmental triggers of anaphylaxis, develop this kind of reactivity. Some subjects who develop anaphylaxis upon challenge with a small amount of the offending allergen can have relatively low levels of total or allergen-specific IgE and/or relatively weak skin test responses to the allergen. By contrast, some patients who have developed IgE reactive with the same kinds of allergens that induce anaphylaxis in others (such as components of bee or wasp venom) do not develop anaphylaxis upon challenge with that allergen [74].

It is well known that some patients who have severe allergic diseases have extremely high levels of total IgE, and patients with certain parasite infections can have even higher IgE levels. The immunological specificity of IgE and allergen-dependent mast cell activation in each of these settings of course depends on which allergens are recognized by allergen-specific IgE. However, high total IgE levels, by having effects that increase levels of FcεRI expressed on the mast cell surface, can make mast cells more potent effector cells. Moreover, the consequences of chronic allergic inflammation in target organs may also predispose such patients to experience extremely severe responses, and to die, when they do develop anaphylaxis. This may explain, at least in part, why young people with severe asthma appear to be particularly susceptible to fatal or near-fatal food-induced anaphylaxis [10, 75]. So, why are some of the individuals who develop IgE antibody-associated immune responses predisposed to anaphylaxis, whereas others are not (despite the suffering they endure as a result of the local signs and symptoms of their IgE-associated allergic disorders)?

The answers(s) to this question might be complex, involving genetic and/or epigenetic contributions [76], as well as the nature of the allergen (e.g., many more subjects develop IgE specific for components of honeybee venom than exhibit anaphylaxis upon being stung [74]). Other contributory factors may include the ratio of allergen-specific to total IgE, the number of IgE-binding epitopes recognized by the individual's IgE, and/or extent of engagement of negative regulatory mechanisms that can diminish the responses of mast cells and other effector cells that are activated by IgE and allergen, and many others [1, 4, 10]. For example, in mice, high allergen-specific IgG levels may inhibit IgE-induced anaphylaxis without inducing immune complex- and FcγRIII-mediated anaphylaxis [77]. Furthermore, it has been shown that other cells, such as dendritic cells, can express FcεRI, and the role of these cells in IgE-dependent human anaphylaxis remains relatively unexplored. Accordingly, we certainly are not proposing here that the 'key' to understanding why some individuals develop anaphylactic reactivity to certain allergens necessarily represents some constellation of features of that subject's mast cells (and/or basophils). However, we do think that it would be interesting to know whether individual variation in aspects of the regulation of mast cell (or basophil) phenotype, signaling or function might represent some of the (potentially many) factors that can contribute to the susceptibility of some individuals to develop this inappropriate and potentially catastrophic immune response.

References

1 Simons FE, Frew AJ, Ansotegui IJ, Bochner BS, Golden DB, Finkelman FD, Leung DY, Lotvall J, Marone G, Metcalfe DD, Muller U, Rosenwasser LJ, Sampson HA, Schwartz LB, van Hage M, Walls AF: Risk assessment in anaphylaxis: current and future approaches. J Allergy Clin Immunol 2007;120:S2–S24.

2 Peavy RD, Metcalfe DD: understanding the mechanisms of anaphylaxis. Curr Opin Allergy Clin Immunol 2008;8:310–315.

3 Bochner BS, Lichtenstein LM: Anaphylaxis. N Engl J Med 1991;324:1785–1790.

4 Finkelman FD: Anaphylaxis: lessons from mouse models. J Allergy Clin Immunol 2007;120:506–515.

5 Galli SJ: Pathogenesis and management of anaphylaxis: current status and future challenges. J Allergy Clin Immunol 2005;115:571–574.

6 Galli SJ, Kalesnikoff J, Grimbaldeston MA, Piliponsky AM, Williams CM, Tsai M: Mast cells as 'tunable' effector and immunoregulatory cells: recent advances. Annu Rev Immunol 2005;23:749–786.

7 Gould HJ, Sutton BJ: IgE in allergy and asthma today. Nat Rev Immunol 2008;8:205–217.

8 Kraft S, Kinet JP: New developments in FcεRI regulation, function and inhibition. Nat Rev Immunol 2007;7:365–378.

9 MacGlashan D Jr: IgE receptor and signal transduction in mast cells and basophils. Curr Opin Immunol 2008;20:717–723.

10 Simons FE: Anaphylaxis. J Allergy Clin Immunol 2008;121:S402–S407.

11 Kitamura Y, Go S, Hatanaka K: Decrease of mast cells in W/W^v mice and their increase by bone marrow transplantation. Blood 1978;52:447–452.

12 Grimbaldeston MA, Chen CC, Piliponsky AM, Tsai M, Tam SY, Galli SJ: Mast cell-deficient W-$sash$ c-kit mutant $Kit^{W-sh/W-sh}$ mice as a model for investigating mast cell biology in vivo. Am J Pathol 2005;167:835–848.

13 Nigrovic PA, Gray DH, Jones T, Hallgren J, Kuo FC, Chaletzky B, Gurish M, Mathis D, Benoist C, Lee DM: genetic inversion in mast cell-deficient W^{sh} mice interrupts $Corin$ and manifests as hematopoietic and cardiac aberrancy. Am J Pathol 2008;173:1693–16701.

14 Wolters PJ, Mallen-St Clair J, Lewis CC, Villalta SA, Baluk P, Erle DJ, Caughey GH: Tissue-selective mast cell reconstitution and differential lung gene expression in mast cell-deficient Kit^{W-sh}/Kit^{W-sh} sash mice. Clin Exp Allergy 2005;35:82–88.

15 Kalesnikoff J, Galli SJ: New developments in mast cell biology. Nat Immunol 2008;9:1215–1223.

16 Musch W, Wege AK, Mannel DN, Hehlgans T: Generation and characterization of α-chymase-Cre transgenic mice. Genesis 2008;46:163–166.

17 Scholten J, Hartmann K, Gerbaulet A, Krieg T, Muller W, Testa G, Roers A: Mast cell-specific Cre/loxP-mediated recombination in vivo. Transgenic Res 2008;17:307–315.

18 Ha TY, Reed ND, Crowle PK: Immune response potential of mast cell-deficient W/W^v mice. Int Arch Allergy Appl Immunol 1986;80:85–94.

19 Oettgen HC, Martin TR, Wynshaw-Boris A, Deng C, Drazen JM, Leder P: Active anaphylaxis in IgE-deficient mice. Nature 1994;370:367–370.

20 Dombrowicz D, Flamand V, Miyajima I, Ravetch JV, Galli SJ, Kinet JP: Absence of FcεRI α chain results in upregulation of FcγRIII-dependent mast cell degranulation and anaphylaxis. Evidence of competition between FcεRI and FcγRIII for limiting amounts of FcR β and γ chains. J Clin Invest 1997; 99:915–925.

21 Tsujimura Y, Obata K, Mukai K, Shindou H, Yoshida M, Nishikado H, Kawano Y, Minegishi Y, Shimizu T, Karasuyama H: Basophils play a pivotal role in immunoglobulin-G-mediated but not immunoglobulin-E-mediated systemic anaphylaxis. Immunity 2008;28:581–589.

22 Miyajima I, Dombrowicz D, Martin TR, Ravetch JV, Kinet JP, Galli SJ: Systemic anaphylaxis in the mouse can be mediated largely through IgG1 and FcγRIII. Assessment of the cardiopulmonary changes, mast cell degranulation, and death associated with active or IgE- or IgG1-dependent passive anaphylaxis. J Clin Invest 1997;99:901–914.

23 Kawakami T, Galli SJ: Regulation of mast-cell and basophil function and survival by IgE. Nat Rev Immunol 2002;2:773–786.

24 Grayson MH, Cheung D, Rohlfing MM, Kitchens R, Spiegel DE, Tucker J, Battaile JT, Alevy Y, Yan L, Agapov E, Kim EY, Holtzman MJ: Induction of high-affinity IgE receptor on lung dendritic cells during viral infection leads to mucous cell metaplasia. J Exp Med 2007;204:2759–2769.

25 Gilfillan AM, Peavy RD, Metcalfe DD: Amplification mechanisms for the enhancement of antigen-mediated mast cell activation. Immunol Res 2008.

26 Rivera J, Fierro NA, Olivera A, Suzuki R: New insights on mast cell activation via the high affinity receptor for IgE. Adv Immunol 2008;98:85–120.

27 Liu Y, Zhu M, Nishida K, Hirano T, Zhang W: An essential role for RasGRP1 in mast cell function and IgE-mediated allergic response. J Exp Med 2007;204: 93–103.

28 Hong H, Kitaura J, Xiao W, Horejsi V, Ra C, Lowell CA, Kawakami Y, Kawakami T: The Src family kinase Hck regulates mast cell activation by suppressing an inhibitory Src family kinase Lyn. Blood 2007;110:2511–2519.

29 Baba Y, Nishida K, Fujii Y, Hirano T, Hikida M, Kurosaki T: Essential function for the calcium sensor STIM1 in mast cell activation and anaphylactic responses. Nat Immunol 2008;9:81–88.

30 Vig M, DeHaven WI, Bird GS, Billingsley JM, Wang H, Rao PE, Hutchings AB, Jouvin MH, Putney JW, Kinet JP: Defective mast cell effector functions in mice lacking the CRACM1 pore subunit of store-operated calcium release-activated calcium channels. Nat Immunol 2008;9:89–96.

31 Vennekens R, Olausson J, Meissner M, Bloch W, Mathar I, Philipp SE, Schmitz F, Weissgerber P, Nilius B, Flockerzi V, Freichel M: Increased IgE-dependent mast cell activation and anaphylactic responses in mice lacking the calcium-activated nonselective cation channel TRPM4. Nat Immunol 2007;8:312–320.

32 Guo Z, Turner C, Castle D: Relocation of the t-SNARE SNAP-23 from lamellipodia-like cell surface projections regulates compound exocytosis in mast cells. Cell 1998;94:537–548.

33 Logan MR, Odemuyiwa SO, Moqbel R: Understanding exocytosis in immune and inflammatory cells: the molecular basis of mediator secretion. J Allergy Clin Immunol 2003;111:923–932.

34 Puri N, Roche PA: Mast cells possess distinct secretory granule subsets whose exocytosis is regulated by different SNARE isoforms. Proc Natl Acad Sci USA 2008;105:2580–2585.

35 Tiwari N, Wang CC, Brochetta C, Ke G, Vita F, Qi Z, Rivera J, Soranzo MR, Zabucchi G, Hong W, Blank U: VAMP-8 segregates mast cell-preformed mediator exocytosis from cytokine trafficking pathways. Blood 2008;111:3665–3674.

36 Sander LE, Frank SP, Bolat S, Blank U, Galli T, Bigalke H, Bischoff SC, Lorentz A: Vesicle-associated membrane protein (VAMP)-7 and VAMP-8, but not VAMP-2 or VAMP-3, are required for activation-induced degranulation of mature human mast cells. Eur J Immunol 2008;38:855–863.

37 Suzuki K, Verma IM: Phosphorylation of SNAP-23 by IκB kinase 2 regulates mast cell degranulation. Cell 2008;134:485–495.

38 Kalesnikoff J, Rios EJ, Chen CC, Alejandro Barbieri M, Tsai M, Tam SY, Galli SJ: Roles of RabGEF1/Rabex-5 domains in regulating FcεRI surface expression and FcεRI-dependent responses in mast cells. Blood 2007;109:5308–5317.

39 Rios EJ, Piliponsky AM, Ra C, Kalesnikoff J, Galli SJ: Rabaptin-5 regulates receptor expression and functional activation in mast cells. Blood 2008;112: 4148–4157.

40 Leung WH, Bolland S: The inositol 5′-phosphatase SHIP-2 negatively regulates IgE-induced mast cell degranulation and cytokine production. J Immunol 2007;179:95–102.

41 Ong CJ, Ming-Lum A, Nodwell M, Ghanipour A, Yang L, Williams DE, Kim J, Demirjian L, Qasimi P, Ruschmann J, Cao LP, Ma K, Chung SW, Duronio V, Andersen RJ, Krystal G, Mui AL: Small-molecule agonists of SHIP1 inhibit the phosphoinositide 3-kinase pathway in hematopoietic cells. Blood 2007;110:1942–1949.

42 Bansal G, Xie Z, Rao S, Nocka KH, Druey KM: Suppression of immunoglobulin E-mediated allergic responses by regulator of G protein signaling 13. Nat Immunol 2008;9:73–80.

43 Bansal G, DiVietro JA, Kuehn HS, Rao S, Nocka KH, Gilfillan AM, Druey KM: RGS13 controls G protein-coupled receptor-evoked responses of human mast cells. J Immunol 2008;181:7882–7890.

44 Saxon A, Kepley C, Zhang K: 'Accentuate the negative, eliminate the positive': engineering allergy therapeutics to block allergic reactivity through negative signaling. J Allergy Clin Immunol 2008; 121:320–325.

45 Mertsching E, Bafetti L, Hess H, Perper S, Giza K, Allen LC, Negrou E, Hathaway K, Hopp J, Chung J, Perret D, Shields M, Saxon A, Kehry MR: A mouse FcγFcε protein that inhibits mast cells through activation of FcγRIIB, SH2 domain-containing inositol phosphatase 1, and SH2 domain-containing protein tyrosine phosphatases. J Allergy Clin Immunol 2008; 121:441–447.

46 Conroy MC, Adkinson NF Jr, Lichtenstein LM: Measurement of IgE on human basophils: relation to serum IgE and anti-IgE-induced histamine release. J Immunol 1977;118:1317–1321.

47 Malveaux FJ, Conroy MC, Adkinson NF Jr, Lichtenstein LM: IgE receptors on human basophils. relationship to serum IgE concentration. J Clin Invest 1978;62:176–181.

48 Stallman PJ, Aalberse RC: Quantitation of basophil-bound IgE in atopic and nonatopic subjects. Int Arch Allergy Appl Immunol 1977;54:114–120.

49 Furuichi K, Rivera J, Isersky C: The receptor for immunoglobulin E on rat basophilic leukemia cells: effect of ligand binding on receptor expression. Proc Natl Acad Sci USA 1985;82:1522–1525.

50 Quarto R, Kinet JP, Metzger H: Coordinate synthesis and degradation of the α-, β- and γ-subunits of the receptor for immunoglobulin E. Mol Immunol 1985;22:1045–1051.

51 Hsu C, MacGlashan D Jr: IgE antibody up-regulates high affinity IgE binding on murine bone marrow-derived mast cells. Immunol Lett 1996;52:129–134.

52 Yamaguchi M, Lantz CS, Oettgen HC, Katona IM, Fleming T, Miyajima I, Kinet JP, Galli SJ: IgE enhances mouse mast cell FcεRI expression in vitro and in vivo: evidence for a novel amplification mechanism in IgE-dependent reactions. J Exp Med 1997;185:663–672.

53 Matsuda K, Piliponsky AM, Iikura M, Nakae S, Wang EW, Dutta SM, Kawakami T, Tsai M, Galli SJ: Monomeric IgE enhances human mast cell chemokine production: IL-4 augments and dexamethasone suppresses the response. J Allergy Clin Immunol 2005;116:1357–1363.

54 James LC, Roversi P, Tawfik DS: Antibody multi-specificity mediated by conformational diversity. Science 2003;299:1362–1367.

55 Kepley CL, Youssef L, Andrews RP, Wilson BS, Oliver JM: Syk deficiency in nonreleaser basophils. J Allergy Clin Immunol 1999;104:279–284.

56 Vonakis BM, Gibbons S Jr, Sora R, Langdon JM, MacDonald SM: Src homology 2 domain-containing inositol 5′ phosphatase is negatively associated with histamine release to human recombinant histamine-releasing factor in human basophils. J Allergy Clin Immunol 2001;108:822–831.

57 Yamashita Y, Charles N, Furumoto Y, Odom S, Yamashita T, Gilfillan AM, Constant S, Bower MA, Ryan JJ, Rivera J: Cutting edge: genetic variation influences FcεRI-induced mast cell activation and allergic responses. J Immunol 2007;179:740–743.

58 Hernandez-Hansen V, Mackay GA, Lowell CA, Wilson BS, Oliver JM: The Src kinase Lyn is a negative regulator of mast cell proliferation. J Leukoc Biol 2004;75:143–151.

59 Odom S, Gomez G, Kovarova M, Furumoto Y, Ryan JJ, Wright HV, Gonzalez-Espinosa C, Hibbs ML, Harder KW, Rivera J: Negative regulation of immunoglobulin E-dependent allergic responses by Lyn kinase. J Exp Med 2004;199:1491–1502.

60 Hibbs ML, Tarlinton DM, Armes J, Grail D, Hodgson G, Maglitto R, Stacker SA, Dunn AR: Multiple defects in the immune system of Lyn-deficient mice, culminating in autoimmune disease. Cell 1995;83:301–311.

61 Nishizumi H, Yamamoto T: Impaired tyrosine phosphorylation and Ca^{2+} mobilization, but not degranulation, in Lyn-deficient bone marrow-derived mast cells. J Immunol 1997;158:2350–2355.

62 Costa JJ, Demetri GD, Harrist TJ, Dvorak AM, Hayes DF, Merica EA, Menchaca DM, Gringeri AJ, Schwartz LB, Galli SJ: Recombinant human stem cell factor (kit ligand) promotes human mast cell and melanocyte hyperplasia and functional activation in vivo. J Exp Med 1996;183:2681–2686.

63 Brockow K, Jofer C, Behrendt H, Ring J: Anaphylaxis in patients with mastocytosis: a study on history, clinical features and risk factors in 120 patients. Allergy 2008;63;226–232.

64 Akin C, Scott LM, Kocabas CN, Kushnir-Sukhov N, Brittain E, Noel P, Metcalfe DD: Demonstration of an aberrant mast-cell population with clonal markers in a subset of patients with 'idiopathic' anaphylaxis. Blood 2007;110:2331–2333.

65 Tilley SL, Wagoner VA, Salvatore CA, Jacobson MA, Koller BH: Adenosine and inosine increase cutaneous vasopermeability by activating A_3 receptors on mast cells. J Clin Invest 2000;105:361–367.

66 Laffargue M, Calvez R, Finan P, Trifilieff A, Barbier M, Altruda F, Hirsch E, Wymann MP: Phosphoinositide 3-kinase γ is an essential amplifier of mast cell function. Immunity 2002;16:441–451.

67 Feoktistov I, Biaggioni I: Adenosine A2b receptors evoke interleukin-8 secretion in human mast cells. An enprofylline-sensitive mechanism with implications for asthma. J Clin Invest 1995;96:1979–1986.

68 Hua X, Kovarova M, Chason KD, Nguyen M, Koller BH, Tilley SL: Enhanced mast cell activation in mice deficient in the A2b adenosine receptor. J Exp Med 2007;204:117–128.

69 Ryzhov S, Zaynagetdinov R, Goldstein AE, Novitskiy SV, Dikov MM, Blackburn MR, Biaggioni I, Feoktistov I: Effect of A2B adenosine receptor gene ablation on proinflammatory adenosine signaling in mast cells. J Immunol 2008;180:7212–7220.

70 Livingston M, Heaney LG, Ennis M: Adenosine, inflammation and asthma – a review. Inflamm Res 2004;53:171–178.

71 Polosa R, Holgate ST: Adenosine receptors as promising therapeutic targets for drug development in chronic airway inflammation. Curr Drug Targets 2006;7:699–706.

72 Spicuzza L, Di Maria G, Polosa R: Adenosine in the airways: implications and applications. Eur J Pharmacol 2006;533:77–88.

73 Holgate ST, Church MK, Lichtenstein LM. Allergy. New York, Elsevier Health Sciences, 2006.

74 Golden DB: Insect allergy in children. Curr Opin Allergy Clin Immunol 2006;6:289–293.

75 Sampson HA, Mendelson L, Rosen JP: Fatal and near-fatal anaphylactic reactions to food in children and adolescents. N Engl J Med 1992;327:380–384.

76 Vercelli D: Genetic regulation of IgE responses: Achilles and the tortoise. J Allergy Clin Immunol 2005;116:60–64.

77 Strait RT, Morris SC, Finkelman FD: IgG-blocking antibodies inhibit IgE-mediated anaphylaxis in vivo through both antigen interception and FcγRIIb cross-linking. J Clin Invest 2006;116:833–841.

Dr. Stephen J. Galli
Department of Pathology, L-235, Stanford University School of Medicine
300 Pasteur Drive, Stanford, CA 94305–5324 (USA)
Tel. +1 650 723 7975, Fax +1 650 725 6902
E-Mail sgalli@stanford.edu

Ring J (ed): Anaphylaxis. Chem Immunol Allergy. Basel, Karger, 2010, vol 95, pp 67–84

Kinins, Airway Obstruction, and Anaphylaxis

Allen P. Kaplan

Department of Medicine, Medical University of South Carolina, Charleston, S.C., USA

Abstract

Anaphylaxis is a term that implies symptoms that are present in many organs, some of which are potentially fatal. The pathogenic process can either be IgE-dependent or non-IgE-dependent; the latter circumstance may be referred to as anaphylactoid. Bradykinin is frequently responsible for the manifestations of IgE-independent reactions. Blood levels may increase because of overproduction; diseases such as the various forms of C1 inhibitor deficiency (hereditary or acquired) or hereditary angioedema with normal C1 inhibitor are examples in this category. Blood levels may also increase because of an abnormality in bradykinin metabolism; the angioedema due to ACE inhibitors is a commonly encountered example. Angioedema due to bradykinin has the potential to cause airway obstruction and asphyxia as well as severe gastrointestinal symptoms simulating an acute abdomen. Formation of bradykinin in plasma is a result of a complex interaction among proteins such as factor XII, prekallikrein, and high molecular weight kininogen (HK) resulting in HK cleavage and liberation of bradykinin. These proteins also assemble along the surface of endothelial cells via zinc-dependent interactions with gC1qR, cytokeratin 1, and u-PAR. Endothelial cell expression (or secretion) of heat-shock protein 90 or prolylcarboxypeptidase can activate the prekallikrein-HK complex to generate bradykinin in the absence of factor XII, however factor XII is then secondarily activated by the kallikrein that results. Bradykinin is destroyed by carboxypeptidase N and angiotensin-converting enzyme. The hypotension associated with IgE-dependent anaphylaxis may be mediated, in part, by massive proteolytic digestion of HK by kallikreins (tissue or plasma-derived) or other cell-derived kininogenases.

Copyright © 2010 S. Karger AG, Basel

Diseases that are known to be mediated by bradykinin include the various forms of C1 inhibitor deficiency, hereditary angioedema (HAE) with normal C1 inhibitor, and angioedema caused by angiotensin-converting enzyme (ACE) inhibitors. Common to all of these are symptoms of angioedema, in the absence of urticaria, that can include laryngeal edema or tongue and/or pharyngeal edema that are sufficiently severe so as to cause airway obstruction, and potentially, asphyxia. These bradykinin-dependent disorders can also include gastrointestinal symptoms reminiscent of an acute abdomen with severe pain, nausea, vomiting, or diarrhea due to edema of the bowel wall. Acute anaphylaxis can include all of the above symptoms, however the most common cutaneous manifestation is urticaria. Anaphylaxis may also be associated with profound hypotension and bradykinin may contribute to this manifestation. In this chapter I will review those disorders that can cause accelerating airway obstruction and then discuss the possible role of bradykinin in IgE-dependent or IgE-independent anaphylactic-like episodes.

Introduction

The plasma kinin-forming system consists of three essential proteins that interact in a complex fashion once bound to certain negatively charged inorganic surfaces, or to macromolecular complexes formed during an inflammatory response, or to proteins along cell surfaces. These are coagulation factor XII (Hageman factor, HF), prekallikrein, and high molecular weight kininogen (HK). Once factor XII is activated to factor XIIa it converts pre-kallikrein to kallikrein and kallikrein digests HK to liberate bradykinin. Factor XIIa has a second substrate in plasma, namely coagulation factor XI and activation of surface-bound factor XI by factor XIIa initiates the intrinsic coagulation pathway. Thus the interactions of all four of these proteins are known as contact activation and the formation of bradykinin is therefore a cleavage product of the initiating step of the cascade [1]. There is also a tissue pathway [2] by which bradykinin is generated in which there is intracellular conversion of prokallikrein to tissue kallikrein by enzymes that are as yet not well characterized. Tissue kallikrein is secreted into the local milieu where it digests low molecular weight kininogen (LK) to generate lysyl-bradykinin (kallidin) and an aminopeptidase converts kallidin to bradykinin. The bradykinin that is produced by either pathway is then degraded by plasma enzymes as well as enzymes that are active along the surface of endothelial cells (particularly pulmonary vascular endothelial cells) to lower molecular weight peptides. The major plasma enzyme is carboxypeptidase N [3]. This removes the C-terminal arginine from bradykinin to yield an 8-amino-acid peptide (des-arg-9 bradykinin) [4]. The second kininase in plasma is termed kininase II and is identical to ACE [5]. This latter enzyme predominates along the pulmonary vascular endothelial cell surface. Bradykinin is thereby rapidly degraded within one or two circulation times. This enzyme removes the dipeptide phe-arg from the C-terminus of bradykinin to yield a heptapeptide and a second cleavage removes ser-pro to leave a pentapeptide [6]. Bradykinin acts on the B2 receptor on the surface of endothelial cells to cause vasodilatation and to increase vascular permeability. Other vasodilators such as nitric oxide are produced secondarily as a result of B2 receptor stimulation [7]. Des-arg-9 bradykinin, the product of carboxypeptidase N, is active dominantly on B1 receptors [8]. These latter receptors, in contrast to B2 receptors, are not constitutively produced but are induced as a result of inflammation due to the presence of cytokines such as interleukin-1 and tumor necrosis factor-α [8, 9]. The heptapeptide and pentapeptide products of kininase II (ACE) are inactive. Additional enzymes that may contribute to bradykinin degradation are encephalinase and aminopeptidase P; any inhibition of

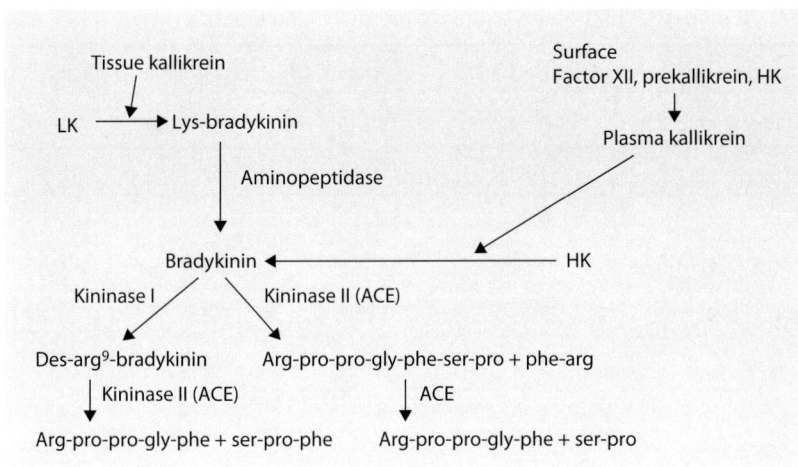

Fig. 1. Pathways for formation and degradation of bradykinin.

these enzymes or polymorphisms that affect their concentration or activity may have a role in angioedema formation due to ACE inhibitors. A schematic diagram of the formation and degradation of bradykinin is shown in figure 1.

Proteins

Factor XII circulates as a single chain zymogen that is devoid of enzymatic activity. It has a molecular weight of approximately 80 kDa on sodium dodecyl sulfate gel electrophoresis, is synthesized in the liver, and circulates in the plasma at a concentration of 30–35 μg/ml. Factor XII is capable of autoactivating once it is bound to initiating surfaces [10] as a result of a conformational change that renders bound factor XII to become a substrate for factor XIIa [11]. Further cleavages can occur at the C-terminal end of the heavy chain to produce a series of fragments the most prominent of which is a 30-kDa species termed factor XIIf [12]. These fragments lack the ability to bind to the surface and therefore are unable to convert factor XI to XIa, but continue to be potent activators of prekallikrein. Thus, formation of factor XIIf allows bradykinin production to continue in the fluid phase until the enzyme is inactivated and the reactions can therefore proceed at sites distant from the initiating surface.

Prekallikrein is also a circulating proenzyme which requires proteolytic cleavage to generate an active protease. On sodium dodecyl sulfate gels it has two bands at 88 and 85 kDa and the heterogeneity observed is not reflected in its amino acid sequence [13]. Thus it appears likely to be due to two variant glycosylated forms that are present in everyone. Activation of prekallikrein by factor XIIa or factor XIIf is the result of cleavage of a single arg-Ile bond within a disulfide bridge such that a heavy chain

Table 1. Physiochemical properties of proteins of the contact activation cascade

Protein	Factor XII	Prekallikrein	Factor XI	HK
Molecular weight, daltons (calculated)	80,427	79,545	140,000	116,643
Carbohydrate (w/w)	16.8%	15%	5%	40%
Isoelectric point	6.3	8.7	8.6	4.7
Extinction coefficient, $E^{1\%}$ 280/nm	14.2	11.7	13.4	7.0
Plasma concentration, µg/ml	30–45	35–50	4–6	70–90
nmol/l (average)	400	534	36	686

of 56 kDa is disulfide linked to light chains of either 33 or 36 kDa. Thus the heterogeneity is reflected in the light chain and the light chain also contains the active site of the enzyme [13]. Prekallikrein circulates in plasma bound to HK in a 1:1 bimolecular complex [14] through a site contained in the prekallikrein heavy chain. It has been shown that 80–90% of prekallikrein is normally complexed in this way and it is the prekallikrein/HK complex that binds to surfaces during contact activation. The surface binding site is located within the light chain of cleaved HK.

HK circulates in plasma as a 115-kDa non-enzymatic glycoprotein with a concentration of 70–90 µg/ml [14, 15]. It forms non-covalent complexes with both prekallikrein and factor XI. The attachment of prekallikrein (or factor XI) to HK occurs within the C-terminal region of HK corresponding to the light chain that forms after cleavage to release bradykinin [14, 16–18]. The isolated light chain (after reduction and alkylation) derived from cleaved HK possesses the same binding characteristics as the whole molecule. HK therefore functions as a coagulation cofactor and this activity resides in the light chain [17–19]. During contact activation kallikrein cleaves HK at two positions within a disulfide bridge. The first is at a C-terminal arg-ser bond followed by cleavage at the N-terminal lys-arg bond to release the nonapeptide bradykinin (arg-pro-pro-gly-phe-ser-pro-phe-arg). The two chain disulfide linked kinin-free HK results, consisting of a heavy chain of 65 kDa disulfide link to a light chain of molecular weight 46–49 kDa [19–23]. The physiochemical properties of these proteins as well as factor XI are shown in table 1.

Mechanisms of Bradykinin Formation (Contact Activation)

The various interactions of the constituents required for the formation of bradykinin are shown in figure 2. The initiating step is a slow autoactivation of factor XII [10]. However, once this has occurred and prekallikrein is converted to kallikrein, there is

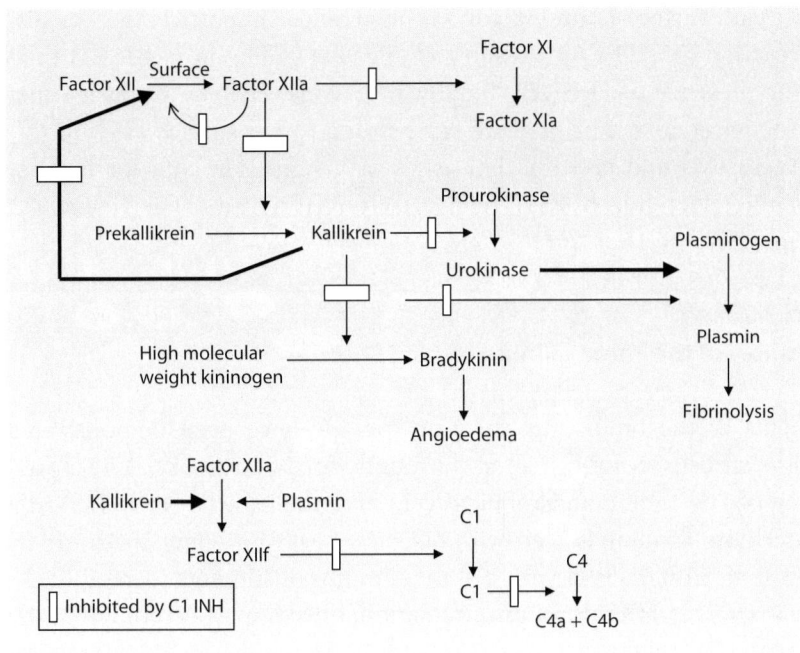

Fig. 2. A diagrammatic representation of the plasma kinin-forming cascade indicating the steps inhibitable by C1 INH. All functions of factor XIIa and kallikrein are affected. The lower figure indicates that further digestion of factor XIIa by kallikrein and plasmin generates factor XII fragment (XIIf), which is an initiator of the complement cascade. Both factor XIIf and C1 are inhibited by C1 INH.

a positive feedback in which the kallikrein generated rapidly activates factor XII to factor XIIa. This reaction is much more rapid than autoactivation is, thus the majority of the factor XIIa generated is due to kallikrein. The presence of a surface plus this reciprocal interaction leads to a tremendously rapid activation of the cascade. It has been calculated that if one molecule each of factor XIIa and kallikrein are present per milliliter in a mixture of factor XII and prekallikrein at plasma concentration, the addition of an initiating surface will lead to a 50% conversion of factor XII to factor XIIa in 13 s [11]. The addition of the cofactor HK (which was not included in the aforementioned kinetic analysis) accelerates these reactions even further. The surface appears to provide a local milieu in the contiguous fluid phase where the concentrations of reactants are greatly increased [24].

One function of HK is to present the substrates of factor XIIa in a conformation that facilitates their activation [25, 26]. More difficult to explain is the effect of HK on the rate of factor XII activation in plasma since HK does not interact with factor XII, nor does it augment the activity of kallikrein. This effect seems to be largely indirect. First, HK is required for efficient formation of kallikrein in surface-activated plasma [26, 27]. Second, since kallikrein can disassociate from surface-bound

HK it can interact with surface-bound factor XII on an adjacent particle thereby disseminating the reaction [25, 28]. As a result the effective kallikrein/factor XII ratio is increased in the presence of HK [25]. Finally, in plasma, HK can displace other adhesive glycoproteins such as fibrinogen from binding to the surface [29]. In this sense, HK, like factor XII and prekallikrein, is also a coagulation cofactor because it is required for the generation of kallikrein (a factor XII activator) as well as the activation of factor XI.

Cell Surface Assembly of the Plasma Kinin-Forming Cascade

All the components of the bradykinin-forming cascade have been demonstrated to bind to endothelial cells. Schmaier et al. [30] and van Iwaarden et al. [31] first described binding of HK to human umbilical vein endothelial cells (HUVEC) in a zinc-dependent fashion. Binding is seen with both the heavy and light chain of HK [32, 33], thus a complex interaction with cell membrane constituents seemed likely. Since prekallikrein binds to HK within the circulation, the complex is brought to the surface of the endothelial cell by virtue of HK binding. When factor XII interaction with HUVEC was studied, it was found to bind with characteristics strikingly similar to those seen with HK including a similar requirement for zinc [34]. We subsequently demonstrated that HK and factor XII can compete for binding at a comparable molar ratio suggesting that they compete for binding to the same receptor sites.

Three endothelial cell binding sites for HK and for factor XII have been described thus far. These include gC1qR (the receptor for the globular heads of the C1q subcomponent of the first component of complement) [35, 36], cytokeratin 1 [37, 38], and the urokinase plasminogen activator receptor (u-PAR) [39]. They exist as bimolecular complexes consisting of gC1qR-cytokeratin 1 and cytokeratin 1-u-PAR, as well as uncomplexed gC1qR [40]. HK binds preferentially to gC1qR-cytokeratin 1 (as well as to free gC1qR) while factor XII binds primarily to u-PAR [K. Joseph and A. Kaplan, unpubl. observations] within the cytokeratin 1-u-PAR complex. gC1qR binds specifically to the light chain of HK and not to the heavy chain. Cytokeratin 1 represents a major site of interaction for the HK heavy chain although it is capable of binding the light chain as well. However, light chain binding to gC1qR appears to predominate because of the affinity of the interaction as well as the much larger number of gC1qR-binding sites.

Affinity chromatography using factor XII as ligand leads to purification of u-PAR rather selectively, with only trace quantities of cytokeratin 1 or gC1qR present [K. Joseph and A. Kaplan, unpubl. observations]. It is of interest that none of these three proteins possesses a transmembrane domain but u-PAR has a phosphatidylinositol linkage within the cell membrane. Nevertheless, each of them has been isolated from purified cell membranes and they have been demonstrated to exist within the cell membrane by immunoelectron microscopy [41] presumably

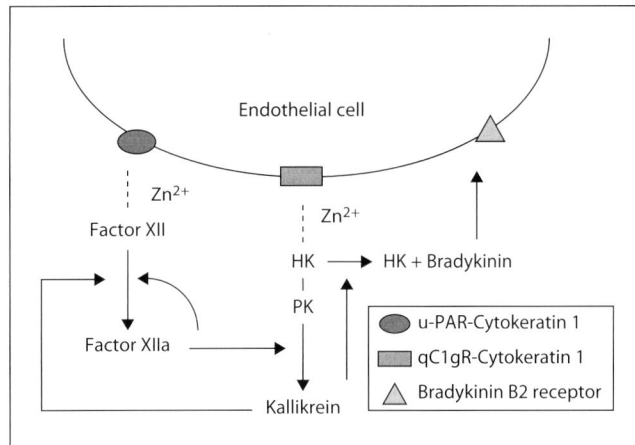

Fig. 3. Diagrammatic representation of the binding of factor XII and the primarily HK-PK complex to endothelial cells indicating that factor XII binds to the u-PAR-cytokeratin 1 complex, HK binds to the gC1qR-cytokeratin 1 complex, and that activation to produce bradykinin can occur along the cell surface.

bound to other membrane constituents. A summary depicting these interactions is shown in figure 3.

Kinin Formation at the Surface of Endothelial Cells

An alternative pathway for activating the cascade has recently been demonstrated in which factor XII is absent from the reaction mixture [42–45]. Two different groups have isolated two different proteins, each of which seems to activate the HK-prekallikrein complex. One is heat-shock protein 90 [46] and the other is a prolylcarboxypeptidase [47]. Neither protein is a direct prekallikrein activator as is factor XIIa or factor XIIf because each activator requires HK to be complexed to the prekallikrein. In addition, the reaction is stoichiometric, thus the amount of prekallikrein converted to kallikrein equals the molar input of heat-shock protein 90 (or prolylcarboxypeptidase). These proteins can be shown to contribute to factor XII-independent prekallikrein activation and antisera to each protein have been shown to inhibit the process. When whole endothelial cells are incubated with normal plasma or factor XII-deficient plasma, the rate of activation of the deficient plasma is very much slower than that of the normal plasma, the latter being factor XII-dependent [45]. Under normal circumstances (with factor XII present), formation of any kallikrein will lead to factor XIIa formation even if the process were initiated by one of these cell-derived factors.

Angioedema

C1 inhibitor deficiency causes angioedema as a result of excessive bradykinin production. Thus the pathways and control mechanisms for bradykinin formation and degradation are variables that one must consider in any patient with angioedema. Activated factor XII as well as factor XIIf are inhibited by C1 INH [48, 49], thus absence of C1 INH facilitates factor XII autoactivation, which augments the ability of factor XIIa to convert both prekallikrein to kallikrein and factor XI to factor XIa. It is estimated that over 90% of plasma inhibition of factor XIIa and factor XIIf is due to C1 INH [49]. The next enzyme in the cascade is kallikrein and it is inhibited by C1 INH and α_2-macroglobulin in approximately equal proportions [50]. Minor inhibitors of kallikrein are antithrombin III and α_1-antitrypsin. Thus if there is any stimulus for activation of the plasma bradykinin-forming cascade, in the absence of functional C1 INH, there is a marked augmentation of bradykinin formation with angioedema as the result. Urticaria is not seen in patients with C1 INH deficiency, but an episode of swelling may begin with a rash resembling erythema marginatum. Hereditary C1 inhibitor deficiency, the most common and best studied presentation of HAE, is an autosomal dominant disorder resulting in low plasma levels or synthesis of a dysfunctional C1 inhibitor. A new form of HAE with normal C1 inhibitor may be due in some families, to a mutant factor XII. Acquired C1 INH deficiency is caused by depletion of functional C1 INH as a result of binding to active enzymes or the presence of antibody to C1 INH, with synthesis being insufficient to maintain a normal level. Disease associations include lymphoma, connective tissue disorder, or autoimmune processes.

C1 Inhibitor Deficiency

Causes and Inheritance

C1 inhibitor deficiency is an important cause of angioedema, which may involve almost any portion of the body. Sometimes local trauma to an extremity can initiate an exaggerated local swelling or a more generalized episode of swelling. However, a triggering event may not be immediately evident, so that swelling appears to occur spontaneously. C1 inhibitor deficiency can be familial (in which there is a mutant C1 inhibitor gene) or it can be acquired. Both the hereditary and acquired forms of C1 inhibitor deficiency have two subgroups. For the hereditary disorder, type 1 HAE is typically an autosomal dominant disorder in which a mutant gene leads to markedly depressed C1 inhibitor levels [51]. Type 2 HAE is also inherited as an autosomal dominant disorder and has a mutation that leads to synthesis of a dysfunctional protein; the C1 inhibitor protein level may then be normal or even elevated [52]. The acquired form of C1 inhibitor deficiency also has two forms. In the first type, there is an association with either a B-cell lymphoma or connective tissue disease in which there is sufficient consumption of C1 inhibitor to cause angioedema [53–55]. The second form of acquired C1 inhibitor deficiency is an autoimmune disorder in which there is a circulating IgG antibody directed to C1 inhibitor itself [56–58]. A positive family history, the presence of a lymphoma, or an underlying connective tissue disease would each suggest C1 inhibitor deficiency when swelling is a manifestation.

The presence of visceral involvement in any patient with angioedema (in the absence of hives) is suggestive. The most severe complication is laryngeal edema, which had been a major cause of mortality in this disorder. Patients can also have abdominal attacks lasting 1–3 days, consisting of vomiting, severe abdominal pain, and guarding in the absence of fever, leukocytosis, or abdominal rigidity. This may nevertheless be difficult to differentiate from an acute surgical abdomen. However, the attacks are self-limited and caused by edema of the bowel wall [59].

Molecular Genetics

HAE is transmitted as an autosomal dominant disorder due, in most instances, to alterations of the C1 INH gene. Its prevalence is 1/50,000 [60]; however, there is a high incidence of de novo mutations accounting for close to 25% of cases. Thus there may not be a family history to guide evaluation of such patients and it is therefore reasonable to obtain a C4 and C1 INH determination in any patient presenting with recurrent angioedema in the absence of urticaria.

Point mutations and deletions or insertions are scattered along the entire C1 INH gene. Missense mutations are found along the entire coding sequence, with the exception of the 100 amino acid long N-terminal segment that is highly glycosylated and has little homology with other plasma proteinase inhibitors. Amino acid substitutions seen in type I HAE often affect intracellular transport of C1 INH (as do other mutations in type I disease) with impairment of protein secretion. Amino acid substitutions, rather than deletions, insertions, stop codons, or frameshift mutations, characterize type II disease in which there is secretion of a dysfunctional protein (i.e. plasma protein levels may appear normal but a large fraction of the secreted protein is dysfunctional). Here the mutations cluster about the reactive site of C1 INH at Arg444 (the protein is cleaved by the enzyme to which it will bind, exposing a reactive site that in turn covalently binds the active site serine of the enzyme, thereby inactivating it). These are sites of spontaneous deamination of methylated cytosines of a CpG dinucleotide which account for most of the type II mutations. It is important to note that in types I and II HAE, there is one normal gene, thus C1INH synthesis should theoretically be at 50% of normal. Yet in type I HAE, the total C1 INH protein is often much less (angioedema typically occurs at levels of 25% or less), and in type II disease normal and dysfunctional proteins circulate side by side. Further depletion of the normal gene product may occur because of hypercatabolism, that is, turnover as a result of binding to plasma proteases [61] or suppression of normal C1 INH protein (transinhibition) by the mRNA or abnormal protein of the dysfunctional allele [52, 62]. An intermediate phenotype encompassing features of type I and II abnormalities may be seen in which an amino acid substitution leads not only to decreased secretion of the protein but it is also dysfunctional. A very rare recessive form of the disease may be seen with mutations in the promotor region of the gene or within the first intron. Homozygosity is required to lower the C1 INH level sufficiently to cause clinical symptoms.

Diagnosis

Patients with HAE have measurable levels of the activated first component of complement (C1) although this protein generally circulates as an unactivated enzyme. The serum level of C4 is diminished, even when the patient is free of symptoms, and is virtually undetectable during an attack [63]. A C4 determination is therefore the simplest way to screen for the hereditary disorder. Rocket immunoelectrophoresis for C4 cleavage products such as C4b is a very sensitive assay, more so than C4 quantitation [64]. It should be noted that 5% of patients have a normal C4 level, so that assays of total and functional inhibitor still need to be done if suspicion of C1 inhibitor deficiency exists. Levels of C2, the other substrate of C1, are usually within normal limits when the patient is asymptomatic, but the concentration is also diminished during an attack of swelling [65]. When a diminished C4 level is obtained, a direct assay of the protein, C1 inhibitor, should always be performed. A diminished or absent level of C1 inhibitor protein would confirm the diagnosis; 80–85% of patients with HAE have this type form of the disorder (type I). However, 15–20% of patients will have a mutant form of C1 inhibitor protein that renders it functionless (type II). Thus an assay for functional C1 inhibitor is necessary to confirm the diagnosis.

Pathogenesis

The pathogenesis of the swelling appears to involve the plasma kinin-forming pathway and bradykinin is now accepted to be the cause of the swelling. The lesions are not pruritic, and administration of antihistamines has no effect on the clinical course of the disease. Complement activation is undoubtedly occurring, perhaps even during quiescent periods to lead to a low level of C4, but the vasoactive consequences of augmented complement activation that occur during attacks of HAE do not appear to be the cause of the swelling. Figure 2 is a diagrammatic representation of the plasma kinin-forming cascade, also indicating the various enzymatic steps including the sites of inhibition by C1 inhibitor.

Factor XIIa converts prekallikrein to kallikrein and kallikrein cleaves HK to generate bradykinin. There is also an important positive feedback in the system in which the kallikrein generated rapidly converts unactivated factor XII to activated factor XII, and the rate of this reaction is hundreds of times faster than the rate of autoactivation [11]. Therefore, much of the unactivated factor XII can be cleaved and activated by kallikrein. C1 inhibitor inhibits all functions of factor XIIa and it is one of two major plasma kallikrein inhibitors. Thus all functions of kallikrein are also inhibited, including the feedback activation of factor XII, the cleavage of HK, and the activation of plasma pro-urokinase [66] to lead to plasmin formation. C1 inhibitor also inhibits the fibrinolytic enzyme plasmin, although it is a relatively minor inhibitor compared to α_2-antiplasmin or α_2-macroglobulin.

Fields et al. [67] first demonstrated evolution of bradykinin in HAE plasma even if an initiating surface is absent indicating seemingly spontaneous activation of the kinin-forming cascade in the absence of this control protein. This work also disproved an earlier theory that a kinin can be generated by activation of complement and concluded that bradykinin is the pathogenic peptide. Curd et al. [68] made a similar observation regarding bradykinin formation in HAE plasma and demonstrated kallikrein-like activity in induced blisters of patients with HAE [69]. Patients with HAE appear to be hyperresponsive to cutaneous injections of kallikrein [70], although it is difficult to control for these observations since any trauma is likely to activate the kinin cascade locally. Elevated levels of bradykinin and cleaved kininogen have been observed during attacks of swelling [71–73]. There is also evidence that C1 activation observed in patients with HAE may also be dependent on factor XII [74]. Thus, a factor XII-dependent enzyme may be initiating the classic complement cascade. Plasmin is capable of activating C1s and may represent one such enzyme [75]. Ghebrehiwet et al. [76, 77] demonstrated that Hageman factor fragment (factor XIIf) can directly activate the classic complement cascade by activating C1. This may represent a critical link between the intrinsic coagulation-kinin cascade and complement activation. More recent data support these earlier observations, favoring bradykinin as the critical pathogenic peptide for HAE and also acquired C1 INH deficiency. One unique family has been described in which there is a point mutation in C1 INH (Ala^{443}→Val) leading to inability to inhibit the complement cascade but normal inhibition of factor XIIa and kallikrein [78, 79]. No family member of this type II mutation has had angioedema. In recent studies, plasma bradykinin levels have been shown to be elevated during attacks of swelling in patients with hereditary and acquired forms of C1 INH deficiency [80]. Local bradykinin generation has been documented at the site of the swelling [73] and swelling seen in a rodent model of C1 INH deficiency is prevented by treatment with a bradykinin B2 receptor antagonist [81].

The role of fibrinolysis also needs to be considered a part of the pathogenesis of the disease, since antifibrinolytic agents such as ε-aminocaproic acid and tranexamic acid appear to be efficacious. As shown in figure 3, kallikrein converts plasminogen to plasmin. Although kallikrein, factor XIa, and even factor XIIa (not shown) have some ability to activate plasminogen directly, the plasma pathway via the pro-urokinase intermediate appears to be the major plasma factor XII-dependent fibrinolytic mechanism. However, bradykinin stimulation of endothelial cells releases tissue plasminogen activation and plasmin may also be formed by this mechanism. Among the functions of plasmin are the activation of C1s, the ability to cleave and activate factor XII just as kallikrein can [82], and digestion of C1 inhibitor [83]. Each of these would serve to augment bradykinin formation and further deplete the levels of C1 inhibitor. Thus, the formation of plasmin may, in this fashion, contribute to the pathogenesis of the disease.

Acquired C1 Inhibitor Deficiency

An acquired form of this disease has been described in patients with lymphoma who have circulating low molecular weight IgM and depressed C1 inhibitor levels. This entity has an unusual complement utilization profile because C1q levels are low and C4, C2, and C3 are depleted. The low C1q level differentiates this condition from the hereditary disorder [53–55]. The depressed C1 inhibitor level may be caused by depletion secondary to C1 activation by circulating immune complexes or C1 interaction with a tumor cell surface antigen. For B-cell lymphoma, the most common associated malignancy, C1 fixation and C1 inhibitor depletion are caused by an anti-idiotypic antibody bound to immunoglobulin on the surface of the B cell [84]. Other B-cell disorders associated with C1 INH depletion are acute and chronic lymphocytic leukemia, multiple myeloma, Waldenström's macroglobulinemia and essential cryoglobulinemia.

Patients with connective tissue disorders such as systemic lupus erythematosus or carcinoma [85, 86] can present with acquired C1 inhibitor deficiency and, like patients with the hereditary form, will respond to androgen therapy, which enhances C1 inhibitor synthesis. A second form of C1 inhibitor deficiency results from the synthesis of an autoantibody directed to C1 inhibitor itself [56, 87]. These patients also have low levels of C4, C1q, and C1 inhibitor protein and function, and no family history. This form of acquired C1 inhibitor deficiency appears to be increasingly recognized. Under normal circumstances, C1 inhibitor is a substrate for the enzymes it inactivates: the active enzyme cleaves C1 inhibitor, which exposes the active site in the inhibitor. The cleaved C1 inhibitor then binds stoichiometrically to the enzyme and inactivates it. When antibody to C1 inhibitor is present, the C1 inhibitor is cleaved but is unable to inactivate the enzyme [58, 88, 89]. Thus, cleaved, functionless C1 inhibitor circulates and unopposed activation of the complement- and kinin-forming cascade takes place. Plasmin is one of the enzymes that is capable of cleaving and inactivating C1 inhibitor, and local C1 inhibitor degradation by plasmin may be a critical event in the loss of protease inhibition during inflammation. In a more general sense, this observation may also explain the efficacy of antiplasmin agents such as ε-aminocaproic acid or tranexamic acid in the treatment of C1 inhibitor deficiency states.

Treatment

Prophylactic treatment of C1 INH deficiency consists of C1 INH replacement infusions, androgens (danazol, stanozolol, oxymethalone) or antifibrinolytic agents. Acute treatment employs C1 INH replacement (where available), fresh-frozen plasma, and placement of an airway when significant airway obstruction is evident. Abdominal attacks require IV fluid, analgesics, and 'watchful waiting'.

This year new agents have reported for the treatment of acute episodes including a B2 receptor antagonist (icatibant) [90, 91] and a kallikrein inhibitor (ecallantide) [92]. These provide a physiologic approach which targets the kallikrein-kinin cascade and might eventually become available in preparations that can also be employed for prophylaxis. Treatment of acquired C1 inhibitor deficiency requires, first, treatment of the underlying disease, if one has been identified, plus treatment with the aforementioned drugs, which is essentially the same as that for treatment of the hereditary disorder. Androgenic agents are typically employed. Treatment of type 2 acquired C1 inhibitor deficiency with an autoantibody directed to C1 inhibitor is indeed more difficult because the ability to replete C1 inhibitor is significantly compromised.

Other Hereditary and Non-Hereditary Angioedemas

Other hereditary forms of angioedema do not relate to C1 inhibitor deficiency, but all of them are rare. Binkley and Davis [93] reported an estrogen-dependent but familial form of angioedema associated with pregnancy or with ingestion of estrogenic compounds. The disorder appears to have dominant inheritance, and was initially thought to be present only in women because of the hormonal dependence. Recent studies of large families with the disorder have revealed occasional males who have symptoms [94]. Peripheral angioedema is very common and gastrointestinal episodes are seen as well. Laryngeal edema, although possible, seems less frequent compared to C1 inhibitor deficiency. Some families have a mutant form of factor XII which when activated, has enhanced activity [95]. Thus, bradykinin may be the mediator and therapy with newer agents that target the kallikrein-kinin system will be of interest.

One of the most prominent causes of non-HAE is the use of ACE inhibitors and this is now the most common cause of angioedema seen in emergency rooms. The angioedema is due to increased bradykinin levels (without urticaria) because the destruction of bradykinin by ACE is then impaired and blood levels gradually rise. It can occur at any time, but is most common within the first few months of therapy, and is particularly common in blacks [96]. There may be polymorphisms of other inhibitors or changes in end-organ responsiveness to bradykinin that determine who becomes symptomatic [97]. These agents are not only employed for treatment of hypertension but are also indicated for congestive heart failure, diabetic neuropathy, and scleroderma renal disease. ACE is identical to kininase II and destroys bradykinin by removing the C-terminal phe-arg dipeptide, followed by removal of ser-pro, leaving the inactive pentapeptide arg-pro-pro-gly-phe [98]. With drug inhibition of ACE, the primary mechanism for bradykinin degradation is eliminated (fig. 1) and bradykinin levels increase. Like C1 inhibitor deficiency, swelling of the tongue, pharynx, and even larynx can be severe, requiring intubation for treatment of airway obstruction. In contrast to patients with C1 INH deficiency, urticaria is occasionally seen accompanying the angioedema, although the angioedema predominates. The reason for this difference is unclear and may relate to a different site of bradykinin action within the skin, or even a concomitant IgE-mediated reaction to the drug.

Kinins and Anaphylactic-Like Reactions

Anaphylaxis that is IgE-dependent is most commonly associated with reactions to foods, drugs, and insect venoms. Anaphylactic-like reactions that are not dependent on IgE antibody (anaphylactoid) include reactions to ACE inhibitors, NSAIDS, and radiocontrast dyes, as well as hypotensive episodes associated with hemodialysis. The properties of bradykinin, including the ability to increase vascular permeability, contract gastrointestinal and uterine smooth muscle, and vasodilate to cause hypotension, lead to manifestations of many of these severe reactions. Many of the membranes employed for hemodialysis have been shown to activate the factor XII-dependent pathway of bradykinin formation which appeared to correlate with hypotensive episodes [99]. In the past, albumin preparations contaminated with factor XIIf caused hypotension upon infusion [1000] and recently, heparin preparations contaminated with oversulfated monopolysaccharides caused anaphylactic-like reactions with hypotension as a major manifestation [101]. All the evidence points to bradykinin as the mediator of these active reactions. However, rigorous studies of the bradykinin-forming cascade in IgE-dependent anaphylaxis in general are lacking (with one exception) and there are no inhibition studies employing bradykinin receptor antagonists. The exception is a study of induced anaphylaxis to bee venom [102] in which severe anaphylaxis was associated with complete digestion of plasma HK. Bradykinin was not measured directly but release of amounts in the micromolar range appears likely, and the partial thromboplastin time was not measurable (essentially infinite) indicating proteolytic digestion of critical coagulant proteins of the intrinsic coagulation pathway.

References

1   Kaplan A, Silverberg M: Contact system and its disorders; in Handin R, Lux S, Stossel T (eds): Blood – Principles Practice of Hematology. Philadelphia, Lippincott Williams & Wilkins, 1995, pp 1131–1155.
2   Margolius H: Tissue kallikreins structure, regulation, and participation in mammalian physiology and disease. Clin Rev Allergy Immunol 1998;16:337–349.
3   Erdos E, Sloane G: An enzyme in human plasma that inactivates bradykinin and kallidins. Biochem Pharmacol 1962;11:585–592.
4   Sheikh IA, Kaplan AP: Studies of the digestion of bradykinin, lysyl bradykinin, and kinin-degradation products by carboxypeptidases A, B, and N. Biochem Pharmacol 1986;35:1957–1963.
5   Yang H, Erdos E: Second kininase in human blood plasma. Nature 1967;215:1402–1403.
6   Sheikh I, Kaplan A: Studies of the digestion of bradykinin, Lys-bradykinin, and des-arg-9 bradykinin by angiotensin-converting enzyme. Biochem Pharmacol 1986;35:1951–1956.
7   Regoli D, Barabe J: Pharmacology of bradykinin and related kinins. Pharmacol Rev 1980;32:1–46.
8   Marceau F: Kinin B1 receptors: a review. Immunopharmacology 1995;30:1–26.
9   Davis A, Perkins M: The involvement of bradykinin B1 and B2 receptor mechanisms in cytokine-induced mechanical hyperalgesia in the rat. Br J Pharmacol 1994;113:63–68.
10 Silverberg M, Dunn J, Garen L, Kaplan A: Auto-activation of human Hageman factor. Demonstration utilizing a synthetic substrate. J Biol Chem 1980;255:7281–7286.
11 Tankersley DL, Finlayson JS: Kinetics of activation and autoactivation of human factor XII. Biochemistry 1984;23:273–279.
12 Kaplan AP, Austen KF: A pre-albumin activator of prekallikrein. J Immunol 1970;105:802–811.
13 Mandle RJ, Kaplan A: Hageman factor substrates. Human plasma prekallikrein: mechanism of activation by Hageman factor and participation in Hageman factor-dependent fibrinolysis. J Biol Chem 1977;252:6097–6104.
14 Mandle R, Colman R, Kaplan A: Identification of prekallikrein and high-molecular-weight kininogen as a complex in human plasma. Proc Natl Acad Sci USA 1976;73:4179–4183.

15 Kerbiriou D, Griffin J: Human high molecular weight kininogen. Studies of structure-function relationships and of proteolysis of the molecule occurring during contact activation of plasma. J Biol Chem 1979;245:12020–12027.

16 Bock P, Shore J, Tans G, Griffin J: Protein-protein interactions in contact activation of blood coagulation. Binding of high molecular weight kininogen and the 5-(iodoacetamido)fluorescein-labeled kininogen light chain to prekallikrein, kallikrein, and the separated kallikrein heavy and light chains. J Biol Chem 1985;260:12434–12443.

17 Thompson RE, Mandle R Jr, Kaplan AP: Studies of binding of prekallikrein and factor XI to high molecular weight kininogen and its light chain. Proc Natl Acad Sci USA 1979;76:4862–4866.

18 Tait JF, Fujikawa K: Primary structure requirements for the binding of human high molecular weight kininogen to plasma prekallikrein and factor XI. J Biol Chem 1987;262:11651–11656.

19 Thompson RE, Mandle R Jr, Kaplan AP: Characterization of human high molecular weight kininogen. Procoagulant activity associated with the light chain of kinin-free high molecular weight kininogen. J Exp Med 1978;147:488–499.

20 Tait JF, Fujikawa K: Identification of the binding site for plasma prekallikrein in human high molecular weight kininogen. A region from residues 185–224 of the kininogen light chain retains full binding activity. J Biol Chem 1986;261:15396–15401.

21 Nakayasu T, Nagasawa S: Studies on human kininogens. I. Isolation, characterization, and cleavage by plasma kallikrein of high molecular weight kininogen. J Biochem 1979;85:249–258.

22 Mori K, Nagasawa S: Studies on human high molecular weight (HMW) kininogen. II. Structural change of HMW kininogen by the action of human plasma kallikrein. J Biochem 1981;89:1465–1473.

23 Reddigari S, Kaplan AP: Cleavage of human high-molecular-weight kininogen by purified kallikreins and upon contact activation of plasma. Blood 1988;71:1334–1340.

24 Griffin JH: Role of surface in surface-dependent activation of Hageman factor (blood coagulation factor XII). Proc Natl Acad Sci USA 1978;75:1998–2002.

25 Silverberg M, Nicoll J, Kaplan A: The mechanism by which the light chain of cleaved HMW-kininogen augments the activation of prekallikrein, factor XI and Hageman factor. Thromb Res 1980;20:173–189.

26 Griffin JH, Cochrane CG: Mechanisms for the involvement of high molecular weight kininogen in surface-dependent reactions of Hageman factor. Proc Natl Acad Sci USA 1976;73:2554–2558.

27 Wiggins RC, Bouma BN, Cochrane CG, Griffin JH: Role of high-molecular-weight kininogen in surface-binding and activation of coagulation factor XI and prekallikrein. Proc Natl Acad Sci USA 1977;74:4636–4640.

28 Cochrane CG, Revak SD: Dissemination of contact activation in plasma by plasma kallikrein. J Exp Med 1980;152:608–619.

29 Schmaier AH, Silver L, Adams AL, Fischer GC, Munoz PC, Vroman L, et al: The effect of high molecular weight kininogen on surface-adsorbed fibrinogen. Thromb Res 1984;33:51–67.

30 Schmaier AH, Kuo A, Lundberg D, Murray S, Cines DB: The expression of high molecular weight kininogen on human umbilical vein endothelial cells. J Biol Chem 1988;263:16327–16333.

31 Van Iwaarden F, de Groot PG, Bouma BN: The binding of high molecular weight kininogen to cultured human endothelial cells. J Biol Chem 1988;263:4698–4703.

32 Nishikawa K, Shibayama Y, Kuna P, Calcaterra E, Kaplan AP, Reddigari SR: Generation of vasoactive peptide bradykinin from human umbilical vein endothelium-bound high molecular weight kininogen by plasma kallikrein. Blood 1992;80:1980–1988.

33 Reddigari SR, Kuna P, Miragliotta G, Shibayama Y, Nishikawa K, Kaplan AP: Human high molecular weight kininogen binds to human umbilical vein endothelial cells via its heavy and light chains. Blood 1993;81:1306–1311.

34 Reddigari SR, Shibayama Y, Brunnee T, Kaplan AP: Human Hageman factor (factor XII) and high molecular weight kininogen compete for the same binding site on human umbilical vein endothelial cells. J Biol Chem 1993;268:11982–11987.

35 Joseph K, Ghebrehiwet B, Peerschke EI, Reid KB, Kaplan AP: Identification of the zinc-dependent endothelial cell binding protein for high molecular weight kininogen and factor XII: identity with the receptor that binds to the globular 'heads' of C1q (gC1q-R). Proc Natl Acad Sci USA 1996;93:8552–8557.

36 Herwald H, Dedio J, Kellner R, Loos M, Muller-Esterl W: Isolation and characterization of the kininogen-binding protein p33 from endothelial cells. Identity with the gC1q receptor. J Biol Chem 1996;271:13040–13047.

37 Hasan AA, Zisman T, Schmaier AH: Identification of cytokeratin 1 as a binding protein and presentation receptor for kininogens on endothelial cells. Proc Natl Acad Sci USA 1998;95:3615–3620.

38 Joseph K, Ghebrehiwet B, Kaplan AP: Cytokeratin 1 and gC1qR mediate high molecular weight kininogen binding to endothelial cells. Clin Immunol 1999;92:246–255.

39 Colman RW, Pixley RA, Najamunnisa S, Yan W, Wang J, Mazar A, et al: Binding of high molecular weight kininogen to human endothelial cells is mediated via a site within domains 2 and 3 of the urokinase receptor. J Clin Invest 1997;100:1481–1487.

40 Joseph K, Tholanikunnel BG, Ghebrehiwet B, Kaplan AP: Interaction of high molecular weight kininogen binding proteins on endothelial cells. Thromb Haemost 2004;91:61–70.

41 Mahdi F, Shariat-Madar Z, Todd RF 3rd, Figueroa CD, Schmaier AH: Expression and colocalization of cytokeratin 1 and urokinase plasminogen activator receptor on endothelial cells. Blood 2001;97:2342–2350.

42 Motta G, Røjkjær R, Hasan AA, Cines DB, Schmaier AH: High molecular weight kininogen regulates prekallikrein assembly and activation on endothelial cells: a novel mechanism for contact activation. Blood 1998;91:516–528.

43 Røjkjær R, Hasan AA, Motta G, Schousboe I, Schmaier AH: Factor XII does not initiate prekallikrein activation on endothelial cells. Thromb Haemost 1998;80:74–81.

44 Schmaier AH: Contact activation: a revision. Thromb Haemost 1997;78:101–107.

45 Joseph K, Ghebrehiwet B, Kaplan AP: Activation of the kinin-forming cascade on the surface of endothelial cells. Biol Chem 2001;382:71–75.

46 Joseph K, Tholanikunnel B, Kaplan A: Heat-shock protein 90 catalyzes activation of the prekallikrein-kininogen complex in the absence of factor XII. Proc Natl Acad Sci USA 2002;99:896–900.

47 Shariat-Madar Z, Mahdi F, Schmaier A: Identification and characterization of prolylcarboxypeptidase as an endothelial cell prekallikrein activator. J Biol Chem 2002;277:17962–17969.

48 Schreiber A, Kaplan A, Austen K: Inhibition by C1INH of Hageman factor fragment activation of coagulation, fibrinolysis, and kinin generation. J Clin Invest 1973;52:1402–1409.

49 Pixley R, Schapira M, Colman R: The regulation of human factor XIIa by plasma proteinase inhibitors. J Biol Chem 1985;260:1723–1729.

50 Harpel P, Lewin M, Kaplan A: Distribution of plasma kallikrein between C-1 inactivator and α_2-macroglobulin in plasma utilizing a new assay for α_2-macroglobulin-kallikrein complexes. J Biol Chem 1985;260:4257–4263.

51 Donaldson V, Evans R: A biochemical abnormality in hereditary angioneurotic edema. Am J Med 1963; 35:37–44.

52 Kramer J, Katz Y, Rosen F, Davis AR, Strunk R: Synthesis of C1 inhibitor in fibroblasts from patients with type I and type II hereditary angioneurotic edema. J Clin Invest 1991;87:1614–1620.

53 Caldwell J, Ruddy S, Schur P, Austen K: Acquired C1 inhibitor deficiency in lymphosarcoma. Clin Immunol Immunopathol 1972;1:39–52.

54 Hauptmann G, Lang J, North M, Oberling F, Mayer G, Lachmann P: Acquired C1-inhibitor deficiencies in lymphoproliferative diseases with serum immunoglobulin abnormalities. A study of three cases. Blut 1976;32:195–206.

55 Schreiber A, Zweiman B, Atkins P, Goldwein F, Pietra G, Atkinson B, et al: Acquired angioedema with lymphoproliferative disorder: association of C1 inhibitor deficiency with cellular abnormality. Blood 1976;48:567–580.

56 Alsenz J, Bork K, Loos M: Autoantibody-mediated acquired deficiency of C1 inhibitor. N Engl J Med 1987;316:1360–1366.

57 Zuraw B, Curd J: Demonstration of modified inactive first component of complement (C1) inhibitor in the plasmas of C1 inhibitor-deficient patients. J Clin Invest 1986;78:567–575.

58 Malbran A, Hammer C, Frank M, Fries L: Acquired angioedema: observations on the mechanism of action of autoantibodies directed against C1 esterase inhibitor. J Allergy Clin Immunol 1988;81:1199–1204.

59 Pearson K, Buchignani J, Shimkin P, Frank M: Hereditary angioneurotic edema of the gastrointestinal tract. Am J Roetgenol Radium Ther Nucl Med 1972;116:256–261.

60 Tosi M: Molecular genetics of C1 inhibitor. Immunobiology 1998;119:358–365.

61 Quastel M, Harrison R, Cicardi M, Alper C, Rosen F: Behavior in vivo of normal and dysfunctional C1 inhibitor in normal subjects and patients with hereditary angioneurotic edema. J Clin Invest 1983; 71:1041–1046.

62 Kramer J, Rosen F, Colten H, Rajczy K, Strunk R: Transinhibition of C1 inhibitor synthesis in type I hereditary angioneurotic edema. J Clin Immunol 1993;91:1258–1262.

63 Ruddy S, Gigli I, Sheffer A, Austen K: The laboratory diagnosis of hereditary angioedema; in Rose N, Richter M, Sehon A (eds): Proceedings of the Sixth International Congress of Allergology. Amsterdam, Excerpta Medica, 1968, pp 351–359.

64 Zuraw B, Sugimoto S, Curd J: The value of rocket immunoelectrophoresis for C4 activation in the evaluation of patients with angioedema or C1-inhibitor deficiency. J Allergy Clin Immunol 1986;78:1115–1120.

65 Austen KF, Sheffer AL: Detection of hereditary angioneurotic edema by demonstration of a reduction in the second component of human complement. N Engl J Med 1965;272:649–656.

66 Ichinose A, Fujikawa K, Suyama T: The activation of pro-urokinase by plasma kallikrein and its inactivation by thrombin. J Biol Chem 1986;261:3486–3489.

67 Fields T, Ghebrehiwet B, Kaplan AP: Kinin formation in hereditary angioedema plasma: evidence against kinin derivation from C2 and in support of 'spontaneous' formation of bradykinin. J Allergy Clin Immunol 1983;72:54–60.

68 Curd J, Yelvington M, Burridge N: Generation of bradykinin during incubation of hereditary angioedema plasma. Mol Immunol 1983;19:1365.

69 Curd J, Prograis LJ, Cochrane C: Detection of active kallikrein in induced blister fluids of hereditary angioedema patients. N Engl J Med 1980;152:742–747.

70 Juhlin L, Michaelsson G: Vascular reactions in hereditary angioneurotic edema. Acta Derm Venereol 1969;40:20–25.

71 Schapira M, Silver L, Scott C, Schmaier A, Prograis LJ, Curd J, et al: Prekallikrein activation and high-molecular-weight kininogen consumption in hereditary angioedema. N Engl J Med 1983;308: 1050–1053.

72 Cugno M, Cicardi M, Coppola R, Agostoni A: Activation of factor XII and cleavage of high molecular weight kininogen during acute attacks in hereditary and acquired C1-inhibitor deficiencies. Immunopharmacology 1996;33:361–364.

73 Nussberger J, Cugno M, Cicardi M, Agostoni A: Local bradykinin generation in hereditary angioedema. J Allergy Clin Immunol 1999;104:1321–1322.

74 Donaldson VH: Mechanisms of activation of C'1 esterase in hereditary angioneurotic edema plasma in vitro. J Exp Med 1968;127:411–429.

75 Ratnoff OD, Naff GB: The conversion of C'1S to C'1 esterase by plasmin and trypsin. J Exp Med 1967; 125:337–358.

76 Ghebrehiwet B, Silverberg M, Kaplan AP: Activation of the classical pathway of complement by Hageman factor fragment. J Exp Med 1981;153:665–676.

77 Ghebrehiwet B, Randazzo B, Dunn J, Silverberg M, Kaplan A: Mechanisms of activation of the classical pathway of complement by Hageman factor fragment. J Clin Invest 1983;71:1450–1456.

78 Zahedi R, Bissler J, Davis AR, Andreadis C, Wisnieski J: Unique C1 inhibitor dysfunction in a kindred without angioedema. II. Identification of an Ala443→Val substitution and functional analysis of the recombinant mutant protein. J Clin Invest 1995;95:1299–1305.

79 Zahedi R, Wisnieski J, Davis AE 3rd: Role of the P2 residue of complement-1 inhibitor (Ala443) in determination of target protease specificity: inhibition of complement and contact system proteases. J Immunol 1997;159:983–988.

80 Nussberger J, Cugno M, Amstutz C, Cicardi M, Pellacani A, Agostoni A: Plasma bradykinin in angioedema. Lancet 1998;351:1693–1697.

81 Han E, MacFarlane R, Mulligan A, Scafidi J, Davis AR: Increased vascular permeability in C1 inhibitor-deficient mice mediated by the bradykinin type 2 receptor. J Clin Invest 2002;8:1057–1063.

82 Kaplan AP, Austen KF: A prealbumin activator of prekallikrein. II. Derivation of activators of prekallikrein from active Hageman factor by digestion with plasmin. J Exp Med 1971;133:696–712.

83 Wallace EM, Perkins SJ, Sim RB, Willis AC, Feighery C, Jackson J: Degradation of C1 inhibitor by plasmin: implications for the control of inflammatory processes. Mol Med 1997;3:385–396.

84 Geha R, Quinti I, Austen K, Cicardi M, Sheffer A, Rosen F: Acquired C1-inhibitor deficiency associated with anti-idiotypic antibody to monoclonal immunoglobulins. N Engl J Med 1985;312:534–540.

85 Donaldson V, Hess E, McAdams A: Lupus-erythematosus-like disease in three unrelated women with hereditary angioneurotic edema. Ann Intern Med 1977;86:312–313.

86 Cohen S, Koethe S, Kozin F, Rodey G, Arkins J, Fink J: Acquired angioedema associated with rectal carcinoma and its response to danazol therapy. Acquired angioedema treated with danazol. J Allergy Clin Immunol 1978;62:217–221.

87 Jackson J, Sim R, Whelan A, Feighery C: An IgG autoantibody which inactivates C1-inhibitor. Nature 1986;323:722–724.

88 Jackson J, Sim R, Whaley K, Feighery C: Autoantibody facilitated cleavage of C1-inhibitor in autoimmune angioedema. J Clin Invest 1989;83:698–707.

89 He S, Sim R, Whaley K: Mechanism of action of anti-C1-inhibitor autoantibodies: prevention of the formation of stable C1s-C1-inh complexes. Mol Med 1998;4:119–128.

90 Bas M, Bier H, Greve J, Kojda G, Hoffmann T: Novel pharmacotherapy of acute hereditary angioedema with bradykinin B2-receptor antagonist icatibant. Allergy 2006;61:1490–1492.

91 Bork K, Frank J, Grundt B, Schlattmann P, Nussberger J, Kreuz W: Treatment of acute edema attacks in hereditary angioedema with a bradykinin receptor-2 antagonist (icatibant). J Allergy Clin Immunol 2007;119:1497–1503.

92 Schneider L, Lumry W, Vegh A, Williams A, Schmalbach T: Critical role of kallikrein in hereditary angioedema pathogenesis: a clinical trial of ecallantide, a novel kallikrein inhibitor. J Allergy Clin Immunol 2007;120:416–422.

93 Binkley K, Davis AR: Clinical, biochemical, and genetic characterization of a novel estrogen-dependent inherited form of angioedema. J Allergy Clin Immunol 2000;106:546–550.

94 Dewald G, Bork K: Missense mutations in the coagulation factor XII (Hageman factor) gene in hereditary angioedema with normal C1 inhibitor. Biochem Biophys Res Commun 2006;343:1286–1289.

95 Martin L, Raison-Peyron N, Nothen M, Cichon S, Drouet C: Hereditary angioedema with normal C1 inhibitor gene in a family with affected women and men is associated with the p.Thr328Lys mutation in the F12 gene. J Allergy Clin Immunol 2007;120:975–977.

96 Kaplan A, Greaves M: Angioedema. J Am Acad Dermatol 2005;53:373–388.

97 Byrd J, Shreevatsa A, Putlur P, Foretia D, McAlexander L, Sinha T, et al: Dipeptidyl peptidase IV deficiency increases susceptibility to angiotensin-converting enzyme inhibitor-induced peritracheal edema. J Allergy Clin Immunol 2007;120:403–408.

98 Sheikh IA, Kaplan AP: Mechanism of digestion of bradykinin and lysylbradykinin (kallidin) in human serum. Role of carboxypeptidase, angiotensin-converting enzyme and determination of final degradation products. Biochem Pharmacol 1989;38:993–1000.

99 Schulman G, Hakim R, Arias R, Silverberg M, Kaplan AP, Arbeit L: Bradykinin generation by dialysis membranes: possible role in anaphylactic reaction. J Am Soc Nephrol 1993;3:1563–1569.

100 Alving BM, Hojima Y, Pisano JJ, Mason BL, Buckingham RE Jr, Mozen MM, et al: Hypotension associated with prekallikrein activator (Hageman-factor fragments) in plasma protein fraction. N Engl J Med 1978;299:66–70.

101 Kishimoto T, Viswanathan K, Ganguly T, Elankumaran S, Smith S, Pelzer K, et al: Contaminated heparin associated with adverse clinical events and activation of the contact system. N Engl J Med 2008;358:2457–2467.

102 Smith P, Kagey-Sobotka A, Bleecker E, Traystman R, Kaplan A, Gralnick H, et al: Physiologic manifestations of human anaphylaxis. J Clin Invest 1980;66:1072–1080.

Prof. Allen P. Kaplan
Department of Medicine, Medical University of South Carolina
96 Jonathan Lucas Street, Charleston, SC 29425 (USA)
Tel. +1 843 792 0264, Fax +1 843 792 0448
E-Mail kaplana@musc.edu

Ring J (ed): Anaphylaxis. Chem Immunol Allergy. Basel, Karger, 2010, vol 95, pp 85–97

Role for Basophils in Systemic Anaphylaxis

Hajime Karasuyama[a,b] · Yusuke Tsujimura[a,c] · Kazushige Obata[a] · Kaori Mukai[a]

[a]Department of Immune Regulation, [b]JST, CREST, Tokyo Medical and Dental University Graduate School of Medical and Dental Sciences, Tokyo, and [c]Tsukuba Primate Research Center, National Institute of Biomedical Innovation, Tsukuba-shi, Japan

Abstract

For more than 100 years since the discovery of basophils by Paul Ehrlich, the functional significance of this rare leukocyte as compared to mast cells has remained an enigma. Studies on basophils have long been hampered by their rarity (less than 1% of peripheral blood leukocytes) and the lack of useful analytical tools such as model animals deficient only in basophils. Recent studies have now defined previously-unrecognized roles for basophils in both allergic responses and immune regulation, and markedly changed our image of basophils, from a neglected minority to a key player in the immune system. We have recently demonstrated that basophils and mast cells play distinct roles in systemic anaphylaxis in mice. Basophils are dispensable for IgE-mediated systemic anaphylaxis unlike mast cells. Instead, basophils play the major role in IgG-mediated systemic anaphylaxis. In vivo depletion of basophils protects mice from anaphylactic death. Upon capture of IgG-allergen complexes, basophils release platelet-activating factor that increases vascular permeability, leading to anaphylactic shock. Thus, there are two major, distinct pathways to allergen-induced systemic anaphylaxis: one mediated by basophils, IgG and platelet-activating factor, and the other 'classical' pathway mediated by mast cells, IgE and histamine.

Biology of Basophils

Basophils represent less than 1% of peripheral blood leukocytes. They have often been regarded as a lesser relative to mast cells, because basophils share several features with mast cells, including the presence of basophilic granules in the cytoplasm, the surface expression of high-affinity IgE receptor FcεRI, and the release of chemical mediators such as histamine in response to various stimuli [1–3]. Therefore, basophils are traditionally analyzed as a surrogate of the less accessible tissue-resident mast cells in clinical settings to assess the allergen sensitization in allergic patients. However, the lineage relationship between basophils and mast cells remains to be clarified. In humans, basophils appear to have a closer lineage relationship with eosinophils than with mast cells [4]. By contrast, common precursors for basophils and mast cells have been identified in mice [5].

In spite of the above-mentioned similarities between basophils and mast cells, they differ in many other aspects [1, 2]. Basophils complete their differentiation within the bone marrow, and mature basophils circulate in the peripheral blood and do not usually infiltrate into peripheral tissues unless inflammation takes place. Mast cells originate from hematopoietic cells in the bone marrow as do basophils, but they mature in peripheral tissues after their bone marrow-derived precursors enter the circulation and migrate into peripheral tissues. Mature mast cells reside in peripheral tissues and do not usually circulate in the peripheral blood. The lifespan of basophils is very short (several days), in contrast to that of mast cells (weeks to months). Basophils do not proliferate once they terminally differentiate whereas mature mast cells keep potential to expand in response to various stimuli. These differences between basophils and mast cells, including distinct anatomical localization, suggest their differential roles in vivo.

In 1970s and 1980s, basophils were extensively studied in the context of a delayed-onset, cutaneous hypersensitivity, termed 'Jones-Mote hypersensitivity' in humans [6] or 'cutaneous basophil hypersensitivity (CBH)' in guinea pigs [7, 8], as well as the acquired immunity against blood-feeding ticks [9, 10]. CBH can be elicited in guinea pigs by immunization of proteins with incomplete Freund's adjuvant or without adjuvant, followed by the skin test with the proteins 7 days later [7]. CBH is characterized by erythema with slight thickening that reaches its maximal intensity 24 h after the antigen challenge, and disappear within 48 h. Importantly, basophils constitute as much as 80% of the dermal infiltrates in guinea pig CBH [8]. Similar basophil-rich skin reactions were detected in the tick-feeding sites of guinea pigs that had already experienced the tick infestation and showed the acquired resistance to the tick feeding [9]. Treatment of guinea pigs with anti-basophil serum before the second tick infestation eliminated basophils at tick-feeding sites and abolished the tick resistance [10], demonstrating that basophils play a critical role in the acquisition of tick resistance. Unfortunately, the studies of basophils in the CBH reaction and the tick resistance faded since then, and have not expanded further.

Compared with extensive investigation on mast cells and advances in our understanding of mast cell functions, the in vivo roles of basophils are far less studied and defined. This could be due to the difficulty of collecting sufficient numbers of basophils for analysis and the lack of animal models suitable for in vivo analysis of basophil functions. Mouse basophils have been notoriously difficult to identify due to their few basophilic granules in contrast to their human counterparts [11], leading to the erroneous conclusion that basophils may not exist in mice. Recent identification of cell surface markers expressed in mouse basophils, such as CD49b (DX5), CD123 (IL-3Rα), CD200R3 and CCR2, together with FcεRI, has made it possible to relatively easily detect and isolate basophils in mice by using flow cytometry [12–14]. However, mice suitable for functional analysis of basophils, such as those deficient for only basophils, have not yet established.

For many years, basophils were thought to release only preformed histamine and newly-synthesized leukotriene C4 in response to a variety of stimuli [3, 15]. However, this view was largely changed after the discovery in the early 1990s that basophils readily generate large quantities of T-helper 2 (Th2) cytokines such as IL-4 and IL-13 in both human and mice [12, 15–17]. These cytokines are the key regulators in conditioning the immune response to the Th2 type [18]. Therefore, basophils were suggested to be involved in mediating allergic diseases and protective immunity against parasites. Nevertheless, further studies on basophil functions have long been hampered by the lack of suitable animal models, as mentioned above.

Newly Identified Roles for Basophils

Recent studies using new analytical tools have defined previously unrecognized roles for basophils in both immune regulation and allergic responses including IgG-mediated systemic anaphylaxis [19–23]. These studies have highlighted that basophils and mast cells have distinct roles in immune and allergic responses [24, 25]. Before we discuss in detail the role for basophils in anaphylaxis, we quickly look through their newly identified roles in immune regulation and chronic allergic inflammation.

Basophils Drive Th2-Cell Differentiation through Secretion of Th2 Cytokines and Antigen Presentation

Effector T cells of the Th2 phenotype produce cytokines such as IL-4, IL-5 and IL-13, and play a pivotal role in many allergic responses. It is well established that IL-4 has an essential role in driving differentiation of naive T cells to Th2 cells. IL-4 can be produced by a panel of hematopoietic cells, including T cells, natural killer T cells, mast cells, basophils and eosinophils. Thus, the cellular source of 'initial IL-4' necessary for Th2-cell differentiation has often been a matter of debate [24]. Basophils are a good candidate for this, since they have been shown to readily secrete large quantities of IL-4 in vitro in response to a variety of stimuli in an IgE-dependent or -independent manner [12, 15–17]. When co-cultured in vitro with basophils, antigen-stimulated naive T cells differentiated into effector cells of the Th2 phenotype [26, 27]. When IL-4-deficient basophils were used for the co-culture, little Th2-cell differentiation was induced, indicating the importance of IL-4 produced by basophils in driving Th2 differentiation. The in vivo relevance of this finding was suggested by the observation that mice deficient for interferon-regulatory factor (IRF2) had an increased number of basophils and showed accelerated Th2 differentiation in vivo as compared with wild-type mice [26]. This was also the case in mice that continuously received exogenous IL-3 [27]. However, it remained to be determined whether basophils and naive T cells indeed meet each other under physiological conditions in lymph nodes, in which Th2 differentiation is thought to take place.

Medzhitov and colleagues [21] recently demonstrated that when protease allergens such as papain are subcutaneously administered, basophils actually migrated to the draining lymph nodes, just before Th2 cells differentiated in the lymph nodes. Of note, the pretreatment of mice with MAR-1, a monoclonal antibody specific to FcεRIα, that depletes basophils when administered in vivo, abolished the papain-induced Th2 differentiation in the draining lymph nodes. Both IL-4 and thymic stromal lymphopoietin (TSLP) produced by papain-stimulated basophils were involved in the Th2 differentiation in vivo. Mast cells were dispensable for the differentiation. Thus, basophils have an essential and non-redundant role in the development of Th2 responses to protease allergens [21]. In addition, recent studies have uncovered that basophils can function as antigen-presenting cells, and therefore promote the Th2 responses even in the absence of dendritic cells [28–30].

Basophils Enhance Humoral Memory Response

Mack et al. [13] previously reported that basophils can function as antigen-capturing cells and trap soluble antigens through antigen-specific IgE that is bound to FcεRI on their surface. They have recently demonstrated that basophils had the antigen-capturing ability even 6 weeks after the first immunization with antigens and increased humoral memory responses by producing IL-4 and IL-6 upon re-exposure to the antigen that had elicited the production of specific IgE in the primary immune response [22]. Importantly, the in vivo depletion of basophils using MAR-1 before the second immunization with antigens resulted in decreased humoral memory responses, including lower serum titers of antigen-specific IgG, compared to untreated mice. Conversely, adoptive transfer of antigen-reactive basophils from antigen-sensitized mice conferred on naive mice a memory-type immune response following the first immunization with antigens. Antigen-stimulated basophils provide support for B-cell proliferation and antibody production, through the secretion of IL-4 and IL-6, in the presence of CD4 T cells that are also stimulated with basophils.

The clinical relevance of this finding was suggested by the observation that mice were more susceptible to sepsis following infection with *Streptococcus pneumoniae* when basophils were depleted before the second vaccination with pneumoccocal antigen [22]. Antigen-specific IgG antibodies produced after the second vaccination were significantly lower in the basophil-depleted mice than in control mice. Thus, basophils are important contributors to humoral memory immune responses.

Basophils Initiate IgE-Mediated Chronic Allergic Inflammation

The recruitment of basophils into the sites of allergic inflammation is often observed. However, no definitive evidence has long been provided that basophils are crucially involved in the pathogenesis of chronic allergic disorders. We have recently identified in a mouse model that basophils play an important role in the development of IgE-mediated chronic allergic inflammation in the skin as an initiator rather than an effector of inflammation [19, 20]. A single subcutaneous administration of antigens in the ear skin induced three waves of ear swelling in antigen-specific IgE transgenic mice or in normal mice that had been passively sensitized with antigen-specific

IgE [19]. The first two waves were typical immediate-type skin reactions, that is, the early-phase ear swelling within 1 h after the antigen challenge followed by the late-phase ear swelling 6–10 h later. The third one was delayed-onset ear swelling, starting on day 2 post-challenge and peaked on day 4. This was much more intense than the first and second ones, and the ear thickness became twice the basal level. Histopathological analysis revealed the massive infiltration of inflammatory cells including eosinophils in the skin lesions, indicating IgE-mediated chronic allergic inflammation. Of note, the immediate- and late-phase responses were mast cell-dependent as expected while the delayed-onset ear swelling was elicited even in the absence of mast cells and T cells. Adoptive transfer of cells from wild-type mice into FcεRI-deficient mice, that could not mount the delayed-onset response, identified basophils as cells responsible for IgE-mediated chronic allergic inflammation [19].

Of note, basophils accounted for only ~2% of infiltrates in the skin lesions while eosinophils and neutrophils were predominant. We have recently established a CD200R3-specific monoclonal antibody Ba103 that selectively depletes basophils when administered in mice [14, 20]. The basophil depletion with Ba103 prior to the antigen challenge completely abolished the development of IgE-mediated chronic allergic inflammation. Importantly, the Ba103 treatment during the progress of the dermatitis showed a therapeutic effect on the inflammation and resulted in decreased numbers of eosinophils and neutrophils in the skin lesions, concomitantly with the elimination of basophils from the site of inflammation. This indicated that basophils function as an initiator or mediator of the recruitment of proinflammatory cells such as eosinophils and neutrophils, rather than an effector of inflammation [20]. Therefore, it would be worthwhile to reassess the role of basophils in human allergic disorders even when the frequency of basophils is low in affected tissues.

A Crucial Role for Basophils in Anaphylaxis

Basophils have been considered to make some contribution to systemic anaphylaxis, because they can release histamine and leukotriene C4 in vitro in response to various stimuli, including IgE-mediated ones. Indeed, basophils are clinically utilized to check the sensitization status of allergic patients by incubating them in vitro with suspected allergens. Activation of sensitized basophils with allergens can be detected by the degranulation assay or the flow cytometric analysis using CD203c and CD63 as activation markers. However, it remains to be determined to what extent basophils contribute to systemic anaphylaxis, particularly IgE-mediated ones, as compared with mast cells. Given the fact that basophils represent less than 1% of peripheral blood leukocytes and do not usually reside in peripheral tissues, it is uncertain that basophils make a great contribution to IgE-mediated systemic anaphylaxis as do mast cells. In this regard, we have recently demonstrated that basophils are dispensable for IgE-mediated anaphylaxis but play a crucial role in IgG-mediated anaphylaxis in the mouse model [23].

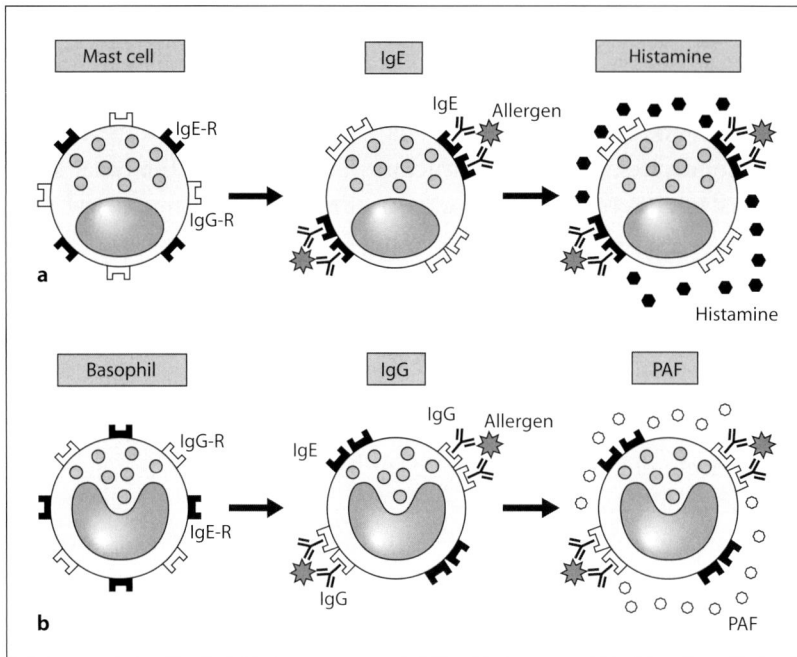

Fig. 1. Two distinct pathways of systemic anaphylaxis: (**a**) in the classical pathway, mast cells, IgE and histamine play important roles, and by contrast (**b**) in the alternative pathway, basophils, IgG and PAF play the major roles.

Systemic Anaphylaxis in the Absence of Mast Cells and IgE

It is well documented that mast cells and IgE are critically involved in systemic ana-phylaxis (fig. 1a) [31–33]. In individuals sensitized with a given allergen, allergen-specific IgE antibodies are produced by B cells, circulate in the peripheral blood and bind to the IgE receptor FcεRI on the surface of mast cells in peripheral tissues. The re-exposure to the same allergen triggers the activation of mast cells by allergen-induced cross-linking of IgE-FcεRI complexes on their surface. The mast cell activa-tion results in the release of chemical mediators such as histamine (fig. 1a), that in turn act on various cells including vascular endothelial cells and bronchial smooth muscle, leading to anaphylactic responses such as hypotension and dyspnea. It has been believed that basophils may also be involved in systemic anaphylaxis through the similar mechanism.

Few prospective studies of induced anaphylaxis have been performed in human subjects to understand the molecular basis of systemic anaphylaxis, because of the potentially rapid, life-threatening outcome. Accordingly, various models of anaphy-laxis have been established in laboratory animals, particularly mice, and extensively studied to clarify the underlying mechanisms. Such studies revealed that the classical pathway utilizing mast cells, IgE and histamine cannot explain all cases of anaphylaxis.

Karasuyama · Tsujimura · Obata · Mukai

Mice deficient for either mast cells or IgE still develop systemic anaphylaxis [34, 35], indicating that an alternative pathway(s) exists [31, 36]. Of note, mice deficient for FcεRI could elicit systemic anaphylaxis whereas those deficient for FcRγ could not [37–39]. Since FcRγ-deficient mice lack not only FcεRI but also stimulatory IgG receptors, these results suggested that IgG instead of IgE is involved in the alternative pathway of systemic anaphylaxis. In accord with this, passive sensitization with allergen-specific IgG, particularly IgG1 subclass, conferred on mice the ability to develop systemic anaphylaxis [37, 38]. The experiments using blocking antibodies indicated that the low-affinity IgG receptor FcγRIII is mainly involved in IgG-mediated systemic anaphylaxis [39]. Thus, beside the classical pathway mediated by mast cells, IgE and FcεRI, the alternative pathway mediated by non-mast cells, IgG and FcγRIII exists to induce systemic anaphylaxis [36]. However, the identity of non-mast cells involved in the alternative pathway remained elusive, although macrophages were demonstrated as responsible cells in a mouse model of IgG-mediated anaphylaxis [39].

A Crucial Role for Basophils in IgG-Mediated Systemic Anaphylaxis

Our finding that basophils play an essential role in IgE-mediated chronic allergic inflammation distinctively from mast cells prompted us to examine whether basophils also play a non-redundant role in systemic anaphylaxis. To identify cells responsible for IgG-mediated systemic anaphylaxis and to clarify its molecular mechanism, we have established a simple model of IgG-mediated penicillin anaphylaxis [23], in that mice were passively sensitized with intravenous injection of penicillin V (PenV)-specific IgG1 monoclonal antibody and then challenged with intravenous injection of PenV-conjugated bovine serum albumin (PenV-BSA). This protocol induced typical anaphylactic manifestations including a drastic drop (–4 to –6°C) in body temperature in both mast cell-sufficient and -deficient mice although the latter mice showed slightly less depression in temperature. This was also true for mice sensitized with another IgG1 with different specificity. Thus, mast cells are dispensable for IgG-mediated systemic anaphylaxis even though they have some minor contribution to it, consistent with previous reports [37, 38]. By contrast, mast cells are essential for the induction of IgE-mediated systemic anaphylaxis.

We next surveyed possible candidate cells responsible for IgG-mediated anaphylaxis by analyzing their ability to capture the allergen-IgG1 immune complexes on their cell surface in vivo. The low-affinity IgG receptor FcγRIII does not efficiently bind free monomeric IgG while it shows high affinity to IgG-antigen immune complexes or IgG aggregates. Therefore, we reasoned that in order to elicit an acute reaction, cells responsible for anaphylaxis should quickly capture immune complexes which are formed in the circulation soon after allergens enter the bloodstream and bind circulating, allergen-specific IgG. Flow cytometric analysis of cells isolated from mice immediately after the allergen challenge revealed that basophils bound the greatest amount of allergen per cell among other cells [23] (fig. 1b, 2a), suggesting basophils are a good candidate for responsible cells.

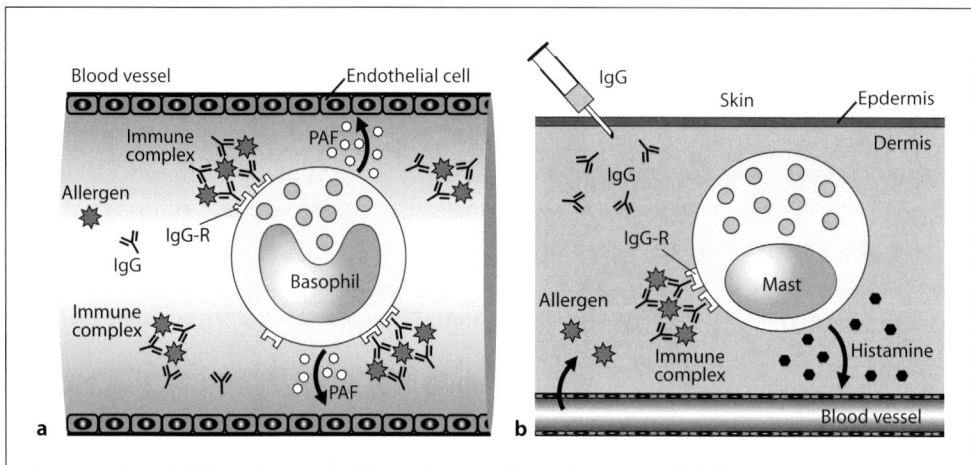

Fig. 2. IgG-mediated systemic versus local anaphylaxis. **a** IgG-mediated systemic anaphylaxis. When allergen-IgG immune complexes are formed in the circulation, basophils immediately capture them through IgG receptors on their surface and are activated to release PAF, that in turn act on vascular endothelial cells, leading to increased vascular permeability. **b** Passive cutaneous anaphylaxis. When allergen-IgG immune complexes are formed in the skin, they stimulate tissue-resident mast cells to release chemical mediators such as histamine, leading to local inflammation.

To clarify the role for basophils in IgG- and IgE-mediated systemic anaphylaxis, we eliminated basophils in vivo before the allergen challenge by treating mice with the basophil-depleting antibody Ba103. The basophil depletion ameliorated IgG-mediated systemic anaphylaxis in both mast cell-sufficient and -deficient mice [23]. By contrast, depletion of macrophages, natural killer cells or neutrophils showed no significant effect on IgG-mediated anaphylaxis in our experimental setting. Notably, the basophil depletion had no apparent impact on IgE-mediated systemic anaphylaxis. These results clearly indicated that basophils are dispensable for IgE-mediated anaphylaxis but play the major role in IgG-mediated one (fig. 1b, 2a). We further examined the role for basophils in a more realistic setting, namely active systemic anaphylaxis, in that mice were immunized with PenV-conjugated ovalbumin and 2 weeks later challenged with intravenous injection of PenV-BSA. This protocol for active anaphylaxis induced severer anaphylaxis compared with passive anaphylaxis, and all mice examined, including mast cell-deficient mice, died from anaphylactic shock. Of note, the basophil depletion with Ba103 before the allergen challenge protected mast cell-deficient mice from anaphylactic death [23], highlighting the important role for basophils in the induction of not only passive but also active systemic anaphylaxis. Intriguingly, the basophil depletion did not protect mast cell-sufficient mice from death. This suggests that both basophils and mast cells make the critical contribution to active systemic anaphylaxis, most likely through distinct mechanisms: IgG-mediated ones utilized by basophils and IgE-mediated ones by mast cells.

IgG1-mediated local anaphylaxis can be induced in mice, by intradermal injection of IgG1 and then intravenous injection of corresponding allergens [40] (fig. 2b). This passive cutaneous anaphylaxis (PCA) is also FcγRIII-dependent [41] but cannot be elicited in mast cell-deficient mice [42], indicating that mast cells are mainly activated in the IgG-mediated PCA unlike in the IgG-mediated systemic anaphylaxis. Indeed, peritoneal mast cells degranulate when incubated ex vivo with allergen-IgG complexes [41]. By contrast, little or no morphological evidence of degranulation of mast cells was detected in the peripheral tissues during IgG1-mediated passive systemic anaphylaxis unlike in IgE-mediated ones [38]. The different modes of action between local and systemic anaphylaxis could be attributed to the difference in the route of antibody delivery and the anatomical localization of mast cells and basophils. In PCA, antibodies are directly delivered into the skin tissue, and therefore immune complexes are formed locally in the skin lesions, leading to activation of tissue-resident mast cells but not circulating basophils (fig. 2b). By contrast, in systemic anaphylaxis, antibodies are delivered into the bloodstream, and thereby form immune complexes in the circulation with intravenously administered allergens, leading to activation of circulating basophils rather than tissue-resident mast cells (fig. 2a).

Basophils Release Platelet-Activating Factor Instead of Histamine to Induce IgG-Mediated Systemic Anaphylaxis

What kind of chemical mediators are involved in IgG-mediated systemic anaphylaxis that is elicited by basophils? Cyproheptadine, an antagonist of histamine and 5-HT, showed little or no inhibitory effect on IgG-mediated passive anaphylaxis in contrast to its prominent effect on IgE-mediated ones. On the other hand, antagonists of platelet-activating factor (PAF) almost completely inhibited IgG-mediated systemic anaphylaxis [23]. Thus, PAF in place of histamine is the major chemical mediator in IgG-mediated systemic anaphylaxis unlike in IgE-mediated ones. PAF is released by a wide variety of cells, including mast cells, eosinophils, basophils, neutrophils, endothelial cells, monocytes and macrophages. When stimulated ex vivo with allergen-IgG1 immune complexes, basophils released much higher amounts of PAF as compared to other types of cells. PAF released from activated basophils acted on human umbilical vein endothelial cells to induce morphological changes [23]. These results strongly suggested that upon stimulation with allergen-IgG immune complexes, basophils release PAF, that in turn stimulates endothelial cells to increase vascular permeability, thereby leading to systemic anaphylaxis (fig. 1b, 2a). When intravenously administered in mice, both PAF and histamine can induce a drastic drop (–5°C) in body temperature as observed in allergen-elicited, IgG-mediated systemic anaphylaxis. Of note, the amounts necessary for inducing such temperature drop greatly differ between two reagents: 100 ng of PAF was sufficient whereas as much as 3 mg of histamine was needed. We estimated that 100 ng of PAF can be released from 3×10^5 basophils, which is close to the total number of basophils per mouse. Taken together, basophils can induce systemic anaphylaxis through the release of the potent vasoamine PAF (30,000 times more potent than histamine) upon stimulation with immune complexes, even though they represent less than 1% of leukocytes in the body [23].

Previous studies reported that macrophages played the major role in a model of IgG-mediated active systemic anaphylaxis [39]. In this model, mice were first immunized with goat anti-mouse IgD antiserum that induced large production of IgE and IgG antibodies specific to goat IgG, and then challenged with intravenous injection of goat IgG to elicit systemic anaphylaxis. The anaphylaxis could be induced even in mast cell-deficient or FcεRI-deficient mice, and the PAF antagonist completely inhibited it. The pretreatment of mice with gadolinium chloride, that is known to inactivate macrophages, also abolished the anaphylaxis [39], suggesting that macrophages induce IgG-mediated systemic anaphylaxis through release of PAF. It remains to be clarified what determines cells responsible for IgG-mediated anaphylaxis, either basophils or macrophages. In addition to the difference in the allergens and immunization protocols, the genetic background of mice might be one of the determinants; our model utilizes C57BL/6 mice because many genetically engineered mice have this background while the other model utilizes BALB/c mice. If the difference between our and the other models is indeed based on the genetic background of mice examined, it would be important to clarify the underlying molecular mechanisms to understand the possible difference in the susceptibility to and the severity of anaphylaxis among individual human subjects with different genetic backgrounds.

Possible Roles for Human Basophils in Anaphylaxis

An important question is whether the alternative pathway mediated by basophils, IgG and PAF is also operative in humans. We know from the mouse studies that higher amounts of both allergens and antibodies are needed to elicit IgG-mediated systemic anaphylaxis than IgE-mediated ones. The exposure to large quantities of allergens followed by production of substantial amounts of specific IgG is very rare in the community setting, but may occur in clinical settings such as administration of therapeutic antibodies including recombinant monoclonal antibodies. Notably, several case reports indicated human anaphylaxis that occurred in the apparent absence of detectable allergen-specific IgE in serum or in the absence of increase in serum tryptase levels [43, 44]. IgG but not IgE antibodies specific to allergens were detected in some individuals who showed systemic anaphylaxis in response to medicines such as protamine, dextran, and recombinant human-mouse chimeric IgG monoclonal antibodies [43, 45–47]. It has been shown that human basophils can release PAF in response to various stimuli [48]. A recent study demonstrated that serum PAF levels are significantly higher in patients with anaphylaxis than in patients in the control groups and are correlated with the severity of anaphylaxis [49]. Therefore, it would be worthwhile to reassess the possible involvement of basophils and PAF in human cases of anaphylaxis, particularly those with high serum titers of IgG but not IgE specific to a relevant allergen.

Karasuyama · Tsujimura · Obata · Mukai

Perspective

Basophils have often been considered to be minor and possibly redundant 'circulating mast cells'. As discussed above, recent studies have uncovered novel roles for basophils in both allergic responses and regulation of acquired immunity that are distinct from those played by mast cells. Basophils are one of the major players in IgG-mediated anaphylaxis, and function as initiators rather than effectors in IgE-mediated chronic allergic inflammation, even though they account for less than 1% of leukocytes in the body. Therefore, basophils and their products might be promising therapeutic targets for immunological disorders. The pretreatment of patients bearing a high risk of anaphylaxis with PAF antagonists together with antihistamine before medications might be beneficial for the prevention of anaphylaxis.

References

1 Galli SJ: Mast cells and basophils. Curr Opin Hematol 2000;7:32–39.
2 Prussin C, Metcalfe DD: 4. IgE, mast cells, basophils, and eosinophils. J Allergy Clin Immunol 2003;111:S486–S494.
3 Falcone FH, Haas H, Gibbs BF: The human basophil: a new appreciation of its role in immune responses. Blood 2000;96:4028–4038.
4 Arock M, Schneider E, Boissan M, Tricottet V, Dy M: Differentiation of human basophils: an overview of recent advances and pending questions. J Leukoc Biol 2002;71:557–564.
5 Arinobu Y, Iwasaki H, Gurish MF, Mizuno S, Shigematsu H, Ozawa H, Tenen TG, Austen KF, Akashi K: Developmental checkpoints of the basophil/mast cell lineages in adult murine hematopoiesis. Proc Natl Acad Sci USA 2005;102:18105–18110.
6 Jones TD, Mote JR: The phases of foreign protein sensitization in human beings. N Engl J Med 1934; 210:120–123.
7 Richerson HB, Dvorak HF, Leskowitz S: Cutaneous basophil hypersensitivity. I. A new look at the Jones-Mote reaction, general characteristics. J Exp Med 1970;132:546–557.
8 Dvorak HF, Dvorak AM, Simpson BA, Richerson HB, Leskowitz S, Karnovsky MJ: Cutaneous basophil hypersensitivity. II. A light and electron microscopic description. J Exp Med 1970;132:558–582.
9 Allen JR: Tick resistance: basophils in skin reactions of resistant guinea pigs. Int J Parasitol 1973;3:195–200.
10 Brown SJ, Galli SJ, Gleich GJ, Askenase PW: Ablation of immunity to Amblyomma americanum by anti-basophil serum: cooperation between basophils and eosinophils in expression of immunity to ectoparasites (ticks) in guinea pigs. J Immunol 1982;129:790–796.
11 Dvorak AM: The mouse basophil, a rare and rarely recognized granulocyte. Blood 2000;96:1616–1617.
12 Voehringer D, Shinkai K, Locksley RM: Type 2 immunity reflects orchestrated recruitment of cells committed to IL-4 production. Immunity 2004;20:267–277.
13 Mack M, Schneider MA, Moll C, Cihak J, Bruhl H, Ellwart JW, Hogarth MP, Stangassinger M, Schlondorff D: Identification of antigen-capturing cells as basophils. J Immunol 2005;174:735–741.
14 Kojima T, Obata K, Mukai K, Sato S, Takai T, Minegishi Y, Karasuyama H: Mast cells and basophils are selectively activated in vitro and in vivo through CD200R3 in an IgE-independent manner. J Immunol 2007;179:7093–7100.
15 Schroeder JT, MacGlashan DW Jr, Lichtenstein LM: Human basophils: mediator release and cytokine production. Adv Immunol 2001;77:93–122.
16 Seder RA, Paul WE, Dvorak AM, Sharkis SJ, Kagey-Sobotka A, Niv Y, Finkelman FD, Barbieri SA, Galli SJ, Plaut M: Mouse splenic and bone marrow cell populations that express high-affinity Fc ε receptors and produce interleukin-4 are highly enriched in basophils. Proc Natl Acad Sci USA 1991;88:2835–2839.
17 Min B, Prout M, Hu-Li J, Zhu J, Jankovic D, Morgan ES, Urban JF Jr, Dvorak AM, Finkelman FD, LeGros G, Paul WE: Basophils produce IL-4 and accumulate in tissues after infection with a Th2-inducing parasite. J Exp Med 2004;200:507–517.

18 Min B, Paul WE: Basophils and type 2 immunity. Curr Opin Hematol 2008;15:59–63.

19 Mukai K, Matsuoka K, Taya C, Suzuki H, Yokozeki H, Nishioka K, Hirokawa K, Etori M, Yamashita M, Kubota T, Minegishi Y, Yonekawa Y, Karasuyama H: Basophils play a critical role in the development of IgE-mediated chronic allergic inflammation independently of T cells and mast cells. Immunity 2005; 23:191–202.

20 Obata K, Mukai K, Tsujimura Y, Ishiwata K, Kawano Y, Minegishi Y, Watanabe N, Karasuyama H: Basophils are essential initiators of a novel type of chronic allergic inflammation. Blood 2007;110:913–920.

21 Sokol CL, Barton GM, Farr AG, Medzhitov R: A mechanism for the initiation of allergen-induced T-helper type 2 responses. Nat Immunol 2008;9:310–318.

22 Denzel A, Maus UA, Rodriguez Gomez M, Moll C, Niedermeier M, Winter C, Maus R, Hollingshead S, Briles DE, Kunz-Schughart LA, Talke Y, Mack M: Basophils enhance immunological memory responses. Nat Immunol 2008;9:733–742.

23 Tsujimura Y, Obata K, Mukai K, Shindou H, Yoshida M, Nishikado H, Kawano Y, Minegishi Y, Shimizu T, Karasuyama H: Basophils play a pivotal role in immunoglobulin-G-mediated but not immuno-globulin-E-mediated systemic anaphylaxis. Immunity 2008;28:581–589.

24 Min B: Basophils: what they 'can do' versus what they 'actually do'. Nat Immunol 2008;9:1333–1339.

25 Karasuyama H, Mukai K, Tsujimura Y, Obata K: Newly discovered roles for basophils: a neglected minority gains new respect. Nat Rev Immunol 2009; 9:9–13.

26 Hida S, Tadachi M, Saito T, Taki S: Negative control of basophil expansion by IRF-2 critical for the regulation of Th1/Th2 balance. Blood 2005;106:2011–2017.

27 Oh K, Shen T, Le Gros G, Min B: Induction of Th2 type immunity in a mouse system reveals a novel immunoregulatory role of basophils. Blood 2007; 109:2921–2927.

28 Sokol CL, Chu NQ, Yu S, Nish SA, Laufer TM, Medzhitov R: Basophils function as antigen-presenting cells for an allergen-induced T-helper type 2 response. Nat Immunol 2009;10:713–720.

29 Yoshimoto T, Yasuda K, Tanaka H, Nakahira M, Imai Y, Fujimori Y, Nakanishi K: Basophils contribute to T_H2-IgE responses in vivo via IL-4 production and presentation of peptide-MHC class II complexes to CD4+ T cells. Nat Immunol 2009; 10:706–712.

30 Perrigoue JG, Saenz SA, Siracusa MC, Allenspach EJ, Taylor BC, Giacomin PR, Nair MG, Du Y, Zaph C, van Rooijen N, Comeau MR, Pearce EJ, Laufer TM, Artis D: MHC class II-dependent basophil-CD4+ T-cell interactions promote T_H2 cytokine-dependent immunity. Nat Immunol 2009;10: 697–705.

31 Galli SJ: Pathogenesis and management of anaphylaxis: current status and future challenges. J Allergy Clin Immunol 2005;115:571–574.

32 Bochner BS, Lichtenstein LM: Anaphylaxis. N Engl J Med 1991;324:1785–1790.

33 Kemp SF, Lockey RF: Anaphylaxis: a review of causes and mechanisms. J Allergy Clin Immunol 2002;110:341–348.

34 Jacoby W, Cammarata PV, Findlay S, Pincus SH: Anaphylaxis in mast cell-deficient mice. J Invest Dermatol 1984;83:302–304.

35 Oettgen HC, Martin TR, Wynshaw-Boris A, Deng C, Drazen JM, Leder P: Active anaphylaxis in IgE-deficient mice. Nature 1994;370:367–370.

36 Finkelman FD: Anaphylaxis: lessons from mouse models. J Allergy Clin Immunol 2007;120:506–515.

37 Dombrowicz D, Flamand V, Miyajima I, Ravetch JV, Galli SJ, Kinet JP: Absence of FcεRI α chain results in upregulation of FcγRIII-dependent mast cell degranulation and anaphylaxis. Evidence of competition between FcεRI and FcεRIII for limiting amounts of FcR β and γ chains. J Clin Invest 1997; 99:915–925.

38 Miyajima I, Dombrowicz D, Martin TR, Ravetch JV, Kinet JP, Galli SJ: Systemic anaphylaxis in the mouse can be mediated largely through IgG1 and FcγRIII. Assessment of the cardiopulmonary changes, mast cell degranulation, and death associated with active or IgE- or IgG1-dependent passive anaphylaxis. J Clin Invest 1997;99:901–914.

39 Strait RT, Morris SC, Yang M, Qu XW, Finkelman FD: Pathways of anaphylaxis in the mouse. J Allergy Clin Immunol 2002;109:658–668.

40 Hirayama N, Hirano T, Kohler G, Kurata A, Okumura K, Ovary Z: Biological activities of anti-trinitrophenyl and antidinitrophenyl mouse monoclonal antibodies. Proc Natl Acad Sci USA 1982;79: 613–615.

41 Hazenbos WL, Gessner JE, Hofhuis FM, Kuipers H, Meyer D, Heijnen IA, Schmidt RE, Sandor M, Capel PJ, Daeron M, van de Winkel JG, Verbeek JS: Impaired IgG-dependent anaphylaxis and Arthus reaction in FcγRIII (CD16)-deficient mice. Immunity 1996;5:181–188.

42 Arimura A, Nagata M, Takeuchi M, Watanabe A, Nakamura K, Harada M: Active and passive cutaneous anaphylaxis in WBB6F1 mouse, a mast cell-deficient strain. Immunol Invest 1990;19:227–233.

43 Cheifetz A, Smedley M, Martin S, Reiter M, Leone G, Mayer L, Plevy S: The incidence and management of infusion reactions to infliximab: a large center experience. Am J Gastroenterol 2003;98:1315–1324.

44 Dybendal T, Guttormsen AB, Elsayed S, Askeland B, Harboe T, Florvaag E: Screening for mast cell tryptase and serum IgE antibodies in 18 patients with anaphylactic shock during general anaesthesia. Acta Anaesthesiol Scand 2003;47:1211–1218.

45 Adourian U, Shampaine EL, Hirshman CA, Fuchs E, Adkinson NF Jr: High-titer protamine-specific IgG antibody associated with anaphylaxis: report of a case and quantitative analysis of antibody in vasectomized men. Anesthesiology 1993;78:368–372.

46 Kraft D, Hedin H, Richter W, Scheiner O, Rumpold H, Devey ME: Immunoglobulin class and subclass distribution of dextran-reactive antibodies in human reactors and non-reactors to clinical dextran. Allergy 1982;37:481–489.

47 Weiss M, Nyhan ED, Peng JK, Horrow JC, Lowenstein E, Hirshman C, Adkinson NF Jr: Association of protamine IgE and IgG antibodies with life-threatening reactions to intravenous protamine. N Engl J Med 1989;320:886–892.

48 Lie WJ, Homburg CH, Kuijpers TW, Knol EF, Mul FP, Roos D, Tool AT: Regulation and kinetics of platelet-activating factor and leukotriene C4 synthesis by activated human basophils. Clin Exp Allergy 2003;33:1125–1134.

49 Vadas P, Gold M, Perelman B, Liss GM, Lack G, Blyth T, Simons FE, Simons JK, Cass D, Yeung J: Platelet-activating factor, PAF acetylhydrolase, and severe anaphylaxis. N Engl J Med 2008;358:28–35.

Dr. Hajime Karasuyama
Department of Immune Regulation, Tokyo Medical and Dental University
Graduate School of Medical and Dental Sciences
1-5-45 Yushima, Bunkyo-ku, Tokyo 113-8519 (Japan)
Tel. +81 3 5803 5162, Fax +81 3 3814 7172, E-Mail karasuyama.mbch@tmd.ac.jp

Ring J (ed): Anaphylaxis. Chem Immunol Allergy. Basel, Karger, 2010, vol 95, pp 98–109

Human Cardiac Mast Cells in Anaphylaxis

Arturo Genovese · Francesca W. Rossi · Giuseppe Spadaro · Maria Rosaria Galdiero · Gianni Marone

Department of Clinical Immunology and Allergy and Center for Basic and Clinical Immunology Research (CISI), University of Naples Federico II, Naples, Italy

Abstract

Human heart mast cells (HHMC), by elaborating vasoactive mediators, cytokines and chemokines, are the main primary effector cells of anaphylaxis. Mast cells have been identified perivascularly, close to myocytes and in the arterial intima in human heart tissue. Mast cells isolated from human heart tissue (HHMC) of patients undergoing cardiac transplantation express high-affinity receptors for IgE (FcεRI) and C5a receptors. Activation of HHMC in vitro with anti-IgE or anti-FcεRI induced the release of preformed mediators (histamine, tryptase, chymase, and renin) and the de novo synthesis of LTC_4 ($\cong$18 ng/10^6 cells) and PGD_2 ($\cong$18 ng/10^6 cells). Complement is activated and anaphylatoxin forms during anaphylaxis. C5a causes rapid release of histamine and tryptase from HHMC. These cells are activated in vitro by therapeutic (general anesthetics, protamine, etc.) and diagnostic agents (radiocontrast media, etc.) which can cause anaphylactoid reactions. Low concentrations of histamine and cysteinyl leukotrienes given to subjects undergoing diagnostic catheterization caused significant systemic and coronary hemodynamic effects. These results indicate that HHMC probably have a role in anaphylactic reactions.

Systemic anaphylaxis is the most dramatic and potentially fatal manifestation of immediate hypersensitivity, accounting for more than 500 deaths annually [1]. Despite these alarming findings, there is surprisingly limited interest and little information on how the cardiovascular system is involved in fatal and near-fatal allergic diseases.

Pathological observations indicate that lesions of the cardiovascular system can be a cause of death in patients with anaphylaxis [2]. Myocardial lesions might be the anatomical basis for the irreversible cardiac failure occasionally associated with systemic anaphylaxis [3]. There is compelling evidence that the heart is directly and/or indirectly involved in several forms of anaphylaxis in man [1, 4, 5].

Systemic anaphylaxis in man is frequently accompanied by electrocardiographic alterations: ischemic ST waves, arrhythmias and atrial fibrillation [6–11]. Anaphylactic reactions after insect stings can lead to coronary spasm or acute myocardial infarction [12, 13]. Myocardial infarction can also occur as a consequence of idiopathic anaphylaxis [14]. In addition, patients with systemic anaphylaxis may present profound myocardial depression presumably because of the negative inotropic effects of mast cell-derived mediators [15].

In this article we will describe the possible roles of cardiac mast cells and their mediators during anaphylactic reactions in man and will briefly review the cardiovascular effects of mast cell-derived mediators in vivo.

Human Heart Mast Cells

We have identified mast cells around blood vessels and between myocardial fibers in all sections of human hearts [16, 17]. These cells are also seen in normal and atherosclerotic human arterial intima [18–21]. In situ electron microscopy of cardiac mast cells revealed a small percentage (about 5%) of activated, i.e. partially degranulated mast cells [16, 22]. This is clinically relevant because it implies that immunologic and non-immunologic stimuli can activate HHMC to release vasoactive and proinflammatory mediators [23].

Mast cells are frequently found close to coronary vessels (see fig. 1) suggesting that circulating antigens, autoantibodies (anti-IgE, anti-FcεRI, etc.), drugs (general anesthetics, protamine, etc.), and diagnostic agents (radiocontrast media, etc.) can easily reach perivascular HHMC. Activated mast cells can in turn release vasoactive substances (histamine, cysteinyl leukotrienes, PGD_2, PAF, etc.) that can affect blood vessels.

Patella and coworkers [16, 17, 24] established an elegant technique to isolate and partially purify mast cells from heart tissue of patients undergoing heart transplantation and victims of traffic accidents. We used this technique to study in vitro various aspects of HHMC biology. We compared the cardiac mast cell density, the concentration of mast cell-derived mediators (histamine and tryptase) and the immunologic and non-immunologic release of mediators from mast cells isolated from failing hearts from patients with idiopathic dilated (DCM) and ischemic cardiomyopathy (ICM) undergoing heart transplantation, and from controls without cardiovascular disease (CH) who had died in accidents [25]. Cardiac mast cell density and the histamine and tryptase contents of DCM and ICM hearts were higher than in CH. Immunologic activation of HHMC induced significantly greater release of mediators (histamine, tryptase and LTC_4) in patients with failing hearts than in CH. The increase in cardiac mast cell density and the greater release of mediators suggest that anaphylactic reactions might be particularly severe in patients with certain underlying cardiovascular diseases.

Preformed Mediators Synthesized by HHMC

The histamine content of isolated HHMC ($\cong 3$ pg/cell) was comparable to lung parenchymal and skin mast cells. The mean tryptase content of HHMC ($\cong 24$ μg/10^6 cells)

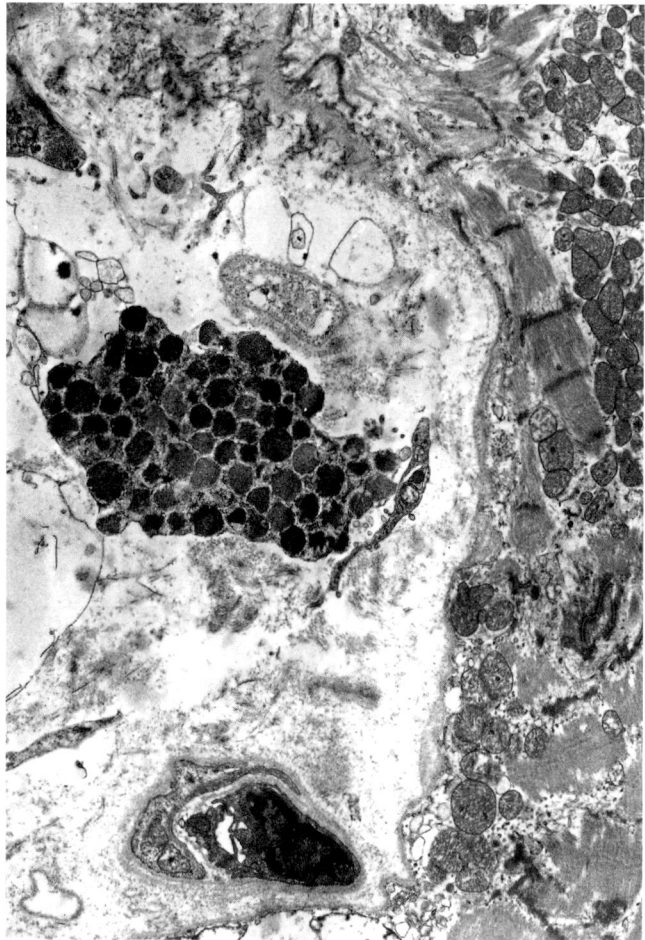

Fig. 1. Electron micrograph of a mast cell in human heart tissue. The cytoplasm contains numerous secretory granules. The mast cell is adjacent to a coronary blood vessel, surrounded by collagen fibers and close to a myocyte. Uranyl acetate and lead citrate stained. Orig. magnif. 10,000×.

was lower than skin mast cells ($\cong 35$ μg/10^6 cells) and higher than lung mast cells ($\cong 10$ μg/10^6 cells). IgE-mediated activation of HHMC caused tryptase release parallel to histamine secretion [16].

Using the immunogold technique and a polyclonal anti-chymase antibody [26], we showed that HHMC contain chymase as well as tryptase [16]. Interestingly, human chymase generates angiotensin II from angiotensin I, acting as an angiotensin-converting enzyme [27]. Supernatants of HHMC challenged in vitro with anti-IgE can convert angiotensin I into angiotensin II, suggesting that chymase released from immunologically challenged HHMC also plays a role in the homeostatic control of blood pressure. The activation of HHMC and release of chymase may therefore serve to control blood pressure during anaphylaxis.

Levi and Silver's groups [28] have shown that mast cells are an additional source of renin and constitute a unique extrarenal renin-angiotensin system; they found

Genovese · Rossi · Spadaro · Galdiero · Marone

that the human mast cell line HMC-1 expressed renin. We have extended their observation by demonstrating that HHMC also contain renin [Marone, unpubl. observation]. These findings imply that the release of renin from activated cardiac mast cells can trigger local formation of angiotensin II. In a subsequent study they reported in the Langendorff-perfused guinea pig heart system that mast cell activation released renin, promoting local angiotensin formation, which was associated with arrhythmias [29]. These studies provided an elegant demonstration that cardiac mast cells contain renin which, when released, activates a local renin-angiotensin system, promoting norepinephrine release and cardiac arrhythmic dysfunction.

Recent evidence from our laboratory shows that the supernatants of HHMC activated by anti-IgE can convert a synthetic substrate of big endothelin to endothelin 1. The latter observation is particularly important because endothelin 1 is a potent bronchoconstrictor in allergic subjects [30].

Lipid Mediators de novo Synthesized by HHMC

Immunologically challenged HHMC synthesize prostaglandin D_2 (PGD_2) ($\cong$18 ng/10^6 cells) de novo through cyclooxygenase activity [16, 17]. The knowledge is useful because PGD_2 is a potent coronary constrictor [31], meaning that the in vivo release of PGD_2 from HHMC can cause coronary vasoconstriction in man. Activation of HHMC with anti-IgE or anti-FcϵRI induced the de novo synthesis of cysteinyl leukotriene (LTC_4) ($\cong$18 ng/10^6 cells).

These studies showed that immunologically activated HHMC release PGD_2 and LTC_4. Interestingly, intravenous and intracoronary injection of traces of LTC_4 and LTD_4 may have several cardiovascular and metabolic effects [32].

Cytokines Synthesized by HHMC

Immunologic responses mediated by cytokines have been implicated in the pathogenesis of heart failure in a variety of diseases [33]. Studies are beginning to focus on the presence and the possible roles of cardiac mast cell-derived cytokines. TNF-α is present in mast cells of human coronary atheromas [34]. We have ultrastructurally located the granule-associated stem cell factor (SCF) in HHMC of patients with dilated cardiomyopathy [25]. SCF is the principal growth, differentiating, chemotactic and activating factor for human mast cells [35, 36]. This raises the possibility that SCF released by HHMC is an autocrine factor that contributes to mast cell hyperplasia in dilated cardiomyopathy.

Cytokines influence several cardiovascular functions through a variety of mechanisms [33, 37, 38]. Additional studies are necessary to clarify the roles of cytokines

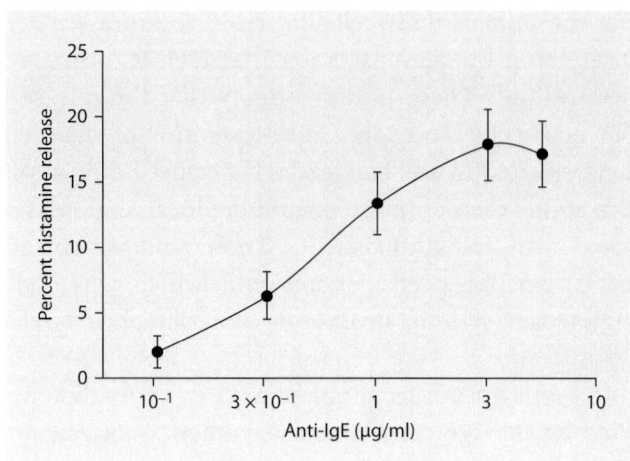

Fig. 2. Effects of increasing concentrations of anti-IgE on histamine secretion from eleven preparations of HHMC from patients undergoing heart transplantation. Each point represents the mean ± SEM.

and chemokines in anaphylactic reactions and the cardiac mast cells contribution to their production.

Immunologic and Non-Immunologic Stimuli that Activate HHMC in vitro

IgE cross-linking on HHMC can be induced by antigen, anti-IgE or anti-FcεRI. Figure 2 shows the effects of increasing concentrations of anti-IgE on histamine release from HHMC from several donors. Activation of HHMC by anti-IgE and by a monoclonal antibody against an epitope of the α-chain of FcεRI may be clinically important. Histamine-releasing autoantibodies against IgE (anti-IgE) or against the α-subunit of FcεRI are present in the circulation of some patients with bronchial asthma, atopic dermatitis and chronic urticaria [39, 40].

Complement is activated and anaphylatoxin forms (C3a and C5a) during cardiac [41] and systemic anaphylaxis [42], and complement deposition has been documented in infarcted areas of the human heart [43]. There is also experimental evidence that C5a causes several cardiovascular derangements directly or through the release of vasoactive mediators [44, 45]. We found that C5a caused rapid, dose-dependent histamine release from HHMC [16]. Interestingly, C5a does not activate human lung mast cells, whereas human skin mast cells (HSMC) are responsive to it [17], suggesting that these are the only mast cells possessing C5a receptors. HHMC are also responsive to SCF [46]. SCF is found in the secretory granules of HHMC and is released after their immunologic activation [47].

HHMC can also be activated by a variety of non-immunological stimuli. Some have clinical relevance because they might explain certain adverse effects observed in vivo when these compounds are used for diagnostic (contrast media, etc.) or therapeutic

Genovese · Rossi · Spadaro · Galdiero · Marone

purposes (general anesthetics, protamine, etc.) [24]. For example, protamine, used to neutralize heparin and certain general anesthetics (propofol and atracurium) can cause histamine release from HHMC [24]. Radiocontrast media, injected into the coronary arteries for diagnostic purposes, can also activate HHMC in vitro [24]. The close proximity of HHMC to coronary blood vessels and the presence of mast cells in human coronary atheromas [20, 21] suggest that intracoronary injection of high doses of contrast media can activate mast cells and induce the in vivo release of vasoactive mediators. This activation may well explain some of the cardiac effects of these agents particularly in patients with underlying cardiovascular diseases [25, 48, 49]. In a multicenter study of 20 patients who experienced immediate reactions to the injection of radiocontrast media, the concentrations of plasma histamine and tryptase rose [50]. Three of these patients had cardiac arrest.

Role of HHMC in Systemic and Cardiac Anaphylaxis

Levi's [44, 51] group has provided convincing evidence that the heart is directly involved in experimental anaphylaxis through the release of chemical mediators from cardiac mast cells. There is evidence of cardiac involvement in human anaphylaxis too [42] and this has been attributed to mediators originating from the lung and reaching the heart. However, there are mast cells around coronary arteries and in human coronary atheromas, particularly in patients with ischemic heart disease [20, 21]. Therefore, the local release of vasoactive mediators by cardiac mast cells can contribute to cardiovascular derangements during anaphylaxis. In addition, complement activation and C5a formation have been documented during anaphylaxis in man [42]. The in vitro immunologic activation of human heart tissue and of isolated mast cells induces the release of preformed and de novo synthesized chemical mediators [16, 17, 52]. HHMC have FcεRI and IgE bound to their membrane surface and C5a receptors. Therefore it is likely that IgE- and C5a-mediated activation of these cells plays some part in systemic and cardiac anaphylaxis in man.

HHMC can also be directly activated by agents injected intravenously for therapeutic (general anesthetics, protamine, etc.) or diagnostic purposes (radiocontrast media, etc.), which can cause non-IgE-mediated anaphylactic reactions in vitro [24, 53] and in vivo [50]. Therefore, the release of vasoactive mediators from perivascular, intimal and interstitial cardiac mast cells may well be involved in anaphylactic reactions related to these agents.

Cardiovascular Effects of Histamine Infusion in Man

In collaboration with our colleagues in the Division of Cardiology at the University of Naples Federico II, we investigated the effects of mast cell-derived preformed (histamine) and de novo synthesized mediators (LTC$_4$ and LTD$_4$) on peripheral and coronary hemodynamics in man. In a first study, histamine (0.4 µg/kg/min) infused in patients with normal left ventricular (LV) function undergoing diagnostic cardiac catheterization [54] induced significant drops in systolic, diastolic, and mean aortic pressure, systemic vascular resistance, LV end-diastolic pressure, and stroke index. There were also significant rises in heart rate, cardiac output, and LV/dP/dt_{max}, with small changes in mean pulmonary vascular resistance. Histamine significantly raised plasma epinephrine and norepinephrine. All hemodynamic changes started 1–2 min after beginning the infusion and reverted to normal within 5 min after the infusion. In 1 subject there was a transient progression from first- to third-degree atrioventricular block, with prompt recovery of 1:1 atrioventricular conduction at the end of the infusion. Thus, exogenous histamine in man causes significant transient hemodynamic changes, mainly systemic hypotension, tachycardia, and increased LV performance. These changes can be partly attributed to the related increase in sympathoadrenergic activity, although it cannot be excluded that histamine has some direct cardiac effect.

Effects of Activation of the H$_1$ Receptor on Coronary Hemodynamics in Man

We examined the effects of selective activation of histamine H$_1$ receptors on coronary hemodynamics in two groups: patients with atypical chest pain and normal coronary arteries, and patients with vasospastic angina [48]. Selective H$_1$ receptor stimulation was achieved by infusing histamine intravenously (0.5 µg/kg/min) for 5 min after pretreatment with cimetidine to antagonize the H$_2$ receptors. Heart rate was kept constant (100 beats/min) by coronary sinus pacing.

In the first group, mean aortic pressure and coronary vascular resistance (CVR) dropped, while coronary blood flow (CBF) and myocardial oxygen consumption remained unchanged during histamine infusion. No patient in this group developed angina during histamine infusion. By contrast, 40% of the second group developed angina during histamine infusion, with a decrease in CBF and an increase in CVR. Circumflex coronary arterial spasm was angiographically demonstrated in 1 of these patients during histamine-induced angina. These findings suggest that stimulation of the H$_1$ receptor in subjects with normal coronary arteries reduces CVR, probably because of vasodilation of small coronary resistance vessels. This response is also seen in approximately 60% of patients with vasospastic angina. However, in a considerable proportion of these patients (40%), H$_1$ receptor activation can cause vasoconstriction of large-capacitance coronary arteries.

These findings may have practical implications in patients taking H$_2$ receptor-blocking drugs. In fact, they support the hypothesis that the endogenous release of histamine, which is a feature of anaphylactic reactions arising during therapeutic or diagnostic interventions [24, 53], may precipitate coronary spasm in a subset of patients with vasospastic angina. This is substantiated by the finding that premedication with an H_2-receptor antagonist increases the risk of heart block in patients who develop anaphylaxis [55].

Studies have now started to clarify the role of histamine H_1 and H_2 receptors in the cardiovascular manifestations of anaphylaxis. However, histamine can activate H_3 and H_4 receptors [56, 57]. Levi and coworkers [58–60] identified H_3 receptors as inhibitory heteroreceptors in cardiac adrenergic nerve endings. This suggests a mechanism by which endogenous histamine can activate norepinephrine release in normal and ischemic conditions [61, 62]. The functional identification of H_3 receptors in the human heart [59] means that these receptors might be directly and/or indirectly involved in the cardiovascular manifestations of anaphylactic reactions.

Hemodynamic Effects of Cysteinyl Leukotrienes in Man

In a third study the time course of the effects of intravenous and intracoronary injections of cysteinyl leukotrienes on metabolic parameters and systemic and coronary hemodynamics was examined in patients with normal coronary arteries [32]. LTD_4 (3 nmol, injected into the left coronary artery) induced an early (20 s), transient fall in mean arterial pressure paralleled by rises in heart rate and plasma levels of epinephrine and norepinephrine, all of which had returned to baseline by 10 min. CVR rose at 10 and 15 min and myocardial oxygen extraction at 15 min. Thus, small doses of cysteinyl leukotrienes may induce both an early, transient fall in mean arterial pressure, with secondary sympathoadrenergic activation, and a later increase in small coronary arteriolar resistance.

Cysteinyl leukotrienes exert potent biological effects through the activation of at least two classes of receptors, $CysLT_1$ and $CysLT_2$. High levels of $CysLT_2$ mRNA were recently detected in the human atrium, ventricles and coronary artery, while $CysLT_1$ mRNA was barely detectable [63]. Although it is not clear which receptor was involved in these cardiovascular and metabolic effects, our findings may contribute to a better understanding of the cardiovascular changes occurring during anaphylaxis associated with leukotriene release.

Conclusions

Anaphylaxis is the most dramatic and potentially catastrophic manifestation of allergic disorders. It can affect virtually any organ including the cardiovascular system. Cardiovascular collapse and hypotensive shock in anaphylaxis have been attributed to peripheral vasodilation, enhanced vascular permeability and plasma leakage, rather than any direct effect on the myocardium. However, there is increasing experimental and clinical evidence that the human heart is a site and target of anaphylaxis.

Mast cells are present in the normal human heart and even more abundant in diseased hearts [16–18, 25, 47]. Within heart tissue, mast cells lie between myocytes and are in close contact with blood vessels. They are also found in the coronary adventitia and in the shoulder regions of coronary atheroma [20, 21]. The density of cardiac mast cells is higher in patients with dilated and ischemic cardiomyopathy than in accident victims without cardiovascular diseases [25]. Importantly, in some of these conditions there is in situ evidence of mast cell activation [16, 34].

HHMC activation by circulating antigens, autoantibodies (anti-IgE, anti-FcεRI, etc.), therapeutic (e.g. protamine, general anesthetics) or diagnostic substances (e.g. radiocontrast media) injected intravenously explains some of the anaphylactic reactions caused by these agents. HHMC have FcεRI and C5a receptors, which could explain the direct involvement of cardiac mast cells in systemic and cardiac anaphylaxis. The increases in cardiac mast cell density and release of vasoactive mediators in patients with dilated cardiomyopathy [25] might also have clinical implications given the marked cardiovascular effects of histamine, cysteinyl leukotrienes and PGD_2 [31, 32, 48, 49, 54].

A series of studies have started to shed light on the cardiovascular and metabolic effects in man caused by such mast cell-derived mediators as histamine and cysteinyl leukotrienes. For instance, exogenous histamine caused a transient fall in blood pressure, a rise in heart rate and cardiac output, and small changes in pulmonary vascular resistance [54]. However, in 1 patient there was a progression from first- to third-degree atrioventricular block. In patients with normal coronary arteries, histamine caused dilation of the small-resistance coronary arteries, which is not completely mediated by H_1 receptors [48, 49]. In contrast, in a significant percentage of patients with vasospastic angina activation of H_1 receptors can cause vasoconstriction of large-capacitance coronary arteries [48].

Interestingly, these studies provided the important information that the hemodynamic effects of mediators depend on both the underlying cardiovascular conditions and the pharmacologic treatment (e.g. H_2 blockade).

Cysteinyl leukotrienes can induce an early, transient fall in arterial pressure associated with sympathoadrenergic activation, plus a late rise in small coronary arteriolar resistance [32]. Using specific antagonists of $CysLT_1$ and $CysLT_2$ [63] it will be possible to assess the each receptor's contribution to the cardiovascular effects of these vasoactive mediators.

In conclusion, these in vitro and in vivo studies clearly indicate that the human heart can be viewed as both a site and a target in anaphylaxis.

Acknowledgements

This work was supported by grants from the Ministero dell'Istruzione, dell'Università e della Ricerca (MIUR), from the Istituto Superiore di Sanità (Rome, Italy) and the Regione Campania (Naples, Italy).

References

1 Bochner BS, Lichtenstein LM: Anaphylaxis. N Engl J Med 1991;324:1785.

2 Carswell F: Thirty deaths from asthma. Arch Dis Child 1985;60:25.

3 Delage C, Irey NS: Anaphylactic deaths: a clinico-pathologic study of 43 cases. J Forensic Med 1972; 17:525.

4 Sampson HA, Mendelson L, Rosen JP: Fatal and near-fatal anaphylactic reactions to food in children and adolescents. N Engl J Med 1992;327:380.

5 Kemp SF, Lockey RF: Anaphylaxis: a review of causes and mechanisms. J Allergy Clin Immunol 2002;110:341.

6 Bernreiter M: Electrocardiogram of patient in anaphylactic shock. JAMA 1959;170:1628.

7 Hanashiro PK, Weil MH: Anaphylactic shock in man. Report of two cases with detailed hemodynamic and metabolic studies. Arch Intern Med 1967;119:129.

8 Booth BH, Patterson R: Electrocardiographic changes during human anaphylaxis. JAMA 1970;211:627.

9 Criep LH, Woehler TR: The heart in human anaphylaxis. Ann Allergy 1971;29:399

10 Sullivan TJ: Cardiac disorders in penicillin-induced anaphylaxis. Association with intravenous epinephrine therapy. JAMA 1982;248:2161.

11 Ferrari S, Pietroiusti A, Galanti A, Compagnucci M, Fontana L: Paroxysmal atrial fibrillation after insect sting. J Allergy Clin Immunol 1996;98:759.

12 Levine HD: Acute myocardial infarction following wasp sting. Am Heart J 1976;91:365.

13 Bristow MR, Ginsburg R, Kantrowitz NE, Baim DS, Rosenbaum JT: Coronary spasm associated with urticaria: report of a case mimicking anaphylaxis. Clin Cardiol 1982;5:238.

14 Wong S, Greenberger PA, Patterson R: Nearly fatal idiopathic anaphylactic reaction resulting in cardiovascular collapse and myocardial infarction. Chest 1990;98:501.

15 Raper RF, Fisher MM: Profound reversible myocardial depression after anaphylaxis. Lancet 1988;1: 386.

16 Patella V, Marinò I, Lamparter B, Arbustini E, Adt M, Marone G: Human heart mast cells. Isolation, purification, ultrastructure and immunologic characterization. J Immunol 1995;154:2855.

17 Patella V, de Crescenzo G, Ciccarelli A, Marinò I, Adt M, Marone G: Human heart mast cells: a definitive case of mast cell heterogeneity. Int Arch Allergy Immunol 1995;106:386.

18 Forman MB, Oates JA, Robertson D, Robertson RM, Roberts LJ, Virmani R: Increased adventitial mast cells in a patient with coronary spasm. N Engl J Med 1985;313:1138.

19 Kamat BR, Galli SJ, Barger AC, Lainey LL, Silverman KJ: Neovascularization and coronary atherosclerotic plaque: cinematographic localization and quantitative histologic analysis. Hum Pathol 1987;18: 1036.

20 Kaartinen M, Penttilä A, Kovanen PT: Accumulation of activated mast cells in the shoulder region of human coronary atheroma, the predilection site of atheromatous rupture. Circulation 1994;90:1669.

21 Kaartinen M, Penttilä A, Kovanen PT: Mast cells of two types differing in neutral protease composition in the human aortic intima. Demonstration of tryptase- and tryptase/chymase-containing mast cells in normal intimas, fatty streaks, and the shoulder region of atheromas. Arterioscler Thromb 1994; 14:966.

22 Laine P, Naukkarinen A, Heikkilä L, Pentillä A, Kovanen PT: Adventitial mast cells connect with sensory nerve fibers in atherosclerotic coronary arteries. Circulation 2000;101:1665.

23 Marone G, de Crescenzo G, Florio G, Granata F, Dente V, Genovese A: Immunological modulation of human cardiac mast cells. Neurochem Res 1999; 24:1195.

24 Patella V, Ciccarelli A, Lamparter-Schummert B, de Paulis A, Adt M, Marone G: Heterogeneous effects of protamine on human mast cells and basophils. Br J Anaesth 1997;78:724.

25 Patella V, Marinò I, Arbustini E, Lamparter-Schummert B, Verga L, Adt M, Marone G: Stem cell factor in mast cells and increased mast cell density in idiopathic and ischemic cardiomyopathy. Circulation 1998;97:971.

26 Schechter NM, Irani AM, Sprows JL, Abernethy J, Wintroub B, Schwartz LB: Identification of a cathepsin G-like proteinase in the MC_{TC} type of human mast cell. J Immunol 1990;145:2652.

27 Urata H, Kinoshita A, Misono KS, Bumpus FM, Husain A: Identification of a highly specific chymase as the major angiotensin II-forming enzyme in the human heart. J Biol Chem 1990;265:22348.

28 Silver RB, Reid AC, Mackins CJ, Askwith T, Schaefer U, Herzlinger D, Levi R: Mast cells: a unique source of renin. Proc Natl Acad Sci USA 2004;101:13607.

29 Mackins CJ, Kano S, Sevedi N, Schafer U, Reid AC, Machida T, Silver RB, Levi R: Cardiac mast cell-derived renin promotes local angiotensin formation, norepinephrine release, and arrhythmias in ischemia/reperfusion. J Clin Invest 2006;116:1063.

30 Advenier C, Sarria B, Naline E, Bybasset L, Lagente V: Contractile activity of three endothelins (ET-1, ET-2 and ET-3) on the human isolated bronchus. Br J Pharmacol 1990;100:168.

31 Hattori Y, Levi R: Effect of PGD_2 on cardiac contractility: a negative inotropism secondary to coronary vasoconstriction conceals a primary positive inotropic action. J Pharmacol Exp Ther 1986;237: 719.

32 Vigorito C, Giordano A, Cirillo R, Genovese A, Rengo F, Marone G: Metabolic and hemodynamic effects of peptide leukotriene C_4 and D_4 in man. Int J Clin Lab Res 1997;27:178.

33 Sasayama S, Matsumori A, Kihara Y: New insights into the pathophysiological role for cytokines in heart failure. Cardiovasc Res 1999;42:557.

34 Kaartinen M, Penttilä A, Kovanen PT: Mast cells in rupture-prone areas of human coronary atheromas produce and store TNF-α. Circulation 1996;94:2787.

35 Tsai M, Takeishi T, Thompson H, Langley KE, Zsebo KM, Metcalfe DD, Geissler EN, Galli SJ: Induction of mast cell proliferation, maturation, and heparin synthesis by the rat c-kit ligand, stem cell factor. Proc Natl Acad Sci USA 1991;88:6382.

36 Columbo M, Horowitz EM, Botana LM, MacGlashan DW Jr, Bochner BS, Gillis S, Zsebo KM, Galli SJ, Lichtenstein LM: The human recombinant c-kit receptor ligand, rhSCF, induces mediator release from human cutaneous mast cells and enhances IgE-dependent mediator release from both skin mast cells and peripheral blood basophils. J Immunol 1992;149:599.

37 Ferrari R, Bachetti T, Confortini R, Opasich C, Febo O, Corti A, Cassani G, Visioli O: Tumor necrosis factor-soluble receptors in patients with various degrees of congestive heart failure. Circulation 1995; 92:1479.

38 Torre-Amione G, Kapadia S, Lee J, Durand JB, Bies RD, Young JB, Mann DL: Tumor necrosis factor-α and tumor necrosis factor receptors in the failing human heart. Circulation 1996;93:704.

39 Marone G, Casolaro V, Paganelli R, Quinti I: IgG anti-IgE from atopic dermatitis induces mediator release from basophils and mast cells. J Invest Dermatol 1989;93:246.

40 Hide M, Francis DM, Grattan CEH, Hakimi J, Kochan JP, Greaves MW: Autoantibodies against the high-affinity IgE receptor as a cause of histamine release in chronic urticaria. N Engl J Med 1993;328:1599.

41 del Balzo U, Polley MJ, Levi R: Activation of the third complement component (C3) and C3a generation in cardiac anaphylaxis: histamine release and associated inotropic and chronotropic effects. J Pharmacol Exp Ther 1988;246:911.

42 Smith PL, Kagey-Sobotka A, Bleecker ER, Traystman R, Kaplan AP, Gralnick H, Valentine MD, Permutt S, Lichtenstein LM: Physiologic manifestations of human anaphylaxis. J Clin Invest 1980;66:1072.

43 Schäfer H, Mathey D, Hugo F, Bhakdi S: Deposition of the terminal C5b-9 complement complex in infarcted areas of human myocardium. J Immunol 1986;137:1945.

44 Hachfeld del Balzo U, Levi R, Polley MJ: Cardiac dysfunction caused by purified human C3a anaphylatoxin. Proc Natl Acad Sci USA 1985;82:886.

45 del Balzo U, Polley MJ, Levi R: Cardiac anaphylaxis. Complement activation as an amplification system. Circ Res 1989;65:847.

46 de Paulis A, Ciccarelli A, Cirillo R, de Crescenzo G, Columbo M, Marone G: Modulation of human lung mast cell function by the c-kit receptor ligand. Int Arch Allergy Immunol 1992;99:326.

47 de Paulis A, Minopoli G, Arbustini E, de Crescenzo G, Dal Piaz F, Pucci P, Russo T, Marone G: Stem cell factor is localized in, released from, and cleaved by human mast cells. J Immunol 1999;163:2799.

48 Vigorito C, Poto S, Picotti GB, Triggiani M, Marone G: Effect of activation of the H_1 receptor on coronary hemodynamics in man. Circulation 1986;73: 1175.

49 Vigorito C, Giordano A, De Caprio L, Vitale DF, Maurea N, Silvestri P, Tuccillo B, Ferrara N, Marone G, Rengo F: Effects of histamine on coronary hemodynamics in man: role of H_1 and H_2 receptors. J Am Coll Cardiol 1987;10:1207.

50 Laroche D, Aimone-Gastin I, Dubois F, Huet H, Gérard P, Vergnaud MC, Mouton-Faivre C, Guéant JL, Laxenaire MC, Bricard H: Mechanisms of severe, immediate reactions to iodinated contrast material. Radiology 1998;209:183.

51 Capurro N, Levi R: The heart as a target organ in systemic allergic reactions: comparison of cardiac anaphylaxis in vivo and in vitro. Circ Res 1975;36: 520.

52 Marone G, Triggiani M, Cirillo R, Vigorito C, Genovese A, Spampinato N, Condorelli M: Chemical mediators and the human heart. Prog Biochem Pharmacol 1985;20:38.

53 Stellato C, de Crescenzo G, Patella V, Mastronardi P, Mazzarella B, Marone G: Human basophil/mast cell releasability. XI. Heterogeneity of the effects of contrast media on mediator release. J Allergy Clin Immunol 1996;97:838.

54 Vigorito C, Russo P, Picotti GB, Chiariello M, Poto S, Marone G: Cardiovascular effects of histamine infusion in man. J Cardiovasc Pharmacol 1983;5:531.

55 Patterson LJ, Milne B: Latex anaphylaxis causing heart block: role of ranitidine. Can J Anaesth 1999; 46:776.

56 Lovenberg TW, Roland BL, Wilson SJ, Jiang X, Pyati J, Huvar A, Jackson MR, Erlander MG: Cloning and functional expression of the human histamine H_3 receptor. Mol Pharmacol 1999;55:1101.

57 Oda T, Morikawa N, Saito Y, Masuho Y, Matsumoto S: Molecular cloning and characterization of a novel type of histamine receptor preferentially expressed in leukocytes. J Biol Chem 2000;275:36781.

58 Endou M, Poli E, Levi R: Histamine H_3-receptor signaling in the heart: possible involvement of G_i/G_0 proteins and N-type Ca^{2+} channels. J Pharmacol Exp Ther 1994;269:221.

59 Imamura M, Seyedi N, Lander HM, Levi R: Functional identification of histamine H_3-receptors in the human heart. Circ Res 1995;77:206.

60 Imamura M, Lander HM, Levi R: Activation of histamine H_3-receptors inhibits carrier-mediated norepinephrine release during protracted myocardial ischemia. Comparison with adenosine A_1-receptors and α_2-adrenoceptors. Circ Res 1996;78:475.

61 Silver RB, Mackins CJ, Smith NCE, Koritchneva IL, Lefkowitz K, Lovenberg TW, Levi R: Coupling of histamine H_3 receptors to neuronal Na^+/H^+ exchange: a novel protective mechanism in myocardial ischemia. Proc Natl Acad Sci USA 2001;98: 2855.

62 Silver RB, Poonwasi KS, Seyedi N, Wilson SJ, Lovenberg TW, Levi R: Decreased intracellular calcium mediates the histamine H_3-receptor-induced attenuation of norepinephrine exocytosis from cardiac sympathetic nerve endings. Proc Natl Acad Sci USA 2002;99:501.

63 Kamohara M, Takasaki J, Matsumoto M, Matsumoto S-I, Saito T, Soga T, Matsushime H, Furuichi K: Functional characterization of cysteinyl leukotriene $CysLT_2$ receptor on human coronary artery smooth muscle cells. Biochem Biophys Res Commun 2001; 287:1088.

Prof. Gianni Marone
Division of Clinical Immunology and Allergy, University of Naples Federico II
Via S. Pansini 5, IT–80131 Napoli (Italy)
Tel. +39 081 7707492, Fax +39 081 7462271
E-Mail marone@unina.it

Ring J (ed): Anaphylaxis. Chem Immunol Allergy. Basel, Karger, 2010, vol 95, pp 110–124

Mastocytosis

Knut Brockow[a] · Dean D. Metcalfe[b]

[a]Department of Dermatology and Allergy Biederstein, Technical University Munich, Munich, Germany, and [b]Laboratory of Allergic Diseases, National Institute of Allergy and Infectious Diseases, National Institutes of Health, Bethesda, Md., USA

Abstract

It is known that patients with mastocytosis have an increased risk of anaphylaxis. This also appears to be the case with patients with evidence of a clonal mast cell disorder resulting in the monoclonal mast cell activation syndrome (MMAS) who do not express the full mastocytosis phenotype. Most patients with mastocytosis are recognized by their characteristic skin lesions. An increased level of baseline serum mast cell tryptase is also an indicator for a possible clonal mast cell disorder including mastocytosis. Other markers for mast cell clonality and for mastocytosis include abnormal immunostaining of mast cells with CD25 and CD2, clustering of mast cells in tissues, abnormal mast cell morphology, and the presence of a mutation in the proto-oncogene c-kit encoding for the mast cell growth receptor KIT. As recognition depends on an understanding of mastocytosis, and this disease should be considered in patients with recurrent anaphylaxis, we describe the features of mast cell clonality, MMAS and mastocytosis, and review recent findings.

Copyright © 2010 S. Karger AG, Basel

Mast cells express high-affinity IgE Fc receptors (FcεRI) on their surface, contain cytoplasmic granules which are major sources of histamine and other inflammatory mediators, and are activated to release and generate these mediators by IgE-dependent and non-IgE-dependent mechanisms [1]. Disturbances either in the release of mast cell mediators or in mast cell proliferation are associated with clonal mast cell disorders including monoclonal mast cell activation syndrome (MMAS) and mastocytosis respectively, which are in turn associated with some cases of anaphylaxis [2]. Molecular mechanisms have been identified which may link increased releasability of mast cell mediators and conditions leading to increased mast cell numbers [3]. Patients with mastocytosis have an increased risk to develop anaphylaxis [4, 5] and those with anaphylaxis may suffer from unrecognized mastocytosis or may display incomplete features of the disease [6–8].

Description

Mastocytosis is a disorder characterized by increased numbers of mast cells in the skin, bone marrow, gastrointestinal tract, liver, spleen, and lymph nodes [9, 10]. The prevalence is unknown; the incidence has been roughly estimated to be 3–7 new patients per million per year [9]. Most cases are sporadic with only a limited number (50–100) of cases with mastocytosis reported to pass from generation to generation [11]. Mastocytosis presents at any age, although most cases occur during the first 2 years of life (childhood-onset) or after puberty (adult-onset) [9]. Mastocytosis in childhood often is self-limited and involves only the skin, whereas the course in patients with adult-onset disease is normally chronic and includes systemic involvement.

Pathogenesis

The most important survival and growth factor for mast cells is the KIT ligand stem cell factor (SCF) [12]. The hypothesis of early studies, that SCF might be elevated in skin lesions associated with mastocytosis [13], however, was not confirmed by later studies on SCF levels in skin and blood, at least for adult patients [14].

Rather, it is now thought that an associated and early event in the evolution of mastocytosis is the occurrence of an activating mutation in *c-kit*, the gene for KIT [10, 15]. KIT is a transmembrane tyrosine kinase growth receptor expressed on mast cells. Ligation of KIT by SCF promotes dimerization of the receptor and subsequent intrinsic tyrosine kinase activation. The resulting phosphorylated tyrosine residue serves as a docking site for intracellular signaling pathways leading to mast cell proliferation and activation.

In 1995, Nagata et al. [16] identified a point mutation consisting of a substitution of valine for aspartic acid in the catalytic domain of *c-kit* (D816V) in the peripheral blood of patients with mastocytosis and predominately myelodysplastic features. Subsequently, the same mutation was identified in adult patients with different forms of mastocytosis in tissues where mast cells are abundant, such as bone marrow, skin and spleen [17]. It is now believed that more than 90% of adults with mastocytosis have the D816V mutation, if bone marrow mononuclear cells are examined [17]. In a subset of patients, primarily those with more severe disease, the clone expands sufficiently to be detected in peripheral blood [16].

Thus, mastocytosis appears connected with the presence of activated KIT, at least in adult patients. The huge variance of symptomatology and disease severity among patients with mastocytosis, however, appears to depend on secondary or coexisting factors [2]. For example, a gain of function polymorphism in the gene for the IL-4 receptor α chain (Q576R) has been reported to be associated with less extensive mast cell involvement [18]. As early addition of IL-4 to human mast cell cultures decreases mast cell number by downregulating KIT expression, the hypothesis is that the polymorphism in the IL-4 receptor results in increased IL-4-induced signaling, limiting the mast cell proliferation by KIT.

In children, the D816V *c-kit* mutation, and other less common mutations in *c-kit*, such as V560G, D816Y, D816F, D816H, E839K, R815K, D820G, V533D, V559A, del419, K509I, F522C, and A533D, have been detected occasionally in biopsies of lesional skin or bone marrow, mainly in those with more severe forms of mastocytosis [2, 15]. However, overall *c-kit* mutations are untypical in children with infant-onset maculopapular cutaneous mastocytosis (MPCM) [2]. Thus, in many children, mastocytosis appears to have a different basis from that in most adults.

Previous studies have revealed that activation of KIT markedly potentates FcεRI-mediated mast cell degranulation [19]. In a study in human mast cells, it was sought how these pathways were linked and how upstream signals produced by FcεRI and KIT were integrated to produce these downstream synergistic responses in mast cells [3]. It was shown that linker of activation of T cells 2 (LAT2) has a role both in antigen-mediated and KIT-enhanced degranulation. Using knock-out mice deficient in specific tyrosine kinases, it was demonstrated that FcεRI employs the tyrosine kinases Lyn and Syk for LAT2 phosphorylation, whereas KIT directly phosphorylates LAT2 [3]. There was evidence for a role of LAT2 in regulating PLCγ1-dependent calcium mobilization in mast cells. Further, phosphoinositide 3-kinase appeared to be a critical player in the amplification pathway utilized by KIT activation for the potentiation of antigen-mediated responses. These insights provide the molecular basis for the observation that in mastocytosis, where an activating mutation of KIT exists, elevated KIT signaling may further potentate mast cell activation.

Clinical Features

Cutaneous Involvement
MPCM is the presenting feature in most children and the majority of adult patients with systemic mastocytosis [9]. This form has also been termed urticaria pigmentosa. The classical lesion of MPCM is a hyperpigmented macula or slightly elevated papula. In adults, the mean diameter of the lesions is 3 mm [20]. Lesions occur in a symmetric and disseminated distribution; the trunk and thighs tend to have the highest density of lesions (fig. 1a). In some patients the lesions are few and not easily recognized (fig. 1b). When mechanically irritated, the lesions develop an edematous wheal. This reaction is referred to as Darier's sign. In children, lesions of MPCM are larger (mean diameter of 5 mm), and tend to be more hyperpigmented. The trunk is the most affected site. In addition, MPCM may have other clinical presentations that are less typical [10, 21]. Thus, MPCM may be telangiectatic and lack pigment (telangiectasia macularis eruptiva perstans), plaque-like (multiple mastocytomas) or nodular [10, 22].

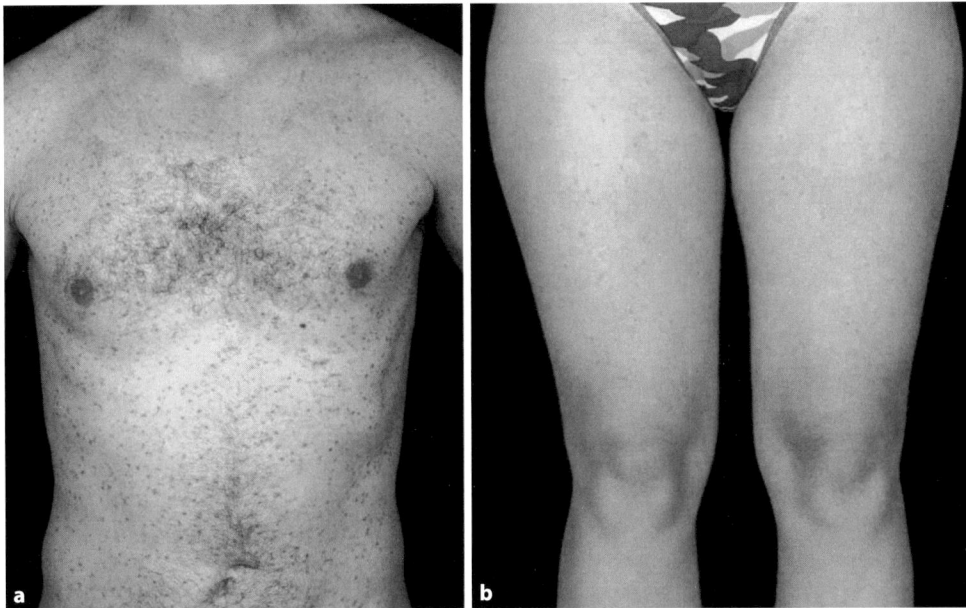

Fig. 1. Typical MPCM (urticaria pigmentosa) is the most common form of cutaneous mastocytosis. **a** In adults, lesions consist of numerous small red-brown macules and slightly elevated disseminated papules. **b** In less obvious cases, however, lesions are few or less well recognizable and may be overlooked.

Mastocytomas and diffuse cutaneous mastocytosis are further manifestations of cutaneous mastocytosis (CM) [9]. Solitary mastocytomas are common in children. Most are present at birth or develop in infancy. These lesions are flat or mildly elevated, well demarcated, solitary yellowish red-brown plaques or nodules, typically 2–5 cm in diameter. Diffuse cutaneous mastocytosis is a rare disorder characterized by diffuse mast cell infiltration of large areas of the skin that presents in infants in the first year of life. Severe edema and leathery indurations of the skin leads to accentuation of skin folds (pseudo-lichenified skin) and a peau-d'orange-like appearance. Systemic complications include hypotension and gastrointestinal hemorrhage. Infants and young children with considerable mast cell infiltration of the skin sometimes exhibit blister formation in the first 3 years of life. MPCM and other forms of CM have been classified in a consensus nomenclature (table 1) [10].

WHO Classification of Systemic Involvement
Whereas in children internal organ involvement (systemic mastocytosis, SM) is unusual, MPCM in adults is associated with SM in the majority of cases [10]. WHO criteria for SM consist of the major criterion of multifocal mast cell infiltrates in the bone marrow or other extracutaneous organ(s) and four minor criteria (table 2) [21]: 25% or more of mast cells in non-cutaneous biopsy sections with spindle-shaped or abnormal morphology, or

Table 1. Classification of cutaneous forms of mastocytosis [adapted from 10]

Maculopapular cutaneous mastocytosis/urticaria pigmentosa
Subvariants
Typical urticaria pigmentosa
Plaque-form
Nodular
Telangiectasia macularis eruptiva perstans
Diffuse cutaneous mastocytosis
Mastocytoma of skin

Table 2. Criteria for the diagnosis of systemic mastocytosis[1] [adapted from 10]

Major criterion
Multifocal dense infiltrates of mast cells in bone marrow and/or other extracutaneous organs
Minor criteria
More than 25% of the mast cells in the bone marrow smears or tissue biopsy sections are spindle shaped or display atypical morphology
Detection of a codon 816 *c-kit* point mutation in blood, bone marrow, or lesional tissue
Mast cells in the bone marrow, blood, or other lesional tissue expressing CD25 or CD2
Baseline total tryptase level persistently >20 ng/ml

[1] One major and one minor, or three minor criteria are needed for the diagnosis of systemic mastocytosis.

>25% of mast cells in bone marrow aspirate smears are immature or atypical; detection of a *c-kit* mutation at codon 816 in non-cutaneous organ(s); mast cells in extracutaneous organs co-expressing KIT with CD2 and/or CD25, and a baseline serum total tryptase persistently of >20 ng/ml. If at least one major and one minor, or at least three minor criteria for SM are fulfilled, the diagnosis is made. If the major criterion is absent and bone marrow mast cells are KIT+ and/or CD2+ and/or CD25+ in the presence of mediator-related symptoms, the findings are consistent with a clonal mast cell disorder MMAS [10]. Criteria defining the mast cell burden, involvement of non-mast cell lineages and aggressiveness of disease subclassify SM in subvariants (table 3) [21].

In children, CM is normally the only manifestation, and resolves in more than 50% of such cases during puberty [23]. Most adults fall into the indolent systemic

Table 3. WHO classification of mastocytosis [adapted from 10]

Cutaneous mastocytosis (CM)
Indolent systemic mastocytosis (ISM)
Subvariants:
Isolated bone marrow mastocytosis
Smouldering systemic mastocytosis
Systemic mastocytosis with an associated clonal hematologic non-mast cell lineage disease (SM-AHNMD)
Aggressive systemic mastocytosis
Subvariant:
Lymphadenopathic mastocytosis with eosinophilia
Mast cell leukemia
Mast cell sarcoma
Extracutaneous mastocytoma

mastocytosis (ISM) category [4, 17]. Although progression of skin involvement may occur, the disease tends to remain stable over many years and evolution of disease into more severe forms is uncommon [10]. Most adults with CM show focal or diffuse accumulations of mast cells in the bone marrow [9, 10]. Osteoporosis is not uncommon, and in occasional cases, osteopenia, sclerosis, cystic lesions and, in severe disease, pathologic fractures are reported [9, 10]. Patients with extensive disease may exhibit hepatomegaly, splenomegaly or lymphadenopathy caused by accumulation of mast cells in these organs. Anemia, thrombocytopenia and eosinophilia are less common.

Patients in the more aggressive categories are less likely to exhibit involvement of the skin and have a less favorable prognosis [10]. Those patients may have a definable hematological disorder such as a myelodysplastic syndrome, myeloproliferative disorder, acute leukemia, or a malignant lymphoma. In aggressive mastocytosis and mast cell leukemia, the clinical course is determined by the rapidity of the increase in mast cell numbers.

Mast Cell Mediator-Induced Symptoms
Some patients with mastocytosis report flushing, shortness of breath, palpitations, nausea, diarrhea, hypotension or even syncope [9, 24]. Lethargy and fatigue lasting several hours may follow. Gastrointestinal complaints are common in patients with SM [9, 24]. Abdominal pain is the most frequent symptom, followed by nausea,

diarrhea, and vomiting. Diarrhea is not generally related to gastric hypersecretion and has been attributed to altered intestinal secretion, structural mucosal abnormalities, and hypermotility [25]. These symptoms are believed to result in part from an excess release of mast cell mediators.

Patients sometimes describe recurrent spontaneous episodes with a single symptom or a combination of symptoms, and where findings sometimes resemble anaphylaxis. The presence, frequency and severity of these symptoms cannot be predicted by the degree of organ involvement, although such symptoms are considerably more frequent with systemic disease [25]. Severe or protracted anaphylaxis may occur in patients with extensive disease, and even fatal reactions have been described [26]. Those episodes may be IgE-mediated, as following a bee sting in a sensitized individual; although anaphylaxis in a patient with MMAS or SM may occur in the absence of demonstrable allergic sensitivity.

Mastocytosis and Anaphylaxis

Frequency of Anaphylaxis in Patients with Mastocytosis

The cumulative prevalence of anaphylaxis in adults with the diagnosis of mastocytosis has been reported to be as high as 49%, and thus is considerably higher than expected in the general population [4]. In another study, the frequency of anaphylaxis in adults with mastocytosis was reported to be 22% [5]. In children with CM, the prevalence was significantly lower and was reported to be 6 and 9%, respectively [4, 5]. One difference between these studies was the definition of anaphylaxis, for which there is yet no universal agreement. In addition to different patient populations, in the first study, anaphylaxis was more broadly defined according to World Allergy Organization criteria as a severe, life-threatening generalized or systemic hypersensitivity reaction [27]. In the second study, anaphylaxis was diagnosed only when more than one organ system symptoms were present or if there was a laryngeal edema [5], according to the recommendations of a consensus symposium [28]. In adults, those with SM had an increased risk for anaphylaxis as compared to patients with CM only [4]. In children, the risk to develop anaphylaxis was restricted to those with extensive skin involvement and high serum levels of tryptase [4].

Clinical Features of Anaphylaxis

The most frequent symptoms of anaphylaxis in patients with mastocytosis are decreased blood pressure and tachycardia. Also observed are dizziness, dyspnea, flushing, nausea and diarrhea [4]. Severe reactions are typical for patients with mastocytosis. In 55 patients with insect sting allergy and confirmed mastocytosis, 81% of patients experienced severe anaphylaxis with shock or cardiopulmonary arrest, whereas clinical reactions of this severity occurred in only 17% of 504 patients without evidence for mastocytosis and normal tryptase levels [29]. In another study in patients with mastocytosis, where the severity of anaphylaxis was rated, 60% reported severe symptoms and 43% experienced loss of consciousness [4]. In addition, there are reports of fatal anaphylactic reactions in patients with mastocytosis [26]. The risk for anaphylaxis appears not to be strictly associated with the mast cell load. For example, we care for patients with the smouldering variant of SM, which is characterized by a high mast cell load and highly elevated serum tryptase levels, and where we have yet to have a report of anaphylaxis.

Elicitors of Anaphylaxis

As in patients without SM, in patients with mastocytosis the most frequent reported elicitors of anaphylaxis are insect venoms, drugs and foods [4, 5]. Atopic diseases and the prevalence of allergy in patients with mastocytosis are similar to the prevalence in the general population [5]. Specific IgE antibodies were commonly found in patients with insect venom allergy, but not to drugs and foods [5, 7]. Foods were implicated in the onset of an anaphylactic episode by some patients with mastocytosis, but this was not confirmed following clinical evaluation. Specific IgE to relevant foods is seldom found [5]. There is insufficient evidence to conclude that histamine in foods can elicit systemic reactions in patients with mastocytosis. The hypothesis that patients with reduced levels of diaminooxidase (a histamine-degrading enzyme) may experience anaphylaxis following histamine intake is not supported by the observation that diaminooxidase levels were no different in patients with mastocytosis with and without anaphylaxis [4].

Some drugs reported to elicit anaphylaxis in patients with mastocytosis [4, 5], such as opiates (including morphine and codeine) and muscle relaxants, may in some instances, directly activate mast cells in some, but not all, patients. Severe anaphylactoid reactions as well as coagulopathy have been reported in a few patients with mastocytosis undergoing general anesthesia, or following upper gastrointestinal endoscopy [9]. Other pharmaceutical agents, such as aspirin (acetylsalicylic acid) and other NSAIDs and alcohol, are described to elicit pseudo-allergic reactions in a subset of patients with mastocytosis and have been reported to be augmentation factors for IgE-mediated allergic reactions. Antibiotics (such as betalactams) and radiocontrast media are also associated with episodes of anaphylaxis in some patients with and without mastocytosis [4].

Hymenoptera venom is a prominent trigger of systemic reactions. Severe and fatal reactions have been described in patients with mastocytosis [9, 30, 31]. In few cases with urticaria pigmentosa and Hymenoptera venom anaphylaxis, no sensitization could be detected by means of skin tests and determination of specific IgE antibodies [32]. However, larger series found evidence that these systemic reactions are normally IgE-mediated insect sting allergies [7, 33].

Physical factors, such as heat, mechanical stimulation and exercise, may sometimes lead to mast cell degranulation and whealing in the skin, but rarely provoke systemic anaphylaxis [4, 26]. Patients do report that these and other factors in combination (such as exercise, heat and alcohol) may elicit anaphylaxis in summation.

In one study, 26% of anaphylactic reactions were reported to have developed after a combination of elicitors [4]. In other patients with mastocytosis, anaphylaxis remains idiopathic despite an extensive search for an allergic basis.

Diagnosis

Mastocytosis is recognized in most patients because of the presence of characteristic cutaneous lesions [10]. A positive Darier's sign and/or histological examination of the skin using metachromatic stains, or by immunohistochemistry using antibodies to mast cell tryptase, helps confirm the diagnosis of cutaneous disease.

Different forms of precursor and mature forms of mast cell tryptase have been described, namely α-, β-, γ-, and δ-tryptase [34]. The monoclonal antibodies prepared against tryptase used in the assay commercially available (Phadia, Uppsala, Sweden) recognize mature and precursor forms of α- and β-tryptases only, whereas the other forms are either not recognized or not present in human mast cells. This is clinically relevant, because α/β-tryptase precursors seem to be continuously secreted by human mast cells, their level in the serum probably providing a measure of systemic mast cell involvement, whereas mature tryptase, presumably β-tryptase, is stored in secretory granules and is released only during granule exocytosis, with levels thereby reflecting mast cell activation.

Thus, whereas biochemical demonstration of elevated serum levels of total (α/β-) mast cell tryptase (>20 ng/ml) raises the suspicion of SM, in CM, tryptase levels tend to be within the normal range. Particularly in adults with CM and elevated serum tryptase, bone marrow biopsy and aspiration should be considered for staging of disease and for exclusion of associated hematological abnormalities. The most sensitive method to support the diagnosis of SM in the bone marrow aspirate is to identify the co-expression of CD2 and/or CD25 in CD117 (KIT)-positive mast cells by flow cytometry or by immunohistochemical analysis of bone marrow biopsies [35, 36]. In addition, a c-*kit* mutational analysis should be performed [37]. The D816V point mutation is best detected in bone marrow tissues, where the number of malignant mast cells is high. The diagnosis of SM and determination of the subcategory is made according to WHO criteria [21]. In patients with SM, the size of the liver and spleen may be evaluated by ultrasound or CT. Bone density is determined by the DXA method because of the risk of osteoporosis.

If patients have experienced anaphylaxis, the identification of any possible elicitor is important to help avoid further episodes. With skin tests and specific IgE antibodies combined with history, a relevant allergy may be detected. Cellular tests monitoring basophil histamine release or basophil activation may be helpful in some patients who resist diagnosis by standard means [26, 31].

Mastocytosis may present as anaphylaxis [9]. Sometimes the diagnosis of MPCM is made during the course of the evaluation of an anaphylactic episode. Thus in all patients with anaphylaxis, a skin examination should be performed to exclude CM [26]. Basal serum tryptase level should be determined. As serum tryptase levels may stay elevated for several hours after severe anaphylaxis, it is important to repeat the determination after some days. In cases with anaphylaxis and basal tryptase values >20 ng/ml, a bone marrow biopsy to exclude SM may be warranted. This examination may also be considered in patients with recurrent anaphylactic episodes even without clearly elevated tryptase levels. There have been cases with idiopathic anaphylaxis in whom the diagnosis of SM was made by bone marrow biopsy [26, 32].

The activating D816V KIT mutation and other minor criteria for the diagnosis of mastocytosis have been reported in some patients with anaphylaxis who do not meet the full diagnostic criteria for mastocytosis [8]. In a report on 12 patients with unexplained anaphylaxis, who neither exhibited urticaria pigmentosa nor the characteristic bone marrow biopsy finding of multifocal mast cell aggregates for SM, 5 patients had evidence of one or more minor criteria for mastocytosis [6]. The D816V KIT mutation was found in all 3 patients in CD25+ bone marrow cells where the analysis was performed. This report and others led a consensus conference to conclude that if the major criterion for the diagnosis of mastocytosis is absent and bone marrow mast cells are KIT+ and/or CD2+ and/or CD25+ in the presence of mediator-related symptoms, the diagnosis should be MMAS [10].

In a later study, the incidence of a clonal mast cell disorder (either mastocytosis or MMAS) was assessed in 44 subjects with a serum baseline total tryptase level >11.4 ng/ml who were among 379 patients with a prior systemic immediate hypersensitivity reaction to a Hymenoptera sting. Resultant data indicated that the majority of these patients had an underlying clonal mast cell disorder, either SM or MMAS, by assessing the bone marrow for mast cell granulomas, spindle-shaped mast cells and mast cells expressing surface CD2 or CD25, and the serum for an elevated tryptase level [7]. These results demonstrate the presence of an aberrant mast cell population carrying clonal markers in patients diagnosed with idiopathic or Hymenoptera venom anaphylaxis. In patients with anaphylaxis and increased serum tryptase levels, a BM examination may thus be indicated for the diagnosis of a clonal mast cell disease.

Therapy

There is no cure for mastocytosis and treatment remains largely symptomatic [2, 9, 10]. All patients with mastocytosis should be informed about the disease, including prognosis and complications. Therapy for mastocytosis encompasses avoidance of trigger factors, targeting symptoms of mast cell mediator release and therapy of skin lesions. Cytoreductive forms of treatment are only indicated in patients with aggressive mastocytosis, or an associated hematological disorder, including mast cell leukemia.

Table 4. Triggers for mast cell mediator release[1]

Mechanical irritation of the skin (rubbing, scratching, friction)
Heat (e.g. hot shower), cold, sudden change of temperature
Physical exercise
Insect stings (e.g. bee and wasp stings)
Drugs (radiocontrast media, drugs used in general anesthesia, codeine morphine, dextromethorphan, aspirin, and other analgesics)
Infection
Alcohol

[1] Note not all patients with mastocytosis have reactions provoked by all factors. For example, many patients with mastocytosis tolerate radiocontrast media, anesthesia, morphine, dextrometorphan, aspirin, and other analgesics. When in question, patients should undergo graded challenges to determine sensitivity.

Avoidance of Trigger Factors and Treatment of Anaphylaxis

Specific information on trigger factors and signs of mast cell degranulation, potentially leading to anaphylactic reactions, should to be provided. A list of trigger factors known to induce symptoms in patients is given in table 4 [9]. Not all patients with mastocytosis have reactions provoked by all factors. For example, many patients with mastocytosis tolerate radiocontrast media, anesthesia, morphine, dextrometorphan, aspirin, and other analgesics. When in question, patients should undergo graded challenges to determine sensitivity.

It has been stated that adults with mastocytosis as well as children with bullous lesions and with more severe involvement, and especially those with previous reactions, are at increased risk for anaphylaxis [4]. Thus, we recommend that patients at risk carry an emergency kit for self-medication which includes epinephrine and, as warranted, an antihistamine and a corticosteroid [38].

Patients with mastocytosis also have to be considered at increased risk when administered iodinated contrast media, when undergoing general anesthesia, or during endoscopic procedures. Protocols aiming at ameliorating these reactions employ premedication with H_1- and H_2-antihistamines, sometimes corticosteroids depending upon the procedure, and availability of means of resuscitation [26]. In 22 children with mastocytosis, the frequency and adverse reactions to routine anesthesia was assessed [39]. In 29 anesthetic procedures, including 24 cases with general anesthesia, these procedures were tolerated with the exception of 2 cases with flushing and 4 cases with nausea and/or vomiting even without specific premedication. Thus, as long as the anesthetist is informed about the patient and regular stabilizing medications are continued, at least in children, a premedication may not be routinely necessary before general anesthesia.

Diet should be modified only in cases where foods have been proven to elicit symptoms. Patients with mastocytosis and Hymenoptera venom exposure are at risk for severe anaphylaxis. Thus, specific immunotherapy should be considered in patients with Hymenoptera venom allergy and then administered under close supervision [31]. The majority of patients with mastocytosis reportedly tolerate immunotherapy without significant side effects and appear protected following this approach [33, 40]. However, there does appear to be some increased risk for adverse reactions during initiation of immunotherapy, as well as for therapy failures [31, 33]. An increased maintenance dose of insect venom has been reported to carry better success rates by sting provocation [41]. Also, in the light of 2 fatal cases of anaphylaxis after discontinuation of SIT in patients with mastocytosis [30], lifelong immunotherapy should be considered [26].

In rare cases, initiation of specific immunotherapy with insect venom leads to recurrent anaphylaxis, even with antihistamine premedication. In those cases, co-medication with omalizumab (anti-IgE) has been reported to induce tolerance. In a case of recurrent anaphylaxis to induction of specific immunotherapy, the injection of 300 mg of omalizumab between 4 days and 1 h reportedly led to tolerance [42]. This approach also appears worthy of consideration in patients with both idiopathic recurrent anaphylaxis and mastocytosis who do not respond to standard antimediator therapy, as has been described in 2 atopic patients with ISM [43]. Most patients with mastocytosis and idiopathic anaphylaxis, however, are sufficiently controlled by standard antimediator therapy with antihistamines with or without low-dose corticosteroids.

Therapy of Mast Cell Mediator-Induced Symptoms
Recommendations for the treatment of mastocytosis have been published [10]. In brief, non-sedating H_1-antihistamines are the agents of choice for pruritus and associated wheal and flare of skin lesions. For prophylaxis of recurrent episodes of anaphylaxis or persistent pruritus, antihistamines should be administered daily. Gastric acid hypersecretion, peptic ulcer disease, and reflux esophagitis may be managed with H_2-receptor blockers and/or proton pump inhibitors. Cromolyn sodium may be helpful for gastrointestinal symptoms, particularly in children. Anticholinergics may be tried to control diarrhea. Systemic corticosteroids are used restrictedly in cases of malabsorption or ascites. Calcium, vitamin D and bisphosphonates are the drugs of choice for osteoporosis.

Therapy of Skin Lesions
Application of topical corticosteroids under occlusion, or UV therapy (PUVA, UVA1) has been reported to lead to dermatologic improvement in patients with CM [9]. Both are effective in reducing pruritus and urtication, but relapse typically occurs

a few months after therapy is discontinued. The benefits of these forms of therapy have to be weighed against the potential for inducing side effects. Thus, topical corticosteroids should be considered primarily for the treatment of localized skin lesions, such as mastocytomas causing flushing or blistering. Topical treatment with the raft modulator miltefosine has been tried as a novel therapeutic option for mastocytosis [44]. However, twice daily application of miltefosine solution led to irritation rather than reduction of skin swelling and skin numbers, possibly due to the presence of potentially irritating alkanol propandiol as a vehicle.

Therapy of Aggressive Forms of Mastocytosis

Patients with SM-AHNMD are managed using therapy appropriate for the associated hematological disorder [2, 10]. Chemotherapy has not been shown to produce remission or to effectively prolong survival in patients with mast cell leukemia, and is not indicated in the management of ISM, as it may lead to bone marrow suppression without improving the symptoms of mastocytosis. A partial response to interferon-α_{2b}, often in combination with corticosteroids, has been reported in some patients with aggressive disease [2]. Cladribine (2-cholorodeoxyadenosine) has been reported to reduce the mast cell burden in case reports and may be used in aggressive mastocytosis [2]. It should be considered however that cladribine can induce pancytopenia, and has an unknown potential oncogenicity. Splenectomy may be performed in the management of patients with aggressive mastocytosis and hypersplenism leading to portal hypertension.

Newer therapeutic approaches being investigated target neoplastic mast cells bearing CD25, or inhibit tumor necrosis factor (thalidomide, lenalidomide) [2]. Bone marrow transplantation is under investigation, although results to date have been disappointing or have to be reproduced [2].

The tyrosine kinase inhibitor imatinib is not generally indicated in patients with typical D816V mutations in KIT, as steric conformations of the receptor interfere with the action of the drug [45]. The drug has been reported to reduce mast cell load and symptoms in patients with mutations in *c-kit* at other sites [46]. Other tyrosine kinase inhibitors, such as dasatinib, PKC412 and AMN 107, inhibit KIT with mutations at codon 816. Data available indicate a somewhat limited effect of these drugs on aggressive mast cell disease and/or significant toxicity [2]. It has been proposed that a multiple drug approach using combination therapy with targeted agents that have different mechanisms of action be considered [2].

Acknowledgement

This work was in part supported by the Division of Intramural Research, NIAID/NIH.

References

1 Metz M, Brockow K, Metcalfe DD, Galli SJ: Mast cells, basophils and mastocytosis; in Rich, Fleisher, Shearer, et al (eds): Clinical Immunology – Principles and Practice. New York, Mosby, 2008, pp 22.21–22.16.

2 Metcalfe DD: Mast cells and mastocytosis. Blood 2008;112:946–956.

3 Tkaczyk C, Horejsi V, Iwaki S, et al: NTAL phosphorylation is a pivotal link between the signaling cascades leading to human mast cell degranulation following Kit activation and Fc epsilon RI aggregation. Blood 2004;104:207–214.

4 Brockow K, Jofer C, Behrendt H, Ring J: Anaphylaxis in patients with mastocytosis: a study on history, clinical features and risk factors in 120 patients. Allergy 2008;63:226–232.

5 Gonzalez de Olano D, de la Hoz Caballer B, Nunez Lopez R, et al: Prevalence of allergy and anaphylactic symptoms in 210 adult and pediatric patients with mastocytosis in Spain: a study of the Spanish Network on Mastocytosis (REMA). Clin Exp Allergy 2007;37:1547–1555.

6 Akin C, Scott LM, Kocabas CN, et al: Demonstration of an aberrant mast-cell population with clonal markers in a subset of patients with 'idiopathic' anaphylaxis. Blood 2007;110:2331–2333.

7 Bonadonna P, Perbellini O, Passalacqua G, et al: Clonal mast cell disorders in patients with systemic reactions to Hymenoptera stings and increased serum tryptase levels. J Allergy Clin Immunol 2009;123:680–686.

8 Sonneck K, Florian S, Mullauer L, et al: Diagnostic and subdiagnostic accumulation of mast cells in the bone marrow of patients with anaphylaxis: monoclonal mast cell activation syndrome. Int Arch Allergy Immunol 2007;142:158–164.

9 Brockow K: Urticaria pigmentosa. Immunol Allergy Clin North Am 2004;24:287–316.

10 Valent P, Akin C, Escribano L, et al: Standards and standardization in mastocytosis: consensus statements on diagnostics, treatment recommendations and response criteria. Eur J Clin Invest 2007;37:435–453.

11 Brockow K, Metcalfe DD: Mastocytosis. Curr Opin Allergy Clin Immunol 2001;1:449–454.

12 Akin C, Metcalfe DD: The biology of Kit in disease and the application of pharmacogenetics. J Allergy Clin Immunol 2004;114:13–19.

13 Longley BJ Jr, Morganroth GS, Tyrrell L, et al: Altered metabolism of mast-cell growth factor (c-kit ligand) in cutaneous mastocytosis. N Engl J Med 1993;328:1302–1307.

14 Brockow K, Akin C, Huber M, et al: Levels of mast-cell growth factors in plasma and in suction skin blister fluid in adults with mastocytosis: correlation with dermal mast- cell numbers and mast-cell tryptase. J Allergy Clin Immunol 2002;109:82–88.

15 Orfao A, Garcia-Montero AC, Sanchez L, Escribano L: Recent advances in the understanding of mastocytosis: the role of KIT mutations. Br J Haematol 2007;138:12–30.

16 Nagata H, Worobec AS, Oh CK, et al: Identification of a point mutation in the catalytic domain of the protooncogene c-kit in peripheral blood mononuclear cells of patients who have mastocytosis with an associated hematologic disorder. Proc Natl Acad Sci USA 1995;92:10560–10564.

17 Garcia-Montero AC, Jara-Acevedo M, Teodosio C, et al: KIT mutation in mast cells and other bone marrow hematopoietic cell lineages in systemic mast cell disorders: a prospective study of the Spanish Network on Mastocytosis (REMA) in a series of 113 patients. Blood 2006;108:2366–2372.

18 Daley T, Metcalfe DD, Akin C: Association of the Q576R polymorphism in the interleukin-4 receptor α chain with indolent mastocytosis limited to the skin. Blood 2001;98:880–882.

19 Gilfillan AM, Peavy RD, Metcalfe DD: Amplification mechanisms for the enhancement of antigen-mediated mast cell activation. Immunol Res 2009;43:15–24.

20 Brockow K, Akin C, Huber M, Metcalfe D: Assessment of the extent of cutaneous involvement in children and adults with mastocytosis: relationship to symptomatology, tryptase levels, and bone marrow pathology. J Am Acad Dermatol 2003;48:508–516.

21 Valent P, Horny H, Li C, et al: Mastocytosis; in Jaffe E, Harris N, Stein H, Vardiman J (eds): World Health Organization Classification of Tumors. Pathology and Genetics of Tumors of Hematopoietic and Lymphoid Tissue. Lyon, IARC Press, 2001, pp 293–302.

22 Simpson JK, Brockow K, Turner ML, et al: Generalized erythematous macules and plaques associated with flushing, repeated syncope, and refractory anemia. J Am Acad Dermatol 2002;46:588–590.

23 Caplan RM: The natural course of urticaria pigmentosa. Arch Dermatol 1963;87:146–157.

24 Horan RF, Austen KF: Systemic mastocytosis: retrospective review of a decade's clinical experience at the Brigham and Women's Hospital. J Invest Dermatol 1991;96:5S–13S.

25 Travis WD, Li CY, Bergstralh EJ, et al: Systemic mast cell disease. Analysis of 58 cases and literature review Medicine (Baltimore) 1988;67:345–368 Published erratum appears in Medicine (Baltimore) 1990;69:34.

26 Brockow K, Ring J, Przybilla B, Ruëff F: Klinik und Therapie der Anaphylaxie bei Mastozytose. Allergo J 2008;17:556–562.

27 Johansson SG, Bieber T, Dahl R, et al: Revised nomenclature for allergy for global use: report of the Nomenclature Review Committee of the World Allergy Organization, October 2003. J Allergy Clin Immunol 2004;113:832–836.

28 Sampson HA, Munoz-Furlong A, Campbell RL, et al: Second symposium on the definition and management of anaphylaxis: summary report–Second National Institute of Allergy and Infectious Disease/ Food Allergy and Anaphylaxis Network symposium. J Allergy Clin Immunol 2006;117:391–397.

29 Ludolph-Hauser D, Rueff F, Fries C, et al: Constitutively raised serum concentrations of mast-cell tryptase and severe anaphylactic reactions to Hymenoptera stings. Lancet 2001;357:361–362.

30 Oude Elberink JN, de Monchy JG, Kors JW, et al: Fatal anaphylaxis after a yellow jacket sting, despite venom immunotherapy, in two patients with mastocytosis. J Allergy Clin Immunol 1997;99:153–154.

31 Rueff F, Placzek M, Przybilla B: Mastocytosis and Hymenoptera venom allergy. Curr Opin Allergy Clin Immunol 2006;6:284–288.

32 Florian S, Krauth MT, Simonitsch-Klupp I, et al: Indolent systemic mastocytosis with elevated serum tryptase, absence of skin lesions, and recurrent severe anaphylactoid episodes. Int Arch Allergy Immunol 2005;136:273–280.

33 Gonzalez de Olano D, Alvarez-Twose I, Esteban-Lopez MI, et al: Safety and effectiveness of immunotherapy in patients with indolent systemic mastocytosis presenting with Hymenoptera venom anaphylaxis. J Allergy Clin Immunol 2008;121:519–526.

34 Schwartz LB: Diagnostic value of tryptase in anaphylaxis and mastocytosis. Immunol Allergy Clin N Am 2006;451–463.

35 Escribano L, Orfao A, Diaz-Agustin B, et al: Indolent systemic mast cell disease in adults: immunophenotypic characterization of bone marrow mast cells and its diagnostic implications. Blood 1998;91:2731–2736.

36 Horny HP, Valent P: Histopathological and immunohistochemical aspects of mastocytosis. Int Arch Allergy Immunol 2002;127:115–117.

37 Sotlar K, Escribano L, Landt O, et al: One-step detection of c-kit point mutations using peptide nucleic acid-mediated polymerase chain reaction clamping and hybridization probes. Am J Pathol 2003;162:737–746.

38 Ring J, Brockow K, Duda D, et al: Akuttherapie anaphylaktischer Reaktionen. Allergo J 2007;16:420–434.

39 Carter MC, Uzzaman A, Scott LM, et al: Pediatric mastocytosis: routine anesthetic management for a complex disease. Anesth Analg 2008;107:422–427.

40 Bonadonna P, Zanotti R, Caruso B, et al: Allergen-specific immunotherapy is safe and effective in patients with systemic mastocytosis and Hymenoptera allergy. J Allergy Clin Immunol 2008;121:256–257.

41 Rueff F, Wenderoth A, Przybilla B: Patients still reacting to a sting challenge while receiving conventional Hymenoptera venom immunotherapy are protected by increased venom doses. J Allergy Clin Immunol 2001;108:1027–1032.

42 Kontou-Fili K: High omalizumab dose controls recurrent reactions to venom immunotherapy in indolent systemic mastocytosis. Allergy 2008;63:376–378.

43 Carter MC, Robyn JA, Bressler PB, et al: Omalizumab for the treatment of unprovoked anaphylaxis in patients with systemic mastocytosis. J Allergy Clin Immunol 2007;119:1550–1551.

44 Hartmann K, Siebenhaar F, Belloni B, et al: Topical treatment with the raft modulator miltefosine – a novel therapeutic option for mastocytosis? Br J Dermatol, in press.

45 Akin C, Brockow K, D'Ambrosio C, et al: Effects of tyrosine kinase inhibitor STI571 on human mast cells bearing wild-type or mutated c-kit. Exp Hematol 2003;31:686–692.

46 Akin C, Fumo G, Yavuz AS, et al: A novel form of mastocytosis associated with a transmembrane c-kit mutation and response to imatinib. Blood 2004;103:3222–3225.

Dr. Knut Brockow
Department of Dermatology and Allergy Biederstein, Technische Universität München
Biedersteiner Strasse 29, DE–80802 Munich (Germany)
Tel. +49 89 41400, Fax +49 89 4140 3171
E-Mail knut.brockow@lrz.tum.de

Ring J (ed): Anaphylaxis. Chem Immunol Allergy. Basel, Karger, 2010, vol 95, pp 125–140

In vitro Diagnosis of Anaphylaxis

María L. Sanz[a] · P.M. Gamboa[b] · B.E. García-Figueroa[c] · M. Ferrer[a]

[a]Department Allergology and Clinical Immunology, Clinica Universidad de Navarra, Pamplona; [b]Allergy Service Basurto Hospital, Bilbao, and [c]Allergy Section, Virgen del Camino Hospital, Pamplona, Spain

Abstract

The application and development of new in vitro techniques aims to enable a diagnosis to be reached while incurring no risk for the patient, a situation which is particularly desirable in the case of severe reactions like anaphylaxis. The in vitro diagnosis of anaphylaxis includes, among other aspects, the serial measurement of mediators which are released in the course of an anaphylactic reaction such as tryptase, histamine, chymase, carboxypeptidase A3, platelet-activating factor and other products from mastocytes. The detection of agents which trigger the anaphylactic reaction can be made with the use of serologic methods: serum-specific IgE or with cellular tests which measure the release of basophil mediators (leukotrienes, histamine) or with the analysis of the expression of basophil markers, a technique known as the basophil activation test. These techniques offer interesting alternatives in the diagnosis of anaphylaxis. The basophil activation test provides important advantages in patients with anaphylaxis to β-lactams, non-steroidal anti-inflammatory drugs, neuromuscular blocking agents and drugs where there is no technique to measure specific IgE.

The application and development of new in vitro diagnostic techniques aims to enable physicians to reach an allergy diagnosis with no risk for the patient. This is particularly desirable in the case of serious reactions such as anaphylaxis, by confirming the existence of an anaphylactic reaction and differentiating between individuals which present with sensitization but no clinical symptoms following exposure to the allergen from those that show a serious clinical reaction.

In general, the in vitro diagnosis of anaphylaxis includes, amongst others, the serial measurement of mediators such as tryptase, as well as other mediators such as histamine, chymase, carboxypeptidase A3, platelet-activating factor and other products of mastocytes. The identification of the allergens triggering such reactions occupies an important place in this chapter on the in vitro diagnosis of anaphylaxis and together with the determination of specific IgE or the quantification of basophil activation markers following their activation by the allergen using flow cytometry or the production of mediators following cell activation offer us interesting alternatives in the diagnosis of anaphylaxis.

Over the last decade, new perspectives have been opened up with the use of natural purified and/or recombinant allergens for the molecular diagnosis of allergy which will provide us with precise information for the diagnosis of clinical reactions experienced by patients and which are particularly applicable to the diagnosis of anaphylaxis.

Diagnosis of Anaphylactic Reaction

Mediators in Anaphylaxis

The latest consensus on the definition and management [1] of anaphylaxis agrees on the lack of universally accepted diagnostic criteria and reliable laboratory biomarkers to confirm the clinical impression. Sometimes it is not feasible to obtain the samples within the optimum time frame. Moreover, in spite of a correct collection of samples, histamine and/or tryptase are within normal levels. Hence, new markers should be explored and further research into the role of selected mediators is urgently needed. Recently however, studies from animal models have shown promising results. In this chapter we will seek to review our current knowledge on confirmed or putative markers for the in vitro diagnosis of anaphylaxis.

Histamine
Histamine is a critical mediator in anaphylactic reactions. It is a diamine produced by decarboxylation of the amino acid histidine in the Golgi apparatus of mast cells and basophils. Once secreted, it is rapidly metabolized by histamine methyltransferase [2]. Plasma histamine levels are elevated in anaphylaxis, reaching a concentration peak at 5 min and declining to baseline by 30–60 min [3]. Therefore, histamine samples for assessing an anaphylactic reaction should be obtained within 15 min of the onset of the reaction. Urinary metabolites of histamine may be found for up to 24 h.

Tryptase
Tryptase is a serine esterase with a molecular weight of 110–130 kDa. Tryptase binds to heparin or other proteoglycans through its cationic groove. Heparin-stabilized tetramers of tryptase are stored in mast cell granules [4]. It is the principal component of mast cells secretory granules accounting for as much as 25% of cell protein. Basophils are the only other cell type that also contain tryptase but in a much lower amount [5, 6]. Tryptase is secreted as a larger active proteoglycan complex that limits tissue diffusion allowing detection of tryptase in fluids for a longer period than histamine.

Tryptase is at the present moment the main clinical marker for anaphylaxis and mastocytosis. There are two major human mast cells tryptases, α- and β-tryptase, encoded by two genes located at chromosome 16. The haploid genotype for tryptase is βα or ββ. 25% of individuals are α-tryptase-deficient; α-tryptase shows a 90% amino acid sequence identity with β-tryptase.

α/β-Protryptases are spontaneously secreted by resting mast cells. Mature β-tryptase is stored within mast cell granules and is secreted upon mast cell activation. The main biological substrate of tryptase has not been fully described. There is no direct evidence of a role for tryptases in the pathogenesis of asthma and allergic inflammation. It may act by spreading a degranulation signal from mast cell to mast cell.

Two immunoassays have been developed to measure tryptase in human fluids, one that measures mature α/β-tryptases, i.e. total tryptase, available commercially, and one developed by Schwartz et al. [7] that measures both mature β-tryptase and immature α/β-tryptases. This distinction is of clinical relevance since immature tryptases reflect mast cell burden whereas mature tryptases indicate mast cell activation. Thus, for the diagnosis of anaphylaxis it would be extremely important to be able to differentiate between acute anaphylaxis and increases in tryptase due to increase in numbers of mast cells as happens in mastocytosis. Total tryptase would be high in both conditions, whereas mature tryptase will be only high in anaphylaxis but negligible in mastocytosis.

In healthy subjects, mature tryptase levels in serum and plasma are undetectable (<1 ng/ml) whereas total tryptase levels range from 1 to 15 ng/ml. Gender or haplotype does not affect amounts of total tryptase.

After an anaphylactic reaction induced by Hymenoptera sting [8], β-tryptase levels in circulation are maximal between 15 and 120 min. For that reason, sampling is recommended 60–120 min after the reaction. The levels of tryptase correlate with the blood pressure drop, thus reflecting the severity of the reaction. There are also reports that indicate that elevated tryptase levels postmortem serve as an indicator of premortem anaphylaxis [9]. However, high serum tryptase levels in a postmortem specimen by itself might be insufficient for the diagnosis of anaphylaxis since tryptase could increase non-specifically. Interestingly, tryptase levels are much higher with venom-induced anaphylaxis than with food-induced anaphylaxis. This might be the reason why after anaphylaxis induced by food allergens even with severe clinical symptoms, often mature tryptase is not elevated [9]. This may be because mast cells are not the effector cell in such reactions.

Finally, it is worth mentioning that tryptase levels do not differentiate between immunologic and non-immunological mast cell activation and do not contribute to the identification of the cause of the anaphylactic reaction. To date, very few mediators [10] apart from histamine and tryptase have been investigated as markers for anaphylaxis. Recent studies also include other mediators that we will only examine briefly. A more extensive review can be found elsewhere [2, 11].

Chymase

As is the case with tryptase, chymase is also stored in mast cell granules. This mediator can activate the angiotensin system converting angiotensin I to angiotensin II. With this action it compensates the intravascular loss of volume and the permeability increase that occurs in an anaphylaxis reaction. This is why angiotensin-converting enzyme inhibitors could inhibit this compensatory effect and may predispose at-risk patients to anaphylaxis. The first report of the usefulness of chymase [12] was based on the examination of 8 autopsy cases with anaphylaxis and 104 control cases without anaphylaxis. Chymase was detected in all 8 cases with anaphylaxis while it was detected in only 2 of the 104 controls. The authors found a significant correlation with tryptase. Moreover, chymase was quite stable in serum.

More recently, the same group [13] found positive chymase staining in lung mast cells from postmortem samples after fatal anaphylactic drug reactions.

Mast Cell Carboxypeptidase A3
Mast cell protease A3 is less well characterized than tryptase and chymase in terms of physiological substrates. It is involved, among its other functions, in angiotensin metabolism.

Platelet-Activation Factor
This mediator, apart from aggregating platelets and stimulating many cells types, is a very potent mediator in allergic reactions causing bronchoconstriction with a 1,000 times more potency than histamine. It is able to increase vascular permeability and cause chemotaxis and degranulation of eosinophils and neutrophils [14–16].

Finally, other mediators such as leukotrienes and prostaglandins may also play a role. Denzlinger et al. [17] first reported an increase in urinary leukotriene E_4 in anaphylactic reactions. This has been recently confirmed [18], along with an increase in $9\alpha,11\beta$-PGF_2 concentrations during anaphylaxis.

Diagnostic Tools for the Identification of Anaphylaxis-Triggering Allergens

The detection of reactions mediated by specific IgE to agents triggering anaphylaxis may be achieved by means of serological methods: serum-specific IgE, or by means of cellular tests which determine the release of basophil mediators (leukotrienes and histamine) or by means of the analysis of basophil expression markers, a technique known as the basophil activation test (BAT).

The principle underlying the BAT is that the attachment of the antigen to the IgE present on the surface of the basophil leads to the activation of the basophil and the release of its mediators (histamine, leukotrienes, prostaglandins, etc.) and the expression on its membrane of molecules such as CD63, CD203c or others which are markers of basophil activation. The basophils are identified with monoclonal antibodies marked with fluorochromes and anti-IgE and anti-CD63 receptors [for a complete review, we suggest readers read references 19–22].

We will now provide an overview of the results obtained using these technologies for the most common elicitors of anaphylaxis.

Drugs

β-Lactam Antibiotics

The β-lactams (penicillins and their derivatives) are the drugs which most frequently cause IgE-mediated anaphylactic reactions. Diagnosis is based on skin tests. To date, the best validated in vitro diagnostic methods are specific IgE and BAT. As for the determination of specific IgE using ImmunoCap (Phadia AB, Uppsala, Sweden), the sensitivity of the technique in the diagnosis of immediate reaction to β-lactams with positive skin test ranges, according to the study, from 37 to 54% with a specificity of between 83 and 100% [23, 24].

In patients allergic to β-lactams with negative skin tests but positive oral challenge tests, the sensitivity of the technique is 42% according to a study carried out by Blanca et al. [24]. In everyday clinical practice a drop in the sensitivity of CAP to β-lactams has been observed in recent years as a result of changes in the type of β-lactam currently consumed, with a tendency towards greater use of aminopenicillins and cephalosporins, which entails a change in the pattern of specificities recognized by the IgE. This means that the haptens currently available in ImmunoCap, benzylpenicillin, penicillin V and amoxicillin, may give false-negatives because of this change. Thus, it is a proven fact that the antigenic determinants of β-lactams in in vitro tests are inadequate for the evaluation of patients with immediate reactions to these drugs and consequently it is necessary to broaden the number of antigenic determinants in which cephalosporins should also be included [20].

As for the results obtained with BAT for β-lactams, this technique provides four important advantages as compared to the determination of specific IgE: (a) greater specificity: 93% for BAT vs. 86% for specific IgE. (b) Greater sensitivity: depending on the technique used sensitivity for BAT ranges from 48 to 50% vs. 37 to 44% for CAP [23, 25]. (c) The ability of BAT to diagnose sensitization to cephalosporins, where sensitivity ranges from 50 to 77% in the cases studied [23, 25]. (d) Detection of patients sensitized to β-lactams with negative skin tests and negative in vitro specific IgE, thus avoiding the use of potentially dangerous challenge tests. In this type of patient, sensitivity ranges from 14% [25] to 33% [26] (fig. 1–5).

Neuromuscular Blocking Agents (NMBA)

NMBAs are the main agents triggering anaphylactic reactions during anesthesia, both by means of IgE-mediated reactions and anaphylactoid reactions. Commercially, suxamethone is the only NMBD for which the possibility exists of determining specific IgE using ImmunoCap (c202, Phadia AB), with a low sensitivity which ranges from 30 to 60% depending on the study [27–30]. Non-commercial prototypes currently exist which include morphine, rocuronium and pholcodine with high levels of sensitivity (60–80%) and specificity (93–100%) [31]. These excellent results have meant that an important part of studies published on BAT and drug-allergic reactions have focused on the analysis of this type of drug. Since the first validation study in this area

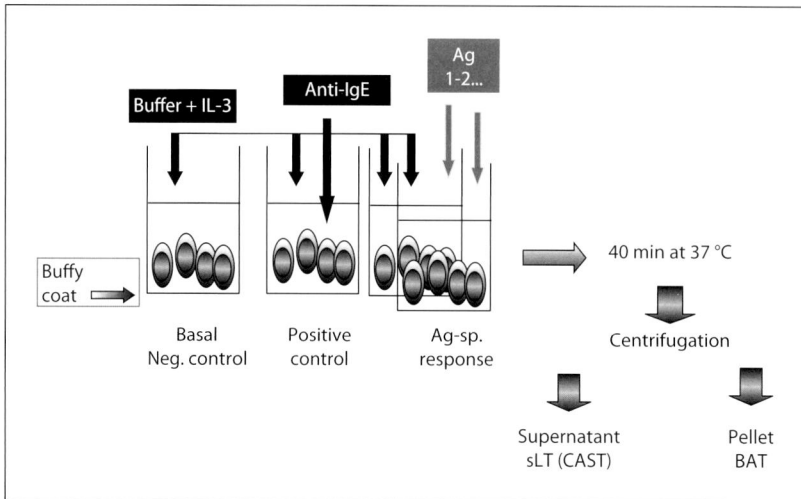

Fig. 1. BAT technique. Stimulation phase.

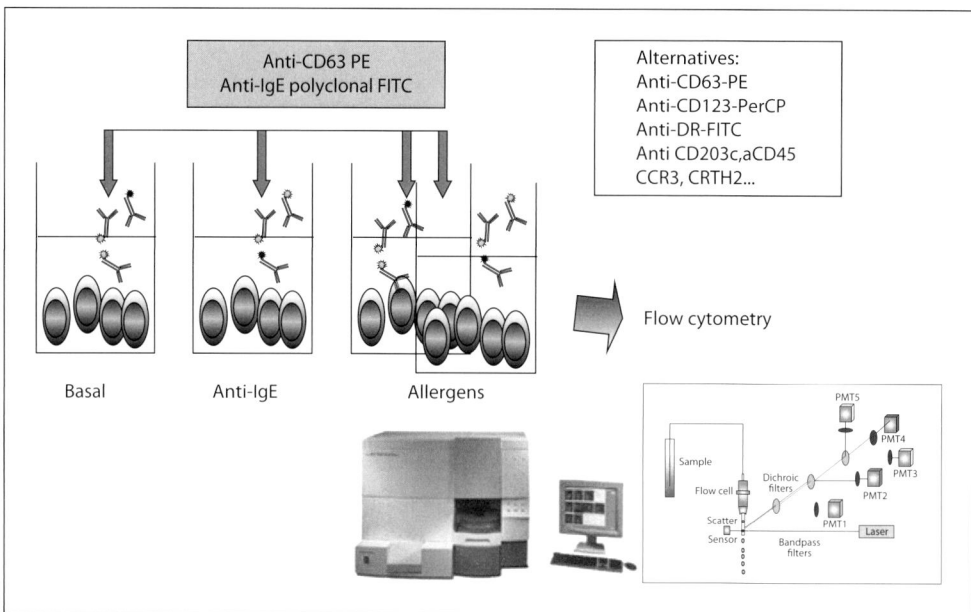

Fig. 2. BAT technique. Labeling phase: basophil capture.

carried out by Abuaf et al. [27] in which the sensitivity of BAT was 64% in patients with immediate reactions due to NMBA, with a specificity of 94%, similar data have been repeated in subsequent studies [28] which have even reported even higher sensitivities for this technique (up to 92%) when the reactions are studied within 3

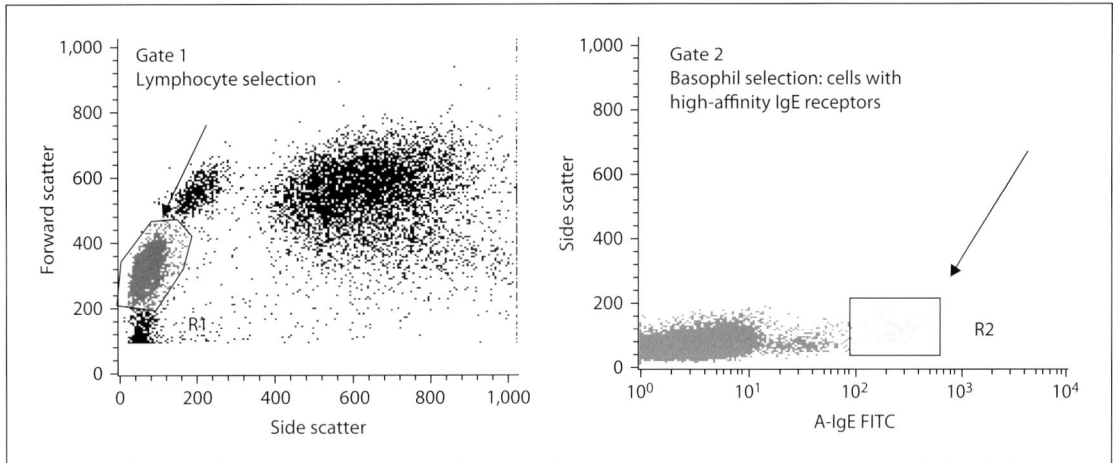

Fig. 3. Flow cytometry analysis. CellQuest software. The fluorescence of 50,000 cells is measured.

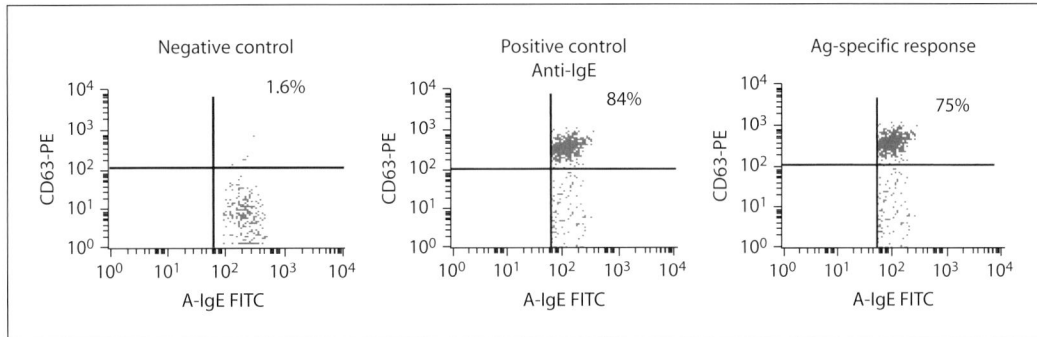

Fig. 4. CellQuest software. Analysis of CD63-expressing cells.

years of their occurrence [29, 31]. Furthermore, with this type of drugs, BAT even proves useful to determine the existence or not of cross-reactivities between different NMBAs and thus is able to indicate the suitable agent in subsequent anesthesias to avoid further reactions.

Non-Steroidal Anti-Inflammatory Drugs (NSAIDs)
Within this group of drugs there are two types of reaction:

(1) Reactions not mediated by IgE but produced by a pharmacologic reaction predominantly by the NSAID inhibitors COX-1 and -2 which can cause respiratory, skin or both types of reaction or severe anaphylaxis. These are the most frequent types of reaction. To date, only BAT has been validated as an in vitro diagnostic test with contrasted usefulness. In the best argued study [32], sensitivity of the test

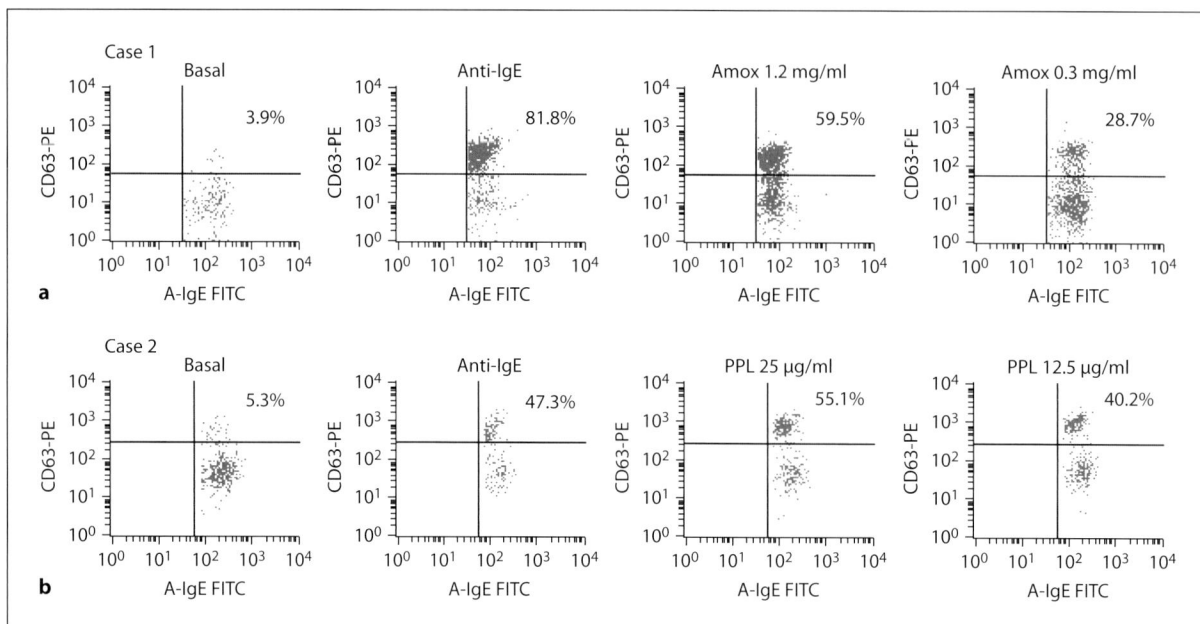

Fig. 5. Two BAT-positive cases (**a**, **b**) in β-lactam-allergic patients.

using only two NSAIDs (acetylsalicylic acid and diclofenac) was 58% with an excellent specificity of 93%, which makes it the in vitro test of choice for this type of disorder.

(2) Allergy mediated by selective IgE to certain types of NSAIDs by which symptoms are caused exclusively by a specific group of NSAIDs and no cross-reactivity exists with the other groups of anti-inflammatories. In a study carried out with 26 methimazole-allergic patients with IgE-mediated reactions [33], 14 of which developed anaphylaxis, BAT showed a sensitivity of 42% with an optimum specificity of 100%. No other validated in vitro test exists to date for the diagnosis of this disorder and so it represents an essential aid to diagnosis.

Other Drugs

In relation to specific IgE, the range available drugs is limited. The reliability of specific IgE determination is good in IgE-mediated reactions to chlorhexidine [34] and also in immediate reactions to tetanus toxoid [35]. BAT has been shown to be useful in the diagnosis of many other allergic reactions caused by drugs, which are less frequently responsible for immediate allergic reactions with an immunologic basis and which in many cases progress to anaphylaxis and for which no specific IgE is available as an in vitro diagnostic aid, such as omeprazole, hyaluronidase, patent blue, etc. [for a complete review, see 19].

Sanz · Gamboa · García-Figueroa · Ferrer

Latex

The determination of specific IgE constitutes an effective method in the diagnosis of latex allergy, with similar results between different commercial immunoassays with levels of sensitivity between 73 and 86% and a specificity of 97% [36, 37].

As far as BAT is concerned, it has been validated by different authors in the diagnosis of latex allergy [36–38] with sensitivity and specificity values near to or higher than 90%. Furthermore, BAT is capable of diagnosing latex-allergic patients with negative skin tests and/or negative specific IgE (BAT positive in the 13 patients studied) and ruling out the existence of latex allergy in non-allergic patients with false-positive specific IgE (20/24 patients) [37].

In any case, BAT is the in vitro technique with the best sensitivity and specificity values without exposing the patient to any kind of risk. The use of natural purified and/or recombinant allergens allows the pattern of sensitization of different groups of patients to be established and the diagnostic yield of both techniques to be increased [39].

Anisakis Allergy

The usual diagnostic methods, both skin tests and specific IgE with whole Anisakis extract, have a good sensitivity but a low specificity to such a degree that in 22% of blood donors specific IgE to the parasite is detected [40] and at least 20% of patients with acute urticaria have positive skin prick tests with whole Anisakis extract [41].As for BAT with whole Anisakis extract, Gonzalez-Muñoz et al. [42] report a sensitivity of 96% with a specificity of 96%, which are clearly higher values than those from specific IgE.

In our experience, BAT with whole Anisakis extract has a sensitivity approaching 100% (with the great majority of the patients studied with anaphylaxis) but with a specificity lower than 70% in patients with acute urticaria with positive skin prick tests and specific IgE with whole Anisakis extract. However, the use of purified allergens native to this parasite (Ani s 1 and Ani s 3) [43] allows a diagnosis to be made in over 90% of patients with immediate allergy to this parasite with a specificity of 100% including among the controls the patients with acute urticaria mentioned above. On the basis of these data, it can be stated that native purified allergens allow a precise diagnosis of Anisakis allergy to be made.

Insect Venom Allergy

Within 1 year of the reaction, between 70 and 90% of patients have specific IgE positive to venoms while only between 10 and 20% of people with a negative history have positive test results. The predictive value of skin tests and the determination of specific IgE is not high in that between 55 and 76% of people with positive specific IgE do not react clinically to a new sting. In contrast, some of the people (between 0 and 28%) with negative IgE do experience a reaction. The negative controls that have positive specific IgE have a risk of suffering reactions following a sting of between 19 and 39%.

One limitation of serum-specific IgE is that given the cross-reactivity between different Hymenoptera venoms, and also due to the presence of anti-carbohydrate antibodies, it is frequent to find several simultaneous positive results in patients with non-identified insect stings, a situation which makes diagnosis of the same difficult. In these cases, RAST inhibition and the release of histamine occasionally provide data on the venom involved and when this is not the case, it is advisable to administer immunotherapy against both [44].

In patients presenting with insect venom allergy, BAT offers sensitivity and specificity values similar to those of CAP. In wasp venom allergy, where the majority of patients have been studied, sensitivity in the different studies ranges from 80 to 100% with specificity values of 100% [45]. In bee venom allergy, the number of patients studied is much lower but the sensitivity values are 100%. In these patients BAT provides added advantages such as its ability to specify the diagnosis in those patients with discrepancies between skin tests and specific IgE, sting by an unknown insect and double positive results in skin tests and/or IgE [46–48]. It may also be useful to determine the success of immunotherapy treatment in these patients [49].

Foods

Although the gold standard in the diagnosis of food allergy is challenge with the food in question, especially within a double-blind placebo-controlled paradigm, in the case of patients who have suffered anaphylaxis the risk involved with re-exposure counter-indicates its use, at least in normal clinical practice. In such cases, the etiologic diagnosis of food allergy is based on the demonstration of the existence of IgE antibodies against the food in question. This demonstration may be carried out in vivo using skin prick tests and in vitro using cellular or serologic techniques by quantifying the levels of specific serum IgE of the food responsible. However, occasionally in highly sensitized patients, skin tests may trigger generalized reactions and as a result in the most serious cases determination of specific serum IgE may be the method of choice to show IgE sensitization as a clearly positive result makes the use of other techniques unnecessary [50].

To date, no studies have been published on the sensitivity and specificity of the determination of specific IgE against foods in series of patients experiencing anaphylaxis as a manifestation of their food allergy. However, in general it is assumed that the determination of specific IgE against animal foods offers better results than the determination of specific IgE against plant foods, both in terms of sensitivity and specificity.

Several studies show that the patients with suspected food allergy in whom clinical reactivity is confirmed in the challenge test have specific IgE concentrations against the respective foods which are greater than those in whom the test was negative [51]. However, the possible relationship between specific IgE concentration against a food and the severity of the reaction remains controversial. No such correlation was found in a European study in patients with soy allergy [52] (children and adults, 97% with another associated atopic disease: 33% atopic dermatitis, 66% asthma and 67% rhinoconjunctivitis) or in the study by Flinterman et al. [53] in which no correlation was found in peanut-allergic children. In contrast, Hourihane et al. [54] found that in adults, and to a lesser degree in children, IgE levels to peanut did correlate with the severity of the reaction observed during challenge with low doses of this food. Similarly, Peeters et al. [55], in a series of adults allergic to peanut, reported that those who reacted at low doses in the challenge had higher IgE levels to peanut than those who reacted at high doses. In any case, the considerable overlap of IgE levels in patients with different clinical expressions of food allergy limits the predictive usefulness of severe reactions.

The allergenic molecules capable of triggering a systemic anaphylactic reaction share certain physical and chemical properties such as being stable to acid pH and the action of digestive proteolytic enzymes. This stability is common among whole food allergens which are capable of both sensitizing and inducing symptoms via the digestive route, thus giving rise to the so-called type 1 food allergy [56]. Most of the food allergens from animal foods belong to this category, such as α-lactalbumin, β-lactoglobulin, casein and bovine milk albumin, ovalbumin, ovomucoid, egg ovotransferrin and lysozyme, fish and amphibian parvalbumins, and shellfish tropomyosins. Given their great stability, other members of this category include plant allergens belonging to the superfamily of the prolamines (cereal prolamines, 2S seed, legume and nut albumins and the ubiquitous lipid transport proteins (LTPs) and the cupins (7S and 11S seed, legume and nut globulins). Especially in plant foods, it is common that in the same food source both whole allergens are present as well as cross-reactivity allergens which sensitize via the airborne route and are generally labile to peptic digestion, thus making systemic clinical reactions unlikely. Therefore, in these food allergies the detection of specific IgE against purified allergens is of prognostic interest as far as the risk of severe reactions is concerned. Thus, for example, sensitization to LTP in patients allergic to rosaceae [57, 58], to ω−5 gliadin in patients allergic to wheat [59] and to class 1 chitinases [60] in patients with latex-fruit syndrome is associated with a high risk of severe reactions. In the case of legumes, seeds and nuts, sensitization to storage proteins (2S albumins and 7S and 11S globulins) is a frequent cause of anaphylaxis. In contrast, sensitization exclusively to homologs of Bet v 1 and/ or prophyllins in the same food sources entails a low risk of a systemic reaction.

To date, few studies have been published on food-induced anaphylaxis which have used BAT as a diagnostic method. In these, whole extracts have been used in the isolated cases of anaphylaxis due to grape [61] and aubergine [62] with positive results. However, native and/or recombinant allergens are those which have shown an excellent diagnostic yield. Thus, in the largest published case series of food-induced anaphylaxis, BAT was capable of diagnosing sensitivity to Pru p 3 from peaches in 7 of the 8 patients studied, with sensitivities and specificities approaching 100% [63]. These same positive results with native extracts have been confirmed in isolated cases of allergies to citrus fruits [64] and lychees [65]. Overall, there have been few studies published on the use of BAT in food allergies and as a result further studies will need to be performed to confirm the usefulness of this technique in the diagnosis of such allergies.

Diagnosis by Components. Microarrays to Determine Specific IgE

Knowledge of the reactivity of IgE to different allergenic molecules from a particular biological source, which is achieved by means of the application of the so-called diagnosis by components, makes it possible to predict if the risk of certain cross-reactivity patterns of known molecular basis exists or not. In this way, diagnosis by purified natural or recombinant allergenic components has passed from being a research tool to form part of the diagnosis of the etiology of food allergy in general [66] and of the diagnosis and prevention of food-induced anaphylaxis.

Microarray technology was first developed for DNA studies in basic biology but now has a real use in in vitro molecular diagnosis of allergic reactions. The combination of this technology with the availability of purified allergens (recombinant or natural) and the possibility of coupling and fixing them to microarrays makes the determination of specific IgE with this methodology a very useful tool in the in vitro diagnosis of allergic reactions to different allergens. Given that it allows several hundred allergens to be analyzed at once with a minimum amount of sample (about 50 μl of serum), its possible application in the in vitro diagnosis of allergies is very interesting, especially in children. A single analysis allows different fluorescences to be analyzed in parallel thus making it feasible to quantify specific IgE and IgG, for example, in the same assay, as has been reported by Flinterman et al. [67]. Another great benefit of this technique is that it facilitates screening in those subjects in which the use of skin tests is not advisable, as is the case in patients with severe atopic dermatitis, dermographism or patients generally with severe reactions.

There is a clear advantage to using molecular components in the form of purified recombinant or natural allergens which allow greater diagnostic accuracy (lower number of false-positives and false-negatives) as well as greater standardization when compared to the use of conventional allergen extracts, avoiding some problems related to the purity of the content of the allergenic and non-allergenic molecules or with the contamination of such extracts or the poor stability of the same [68]. Their application in the diagnosis of allergy to egg and milk, where the majority of anaphylactic reactions occur in children, has recently been evaluated by Ott et al. [69]

in a study undertaken with a large sample of 130 children diagnosed using skin tests, specific IgE using conventional techniques (CAP FEIA, Phadia AB), and a challenge test. These authors found that by analyzing the major allergens of egg and milk present in the microarray (ISAC™, VBC Genomics Bioscience Research, Vienna, Austria), they obtained results similar to those obtained with conventional techniques but with more information (greater number of allergens), and a smaller amount of blood. According to these authors, microarray-based IgE quantification was accurate in predicting clinical reactivity to allergenic proteins.

This technique could allow us to establish the values predicting the severity of symptoms derived from the sensitization to LTP or to tropomyosins, as has been reported in some recently published studies in which recognition patterns were studied using molecular components in food-allergic patients as related to the severity of the clinical picture [70]. The diagnosis of anaphylaxis relies mainly on the clinical picture. An in vitro test for diagnosis is urgently needed. We now have at our disposal more tools to investigate the cause. We should also explore novel mediators. In the mean time, studies on the performance of known markers should be carried out in order to allow us to evaluate the risk of anaphylaxis and to avoid the use challenge tests.

Acknowledgements

M.L.S., P.M.G. and M.F. are supported by grant RD07/0064 from the Spanish Research Network on Adverse Reactions to Allergens and Drugs (RIRAAF: Red de Investigación de Reacciones Adversas a Alérgenos y Fármacos) of the Carlos III Health Institute.

References

1 Sampson HA, Muñoz-Furlong A, Campbell RL, Adkinson NF Jr, Bock SA, Branum A, Brown SG, Camargo CA Jr, Cydulka R, Galli SJ, Gidudu J, Gruchalla RS, Harlor AD Jr, Hepner DL, Lewis LM, Lieberman PL, Melcalfe DD, O'Connor R, Muraro A, Rudman A, Schmitt C, Scherrer D, Simons FE, Thomas S, Wood JP, Decker WW: Second symposium on the definition and management of anaphylaxis: summary report. Second National Institute of Allergy and Infectious Disease/Food Allergy and Anaphylaxis Network Symposium. J Allergy Clin Immunol 2006;117:391–397.

2 Ogawa Y, Grant JA: Mediators of anaphylaxis. Immunol Allergy Clin North Am 2007;2:249–260, vii.

3 Van der Linden PW, Hack CE, Poortman J, Vivie-Kipp YC, Struyvenberg A, van der Zwan JK: Insect-sting challenge in 138 patients: relation between clinical severity of anaphylaxis and mast cell activation. J Allergy Clin Immunol 1992;90:110–118.

4 Schwartz LB: Diagnostic value of tryptase in anaphylaxis and mastocytosis 2. Immunol Allergy Clin North Am 2006;26:451–463.

5 Jogie-Brahim S, Min HK, Fukuoka Y, Xia HZ, Schwartz LB: Expression of α-tryptase and β-tryptase by human basophils. J Allergy Clin Immunol 2004; 113:1086–1092.

6 Foster B, Schwartz LB, Devouassoux G, Metcalfe DD, Prussin C: Characterization of mast-cell tryptase-expressing peripheral blood cells as basophils. J Allergy Clin Immunol 2002;109:287–293.

7 Schwartz LB, Bradford TR, Rouse C, Irani AM, Rasp G, Van der Zwan JK, Van del Linden PW: Development of a new, more sensitive immunoassay for human tryptase: use in systemic anaphylaxis. J Clin Immunol 1994;14:190–204.

8 Schwartz LB, Yunginger JW, Miller J, Bokhari R, Dull D: Time course of appearance and disappearance of human mast cell tryptase in the circulation after anaphylaxis. J Clin Invest 1989;83:1551–1555.

9   Yunginger JW, Nelson DR, Squillace DL, Jones RT, Holley KE, Hyma BA, Biedrzycki L, Sweeney KG, Sturner WQ, Schwartz LB: Laboratory investigation of deaths due to anaphylaxis. J Forensic Sci 1991;36: 857–865.

10 Simons FE, Frew AJ, Ansotegui IJ, Bochner BS, Golden DB, Finkelman FD, Leung DY, Lotvall J, Marone G, Metcalfe DD, Müller U, Rosenwasser LJ, Sampson HA, Schwartz LB, van Hage M, Walls AF: Risk assessment in anaphylaxis: current and future approaches. J Allergy Clin Immunol 2007;120(suppl): 2–24.

11 Pejler G, Abrink M, Ringvall M, Wernersson S: Mast cell proteases. Adv Immunol 2007;95:167–255.

12 Nishio H, Takai S, Miyazaki M, Horiuchi H, Osawa M, Uemura K, Yoshida K, Mukaida M, Ueno Y, Suzuki K: Usefulness of serum mast cell-specific chymase levels for postmortem diagnosis of anaphylaxis. Int J Legal Med 2005;119:331–334.

13 Osawa M, Satoh F, Horiuchi H, Tian W, Kugota N, Hasegawa I: Postmortem diagnosis of fatal anaphylaxis during intravenous administration of therapeutic and diagnostic agents: evaluation of clinical laboratory parameters and immunohistochemistry in three cases. Leg Med (Tokyo) 2008;10:143–147.

14 Okamoto H, Kamatani N: Platelet-activating factor, PAF acetylhydrolase, and anaphylaxis. N Engl J Med 2008;358:1516–1517.

15 Arias K, Baig M, Colangelo M, Chu D, Walker T, Goncharova S, Coyle A, Vadas P, Waserman S, Jordana M: Concurrent blockade of platelet-activating factor and histamine prevents life-threatening peanut-induced anaphylactic reactions. J Allergy Clin Immunol 2009;124:307–314.

16 Korhonen H, Fisslthaler B, Moers A, Wirth A, Habermehl D, Wieland T, Schütz G, Wettschureck N, Fleming I, Offermanns S: Anaphylactic shock depends on endothelial Gq/G11. J Exp Med 2009; 206:411–420.

17 Denzlinger C, Haberl C, Wilmanns W: Cysteinyl leukotriene production in anaphylactic reactions. Int Arch Allergy Immunol 1995;108:158–164.

18 Ono E, Taniguchi M, Mita H, Fukutomi Y, Higashi N, Miyazaki E, Kumamoto T, Akiyama K: Increased production of cysteinyl leukotrienes and prostaglandin D_2 during human anaphylaxis. Clin Exp Allergy 2009;39:72–80.

19 Sanz ML, Gamboa PM, de Weck AL: Cellular tests in the diagnosis of drug hypersensitivity. Curr Pharm Des 2008;14:2803–2808.

20 Ebo DG, Sainte-Laudy J, Bridas CH, Mertens CH, Hagendorens MM, Schuerwegh AJ, De Clerk LS, Stevens WJ: Flow-assisted allergy diagnosis: current applications and future perspectives. Allergy 2006; 61:1028–1039.

21 De Weck AL, Sanz ML, Gamboa PM, Aberer W, Bienvenue J, Blanca M, Demoly P, Ebo DG, Mayorga L, Monneret G, Sainte Laudy J: Diagnostic tests based on human basophils: more potential and perspectives than pitfalls. Int Arch Allergy Appl Immunol 2008;146:177–189.

22 De Weck AL, Sanz ML, Gamboa PM, Aberer W, Bienvenue J, Blanca M, Demoly P, Ebo DG, Mayorga L, Monneret G, Sainte Laudy J: Diagnostic tests based on human basophils: more potential and perspectives than pitfalls. II. Technical issues. J Investig Allergol Clin Immunol 2008;18:143–155.

23 Sanz ML, Gamboa PM, Antepara I, Uasuf C, Vila L, García-Avilés C, Chazot M, De Weck L: Flow cytometric basophil activation test by detection of CD63 expression in patients with immediate-type reactions to β-lactam antibiotics. Clin Exp Allergy 2002; 32:277–286.

24 Blanca M, Mayorga C, Torres MJ, Reche M, Moya MC, Rodriguez JL, Romano A, Juarez C: Clinical evaluation of Pharmacia CAP System RAST FEIA amoxicilloyl and benzylpenicilloyl in patients with penicillin allergy. Allergy 2001;56:862–870.

25 Torres MJ, Padial A, Mayorga C, Fernández T, Sánchez-Sabate E, Cornejo-García A, Antúnez C, Blanca M: The diagnostic interpretation of basophil activation test in immediate allergic reactions to β-lactams. Clin Exp Allergy 2004;34:1768–1775.

26 Gamboa PM, García-Avilés MC, Urrutia I, Antepara I, Esparza R, Sanz ML: Basophil activation and sulfidoleukotriene production in patients with immediate allergy to β-lactam antibiotics and negative skin tests. J Investig Allergol Clin Immunol 2004;14:278–283.

27 Abuaf N, Rajoely B, Ghazouani E, Levy DA, Pecquet C, Chabane H, Leynadier F: Validation of a flow cytometric assay detecting in vitro basophil activation for the diagnosis of muscle relaxant allergy. J Allergy Clin Immunol 1999;104:411–418.

28 Monneret G, Benoit Y, Debard AL, Gutowski MC, Topenot I, Bienvenu J: Monitoring of basophil activation using CD63 and CCR3 in allergy to muscle relaxant drugs. Clin Immunol 2002;102:192–199.

29 Sudheer PS, Hall JE, Read GF, Rowbottom AW, Williams PE: Flow cytometric investigation of peri-anaesthetic anaphylaxis using CD63 and CD203c. Anaesthesia 2005;60:251–256.

30 Kvedariene V, Kamey S, Ryckwaert Y, Rongier M, Bousquet J, Demoly P, Arnoux B: Diagnosis of neuromuscular blocking agent hypersensitivity reactions using cytofluorometric analysis of basophils. Allergy 2006;61:311–315.

31 Ebo DG, Bridts CH, Hagendorens MM, Mertens CH, De Clerk LS, Stevens WJ: Flow-assisted diagnostic management of anaphylaxis from rocuronium bromide. Allergy 2006;61:935–939.

32 Gamboa P, Sanz ML, Caballero MR, Urrutia I, Antepara I, Esparza R, De Weck L: The flow-cytometric determination of basophil activation induced by aspirin and other non-steroidal and anti-inflammatory drugs (NSAIDs) is useful for in vitro diagnosis of the NSAID hypersensitivity syndrome. Clin Exp Allergy 2004;34:1448–1457.

33 Gamboa PM, Sanz ML, Caballero MR, Antepara I, Urrutia I, González G, Dieguez I, De Weck AL: Use of CD63 expression as a marker of in vitro basophil activation and leukotriene determination in methimazole allergic patients. Allergy 2003;58:312–317.

34 Garvey LH, Krogaard M, Poulsen LK, Skov PS, Mosbech H, Venelmalm L, Degerbeck F, Husum B: IgE-mediated allergy to chlorhexidine. J Allergy Clin Immunol 2007;120:409–415.

35 Grüber C, Lau S, Dannemann A, Sommerfeld C, Wahn U, Aalberse RC: Down-regulation of IgE and IgG4 antibodies to tetanus toxoid and diphtheria toxoid by co-vaccination with cellular *Bordetella pertussis* vaccine. J Immunol 2001;15;167:2411–2417.

36 Hemery ML, Arnoux B, Dhivert-Donnadieu H, Rongier M, Barbotte E, Verdier E, Demoly P: Confirmation of the diagnosis of natural rubber latex allergy by the Basotest® method. Int Arch Allergy Immunol 2005;136:53–57.

37 Ebo D, Lehkar B, Schuerwegh, Bridts CH, De Clerk LS, Stevens WJ: Validation of a two-color flow cytometric assay detecting in vitro basophil activation for the diagnosis of IgE-mediated natural rubber latex allergy. Allergy 2002;57:706–712.

38 Sanz ML, Gamboa PM, García-Avilés C, Vila L, Dieguez I, Antepara I, de Weck AL: Fluorocytometric cellular allergen stimulation test in latex allergy. Int Arch Allergy Immunol 2003;130:33–39.

39 Sanz ML, García-Avilés MC, Tabar AI, Anda M, García BE, Barber D, Salcedo G, Rihs HP, Raulf-Heimsoth M: Basophil activation test and specific IgE measurements using a panel of recombinant natural rubber latex allergen to determine the latex allergen sensitization profile in children. Pediatr Allergy Immunol 2006;17:148–156.

40 Del Rey A, Valero A, Mayorga C, Gómez B, Torres MJ, Hernández J, Ortiz M, Lozano J: Sensitization to Anisakis simplex s. l. in a healthy population. Acta Trop 2006;97:265–269.

41 Del Pozo M, Audicana M, Diez JM, Muñoz D, Ansotegui IJ, Fernandez E, Garcá M, Etxenagusia M, Moneo I, Fernández de Corres L: Anisakis simples, a relevant etiologic factor in acute urticaria. Allergy 1997;52:576–579.

42 Gonzalez-Muñoz M, Luque R, Nauwelaers F, Moneo I: Detection of Anisakis simplex-induced basophil activation by flow cytometry. Cytometry B Clin Cytom 2006;68:31–36.

43 Gamboa PM, Urrutia I, Asturias J: BAT with Anisakis purified allergens in diagnosis of Anisakis. J Invest Allergol Clin Immunol 2010, in press.

44 Müller U, Mosbech H: Immunotherapy with Hymenoptera venoms. Allergy 2008;48:37–46.

45 Sainte-Laudy J, Sabbah A, Drouet M, Lauret MG, Loiry M: Diagnosis of venom allergy by flow cytometry. Correlation with clinical history, skin tests, specific IgE histamine and leukotriene C_4 release. Clin Exp Allergy 2000;30:1166–1171.

46 Eberlein-König B, Schmidt-Leidescher C, Rakoski J, Behrendt H, Ring J: In vitro basophil activation using CD63 expression in patients with bee and wasp venom allergy. J Investig Allergol Clin Immunol 2006;16:5–10.

47 Eberlein-König B, Rakoski J, Behrendt H, Ring J: Use of CD63 expression as marker of in vitro basophil activation in identifying the culprit in insect venom allergy. J Investig Allergol Clin Immunol 2004;14:10–16.

48 Ebo D, Hagendorens MM, Bridts CH, De Clerk LS, Stevens WJ: Hymenoptera venom allergy: taking the sting out of difficult cases. J Investig Allergol Clin Immunol 2007;17:357–360.

49 Ebo D, Hagendorens MM, Schuerwegh AJ, Beirens LMN, Bridts CH, De Clerk LS, Stevens WJ: Flow-assisted quantification of in vitro activated basophils in the diagnosis of wasp venom allergy and follow-up of wasp venom immunotherapy. Cytometry B Clin Cytom 2007;72:196–192

50 Bush RK, Taylor SL: Adverse reaction to foods and drug additives; in Middleton E, Reed CE, Ellis EF, Adkinson F, Yunginger JW, Busse WW (eds): Allergy. Principles and Practice, ed 5. St Louis, Mosby, 1998, pp 1183–1198.

51 García-Ara C, Boyano-Martínez T, Díaz-Pena JM, Martín-Muñoz F, Reche-Frutos M, Martín-Esteban M: Specific IgE levels in the diagnosis of immediate hypersensitivity to cows' milk protein in the infant. J Allergy Clin Immunol 2001;107:185–190.

52 Ballmer-Weber BK, Holzhauser T, Scibilia J, Mittag D, Zisa G, Ortolani C, Oesterballe M, Poulsen LK, Vieths S, Bindslev-Jensen C: Clinical characteristics of soybean allergy in Europe: a double-blind, placebo-controlled food challenge study. J Allergy Clin Immunol 2007;119:1489–1496.

53 Flinterman AE, Pasmans SG, Hoekstra MO, Meijer Y, van Hoffen E, Knol EF, Hefle SL, Bruijnzeel-Koomen CA, Knulst AC: Determination of no-observed-adverse-effect levels and eliciting doses in a representative group of peanut-sensitized children. J Allergy Clin Immunol 2006;117:448–454.

54 Hourihane JO, Grimshaw KE, Lewis SA, Briggs RA, Trewin JB, King RM, Kilburn SA, Warner JO: Does severity of low-dose, double-blind, placebo-controlled food challenges reflect severity of allergic reactions to peanut in the community? Clin Exp Allergy 2005;35:1227–1233.

55 Peeters KA, Koppelman SJ, Van Hoffen E, van der Tas CW, den Hartog Jager CF, Penninks AH, Hefle SL, Bruijnzeel-Koomen CA, Knol EF, Knulst AC: Does skin prick test reactivity to purified allergens correlate with clinical severity of peanut allergy? Clin Exp Allergy 2007;37:108–115.

56 Breiteneder H, Ebner C: Molecular and biochemical classification of plant-derived food allergens. J Allergy Clin Immunol 2000;106:27–36.

57 Fernández-Rivas M, Bolhaar S, González-Mancebo E, Asero R, van Leeuwen A, Bohle B, Ma Y, Ebner C, Rigby N, Sancho AI, Miles S, Zuidmeer L, Knulst A, Breiteneder H, Mills C, Hoffmann-Sommergruber K, van Ree R: Apple allergy across Europe: how allergen sensitization profiles determine the clinical expression of allergies to plant foods. J Allergy Clin Immunol 2006;118:481–488.

58 Tabar A, Alvarez-Puebla M, Gómez B, Sánchez-Monge R, García B, Echechipía S, Olaguibel JM, Salcedo G: Diversity of asparagus allergy: clinical and immunological features. Clin Exp Allergy 2004; 34:131–136.

59 Palosuo K, Varjonen E, Kekki OM, Klemola T, Kalkkinen N, Alenius H, Reunala T: Wheat omega–5 gliadin is a major allergen in children with immediate allergy to ingested wheat. J Allergy Clin Immunol 2001;108:634–638.

60 Sánchez-Monge R, Díaz-Perales A, Blanco C, Salcedo G: Latex allergy and plant chitinases; in Mills ENC, Shreffler WG (eds): Plant Food Allergens. Oxford, Blackwell Science, 2004, pp 87–104.

61 Schäd SG, Trcka J, Vieth S, Scheurer S, Conti A, Bröcker EB, Trautmann A: Wine anaphylaxis in a German patient: IgE-mediated allergy against a lipid transfer protein of grapes. Int Arch Allergy Immunol 2005;136:159–164.

62 Gamboa PM, Sánchez-Monge R, Díaz-Perales A, Salcedo G, Ansótegui I, Sanz ML: Latex-vegetable syndrome due to custard apple and aubergine: new variations of the hevein symphony. J Invest Allergol Clin Immunol 2005;15:308–311.

63 Gamboa PM, Cáceres O, Antepara I, Sánchez-Monge R, Ahrazem O, Salcedo G, Barber D, Lombardero M, Sanz ML: Two different profiles of peach allergy in the north of Spain. Allergy 2006;

64 Ebo DG, Ahrazem O, López-Torrejón G, Bridts CH, Salcedo G, Stevens WJ: Anaphylaxis from mandarin (Citrus reticulata): identification of responsible allergens. Int Arch Allergy Appl Immunol 2007;144:39–43.

65 Raap U, Schaefer T, Kapp A, Wedi B: Exotic food allergy: anaphylactic reaction to lychee. J Invest Allergol Clin Immunol 2007;17:199–201.

66 Lidholm J, Ballmer-Weber BK, Mari A, Vieths S: Component-resolved diagnostics in food allergy. Curr Opin Allergy Clin Immunol 2006;6:234–240.

67 Flinterman AE, Knol EF, Lencer DA, Bardina L, Hartog Jager CF, Lin J: Peanut epitopes for IgE and IgG4 in peanut-sensitized children in relation to severity of peanut allergy. J Allergy Clin Immunol 2008;21:737–743.

68 Van der Veen MJ, Mulder M, Witteman AM, van Ree R, Aalberse RC, Jansen HM, van der Zee JS: False-positive skin prick test responses to commercially available dog dander extracts caused by contamination with house dust mite (Dermatophagoides pteronyssimus) allergens. J Allergy Clin Immunol 1996;98:1028–1034

69 Ott H, Baron JM, Heise R, Ocklenburg C, Stanzel S, Merk HF, Niggemann B, Beyer K: Clinical usefulness of microarray-based IgE detection in children with suspected food allergy. Allergy 2008;63:1521–1528.

70 Capobianco F, Butteroni C, Barletta B, Corinti S, Afferni C, Tinghino R, Boirivant M, Di Felice G: Oral sensitization with shrimp tropomyosin induces in mice allergen-specific IgE, T-cell response and systemic anaphylactic reactions. Int Immunol 2008; 20:1077–1086.

Prof. María L. Sanz
Department of Allergology and Clinical Immunology
Clínica Universidad de Navarra, Apartado 4209
ES–31008 Pamplona (Spain)
Tel. +34 94825 5400, Fax +34 94829 6500, E-Mail mlsanzlar@unav.es

Ring J (ed): Anaphylaxis. Chem Immunol Allergy. Basel, Karger, 2010, vol 95, pp 141–156

Insect Venoms

Ulrich R. Müller

Spital Ziegler, Bern, Switzerland

Abstract

Insect venoms applied by stings of social Hymenoptera, like honey bees, vespids or ants are – together with foods and drugs – the most frequent elicitors of anaphylaxis in humans. Besides taxonomy, the biology of the responsible social Hymenoptera is important: guidelines based upon its knowledge allow to reduce the risk of further stings in patients with a history of venom anaphylaxis. Epidemiology of venom anaphylaxis has special aspects with regard to prevalence, fatality and natural history. An estimated 200 individuals die every year in Europe from anaphylaxis following Hymenoptera stings. Most of the relevant venom protein allergens have been identified and many of them have been expressed in recombinant form. Proof of venom sensitization is based on skin tests with venoms and serum venom-specific IgE antibodies as standard diagnostic tests. Allergen-specific immunotherapy with Hymenoptera venoms is highly effective and therefore recommended for all patients with a history of Hymenoptera sting anaphylaxis and positive diagnostic tests with the respective venom. Frequent cross-reactions to venoms of different Hymenoptera species may cause difficulties in identifying the responsible species and the selection of the respective venom for immunotherapy.

Insect venoms, together with foods and drugs, are the most frequent elicitors of anaphylaxis in men. The insect venom is applied by stings which must have occurred for more than 100,000 years, since human beings exist. Conflicts between stinging insects and humans occur while fighting for food, like honey or foods consumed outdoors, or while venomous insects feel threatened by human beings, most often near their nests.

Taxonomy and Biology of Responsible Insects

Venoms causing anaphylaxis or other allergic reactions originate almost exclusively from social Hymenoptera, most often honey bees and vespids (fig. 1) [1], occasionally from bumble bees [2], in America [3] and in Australia [4], also from ants. Stings by other insects like mosquitoes, bedbugs, fleas, horse flies and midges can very rarely also cause systemic allergic reactions. These are however not due to venoms but to

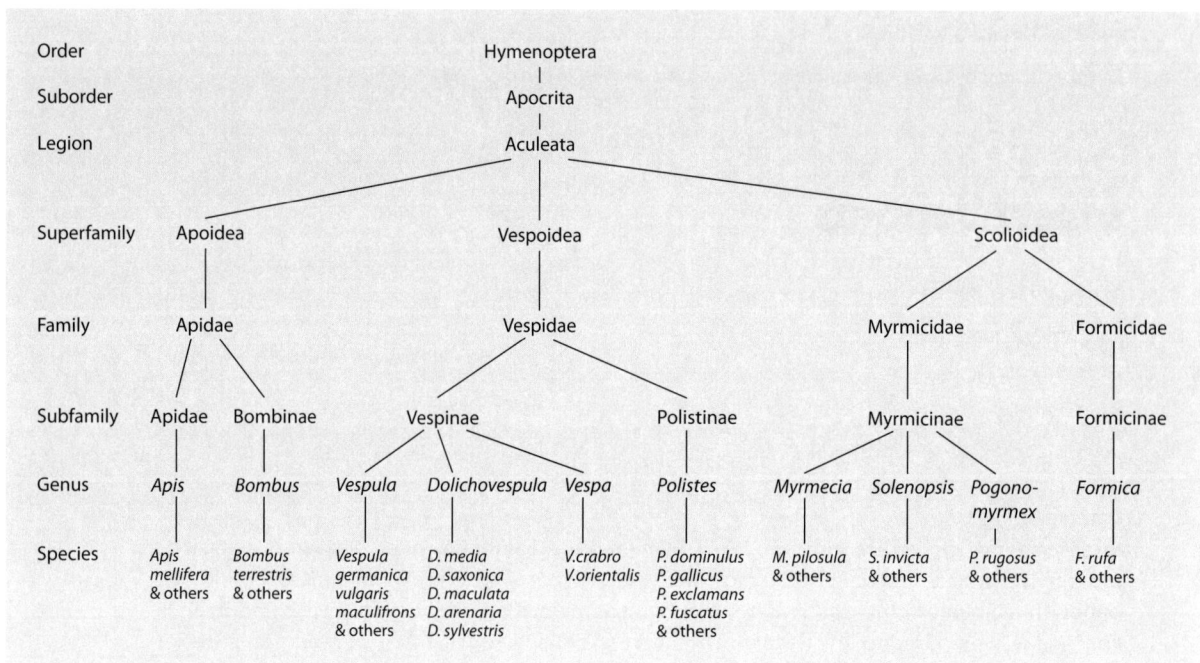

Fig. 1. Taxonomy of Hymenoptera.

salivary proteins, since these insects sting, or better bite, to suck blood and not to defend themselves [5]. Exceptionally, anaphylaxis has also been reported following stings by venomous arthropods like scorpions or arachnids and bites by ticks, which all are of course not insects.

We will concentrate in this chapter on venoms of social Hymenoptera which are certainly responsible for more than 99% of insect sting-induced anaphylaxis.

Apidae

The domesticated honey bee *(Apis mellifera)* (fig. 2a) is the most important species of this family. It is cultured by man all over the world for production of honey and pollination of fruit trees. In contrast to bumble bees and vespids, not only the queen, but the whole bee hive survives during winter. Stings may therefore occur exceptionally also on warm sunny winter days, but are most frequent in spring and early summer. The risk of exposure is highest near bee hives, while gardening, or when walking barefoot on a lawn. After stinging, the sting usually stays in the skin. Bumble bees *(Bombus spp.)* (fig. 2b) are also social Hymenoptera and usually build their nests in the ground. They are increasingly used as pollinators in greenhouses and occasionally cause anaphylaxis in greenhouse workers [2]. Bumble bees are much larger than honey bees, more hairy and most species have distinct yellow or white bands on their abdomen. After stinging, the sting usually does not stay in the skin.

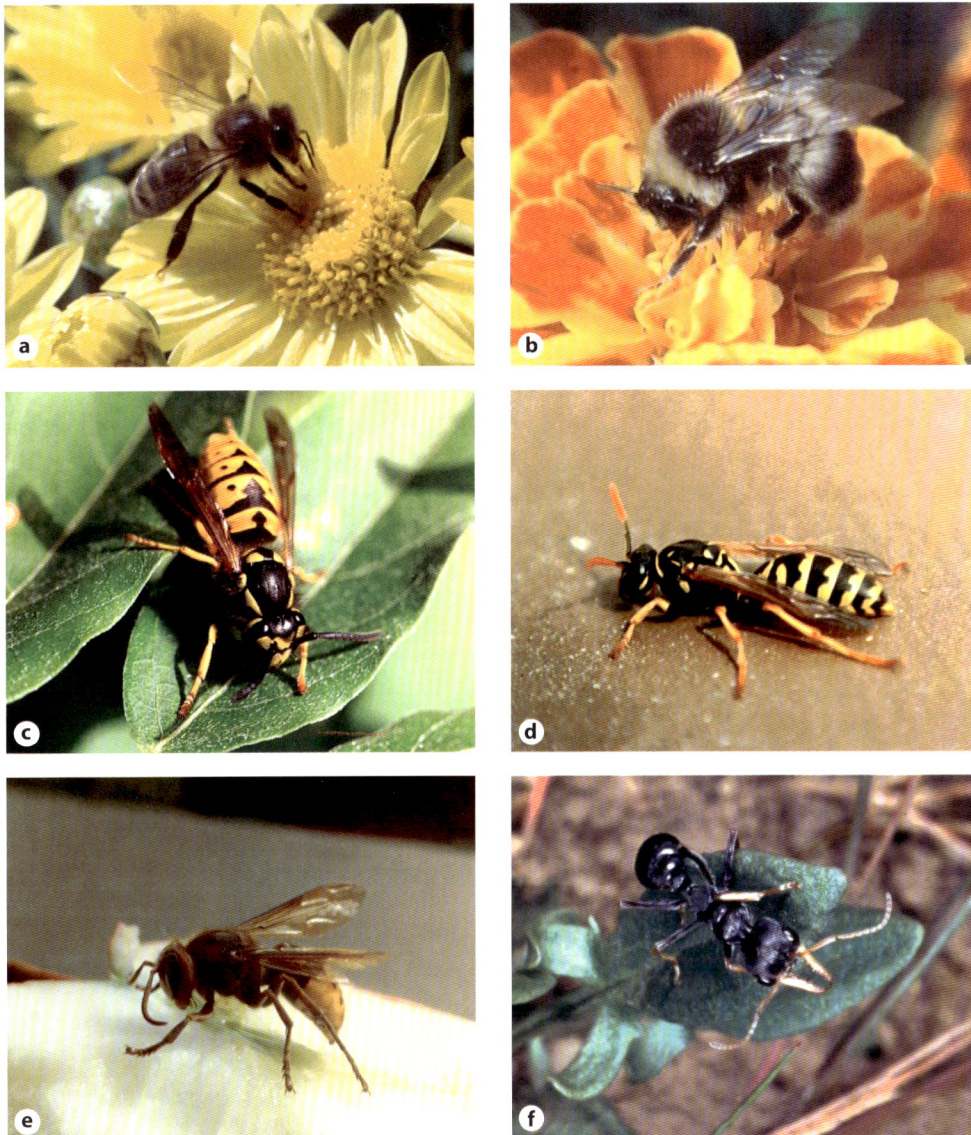

Fig. 2. Species of Hymenoptera responsible for systemic allergic reactions: (**a**) honey bee (*A. mellifera*), (**b**) bumble bee *(Bombus spp.)*, (**c**) wasp, in the USA yellow jacket *(Vespula spp.)*, (**d**) European paper wasp *(P. gallicus)*, (**e**) European hornet *(V. crabro)*, and (**f**) Australian jack jumper ant *(M. pilosula)* [by courtesy of Dr. S.G. Brown, Perth, Australia].

Vespidae

The family Vespidae is divided in subfamilies *Vespinae* and *Polistinae*, which are distinguishable by differences at the junction of thorax and abdomen: The abdomen becomes thicker rapidly after the waist in Vespinae but only gradually in *Polistinae* (fig. 2c, d). *Vespinae* include the genera *Vespula, Dolichovespula* and *Vespa* (fig. 1). While only the queen survives winter, vespid populations reach their maximal size only in summer and stings occur most often in summer and fall. After vespid stings, the sting does not stay in the skin as a rule. It may however stay when the insect is crushed during stinging, and according to one report more often in *Vespula maculifrons* than in other vespids [6].

The most important species of the genus *Vespula,* in Europe called wasps, are *Vespula vulgaris* and *V. germanica* (fig. 2c). In America they are called yellow jackets and besides *V. vulgaris* and *V. germanica* also *V. maculifrons, V. squamosa* and *V. pennsylvanica* are of importance. *Vespula* build their nests most often underground, but also under the roofs or in attics or window shutters. In contrast to honey bees, *Vespula* are prevalent also in urban areas. They like human food and stings most often occur while eating outdoors, under trees with fallen fruits, around garbage bins and of course near their nests.

In the genera *Dolichovespula, D. maculata* and *D. arenaria,* the American hornets, are the most prevalent species in the USA; in Europe, *D. saxonica, D. media* and *D. sylvestris* are important. *Dolichovespula* usually build their nests above ground, either hanging freely in tree branches, or in attics or window shutters. In contrast to *Vespula, Dolichovespula* has not much interest in human foods and stings therefore occur mainly near their nests.

Vespa crabro, the European hornet, *and V. orientalis* are the most important species of the genus *Vespa* in Europe, Asia and Africa, and *V. crabro* has also been imported in the USA. These species are much larger than other vespids (fig. 2e). They build their nest mostly above ground, in hollow tree trunks or in birds' nest boxes. Stings occur almost exclusively near the nests.

Among the subfamily *Polistinae, P. annularis, P. exclamans* and *P. fuscatus* are the most important species in southern US states, *P. dominulus* and *P. gallicus* (fig. 2d) in southern and Mediterranean areas of Europe. Occasional members of these species are however also observed in regions with a temperate climate. Because *Polistes* build their nest mostly around or on human buildings, stings may occur frequently, especially in southern countries of Europe and southern US states.

Ants (Formicidae, Myrmicidae)

In South and Central America as well as in southern US states, the fire ants *(Solenopsis invicta)* are often responsible for allergic sting reactions [7]. Fire ants build their mounds in playgrounds, gardens and fields. The sting does not stay in the skin of the victim. Besides local wheal-and-flare reactions, later pustule formation is characteristic of fire ant stings. Occasional allergic reactions have also been reported on stings by *Pogonomyrmex,* the harvester ant, and to other ant species all over the world [7]. In Southern Australia several species of Myrmicinae, especially the jack jumper ant *Myrmecia pilosula* (fig. 2f), are an important cause of allergic sting reactions [4].

Table 1. Allergens of Hymenoptera venoms

Venom	Allergen	Function/name	MW kDa	Major/minor	Cloned and sequenced	Expressed as recombinant	Glycosylated (n sites)
A.mellifera	Api m1	phospholipase A$_2$	16	major	yes	yes	yes (1)
	Api m2	hyaluronidase	43	major	yes	yes	yes (4)
	Api m3	acid phosphatase	45	major?	yes	yes	yes (4)
	Api m4	melittin	2.9	minor	available as synthetic peptide		no
	Api m5	dipeptidylpeptidase*	102	minor	yes	yes	yes
	Api m6		7.9	minor	yes	yes	no
	Api m7	CUB serine protease	39	major?	partly	partly	yes
V. vulgaris (similar for *V. germanica*, *V. maculifrons*)	Ves v1	phospholipase A$_1$	33.5	major	yes	yes	no
	Ves v2	hyaluronidase	45	minor	yes	yes	yes (4)
	Ves v3	dipeptidylpeptidase**	100	minor	yes	yes	yes
	Ves v5	antigen 5	23	major	yes	yes	no
S. invicta	Sol i1	phospholipase A$_1$	37	major	yes		
	Sol i2		14	minor	yes		
	Sol i3	antigen 5	24	major	yes		
	Sol i4		13.4	minor			
M. pilosula	Myr p1	pilosulin 1	6.1	major			
	Myr p2	pilosulin 3	5.6	minor			
	Myr p3	pilosulin 4.1	8.2	minor			
			25.6	major?			
			89.8	major?			

* allergen C; ** Vmac 3.

Allergens in Hymenoptera Venoms (table 1)

Hymenoptera venoms are composed of biogenic amines and other low molecular weight substances, of basic peptides and of proteins. Injection of venom by Hymenoptera stings has toxic effects, due to biogenic amines, peptides and proteins: biogenic amines such as histamine cause pain, are vasodilatory and increase vascular permeability, allowing the spread of the venom through the body of the victim, as do some of the enzymes, like hyaluronidase. Biogenic amines and peptides are mainly responsible for the local wheal-and-flare reaction after Hymenoptera stings. Cyototoxic and hemolytic effects after multiple, several hundred to over 1,000 stings, with systemic tissue damage, especially renal failure, are caused by basic peptides and phospholipases and responsible for severe toxic and sometimes fatal reactions. Allergic reactions on the other hand can occur after a single sting and are due to specific IgE antibodies, mainly to proteins, occasionally also to peptides. Major allergens are defined as inducing specific IgE antibodies in at least 50% of patients with allergy to the respective venom [1].

Venom collection is done by electrostimulation in honey bees [8] and by venom sac extraction in vespids [9]. While electrostimulation results in pure venom, venom sac extracts may be contaminated by some body proteins. The amount of venom injected by a sting varies from 50 to 140 μg dry weight for the honey bee, but was estimated to be much lower in vespids: 1.7–3.1 μg for *Vespula,* 2.4–5 μg for *Dolichovespula,* and 4.2–17 μg for *Polistes* [10].

Allergens in Apid Venoms (table 1)
Definite major allergens in bee venom are phospholipase A_2 (Api m1), a 16-kDa glycosylated enzyme which cleaves fatty acids at the 2 position of phosphatidylcholine and makes up for 10–15% of dry weight of bee venom [9, 11], and hyaluronidase (Api m2) a 43-kDa glycoprotein, which by cleaving hyaluronic acid increases permeability of connective tissue and makes up for about 1% of dry weight [12]. Specific IgE antibodies have also been identified against acid phosphatase (Api m3) [13], the peptide melittin (Api m4), a 39-kDa-serine protease (Api m7) [9], a 7.9-kDa protein (Api m6) [14], and the high molecular weight protein allergen C (Api m5), recently identified as dipeptidylpeptidase of 102 kDa [15, 16]. Except for melittin and Api m6, all these allergens are glycosylated. Part of the specific IgE antibodies to bee venom are directed to carbohydrate epitopes, so-called cross-reacting carbohydrate determinants, which are not species-specific, occur also in vespids, other insects and in plants, but not in mammals, and probably are of little clinical relevance [17, 18]. The significance of the heavily glycosylated higher molecular weight proteins protease, hyaluronidase, acid phosphatase and allergen C may therefore be overestimated.

Bumble bee venom contains also a phospholipase A_2 with partial identity to bee venom phospholipase A_2 and a protease, but no melittin. Instead there are several small peptides called bombolitins [9]. There is limited cross-reactivity between honey bee and bumblebee venoms [2].

Allergens in Vespid Venoms (table 1)
Major allergens in all vespid venoms are phospholipase A_1, a 33.5-kDa enzyme which digests cell membranes (Ves v1 for *V. vulgaris*) and antigen 5 (Ves v5), a 23-kDa

protein, maybe a neurotoxin. While antigen 5 is non-glycosylated, the situation is unclear for phospholipase A_1, which is not related to phospholipase A_2 of bee venom. Hyaluronidase is also present in vespid venoms but most likely is not a major allergen in the family of *Vespidae*. A dipeptidylpeptidase of 100 kDa (Ves v3), earlier called Vmac 3, with partial identity to Api m5, has been described recently [15, 16]. Sequence identity between different species of the major allergens antigen 5 and phospholipase A_1 is high (above 80–90%) within the genera *Vespula, Dolichovespula and Vespa*, but lower (around 70%) between these genera. It is even lower between these three genera and *Polistes*. Within the genus *Polistes* there is limited sequence identity and cross-reactivity between the European *(P. dominulus, P. gallicus)* and the American species *(P. fuscatus, P. exclamans)*, because a protease, rather than phospholipase A_1 and antigen 5, seems to be the major allergen in European *Polistes* venoms [9]. Hyaluronidase (Ves v2) is a minor allergen in vespids, is glycosylated and shows considerable sequence identity with bee venom hyaluronidase. Part of the cross-reactivity between bee and vespid hyaluronidase is however also due to specific IgE to carbohydrate epitopes [17, 18].

Allergens in Ant Venoms (table 1)

The venom of the American fire ant *S. invicta* consists of 90–95% water-insoluble *n*-alkyl and *n*-alkenyl piperidine alkaloids, which are responsible for early wheal-and-flare and later pustule formation characteristic of fire ant stings, but are not allergenic [5]. The allergens are present in the aqueous phase which contains 10–100 ng/sting of a mixture of four proteins: Sol i1, a 37-kDa phospholipase A_1, cross-reacting with specific IgE from vespid venom-sensitive patients; Sol i2, a 14-kDa protein, is not related to other known Hymenoptera venom allergens; Sol i3, a 24-kDa protein, is a member of the antigen 5 family of vespid venom proteins, but in spite of a 40–50% sequence identity does not exhibit significant cross-reactivity with these, and Sol i4 is a 13.4-kDa protein. Sol i1 and Sol i3 are major allergens [9].

The venom of the Australian jack jumper ant *M. pilosula* has only been analyzed for its allergen composition in recent years. Besides three low molecular weight allergens, Myr p1, Myr p2 and Myr p3 (table 1), six higher molecular weight allergens of 22.8–89.9 kDa have been identified by Western blot [19]. Myr p1, a 25.6- and a 89.9-kDa protein could be major allergens.

Recombinant Venom Allergens

A number of allergens from both honey bee and vespid venoms have been cloned and expressed by either *Escherichia coli* or baculovirus-infected insect cells (table 1): phospholipase A_2 [20], hyaluronidase [21], acid phosphatase [13] and Api m6 [14] from honey bee venom, as well as antigen 5 [22], phospholipase A_1 and hyaluronidase [23] from vespid venom, and dipeptidylpeptidases from both bee and *Vespula* venoms [15, 16]. Their reactivity with human-specific IgE antibodies to the respective allergens has been documented [11–16, 22, 23] and their specificity is superior to natural purified venom proteins or whole venoms. Recombinant species-specific non-glycosylated major allergens like Api m1 and Ves v5 are helpful in distinguishing between cross-reactivity and true double sensitization in the frequent Hymenoptera venom-allergic patients with double positivity to both honey bee and *Vespula* venoms [24].

Clinical Presentation of Anaphylaxis to Hymenoptera Venoms

The symptoms of anaphylaxis following Hymenoptera stings are the same as in anaphylaxis from other causes: cutaneous involvement with flush, urticaria and angioedema; respiratory symptoms include dyspnea, wheezing, cough, hoarseness; gastrointestinal tract involvement is characterized by abdominal pain, vomiting and diarrhea, and cardiovascular symptoms are dizziness, palpitations, arrhythmia, drop in blood pressure, collapse and unconsciousness. The interval between sting and symptoms lies between minutes and half an hour as a rule and is thus usually shorter than in anaphylaxis induced by food or oral medication [1, 25].

Severe or even fatal anaphylaxis to Hymenoptera stings occur most often in elderly patients with preexisting cardiovascular disease [26], not in children or young adults with preexisting asthma, as in food allergy [27]. This is partly explained by the fact that atopy is not more frequent in Hymenoptera venom-allergic patients than in the whole population [1, 25], whereas most patients with severe food-induced anaphylaxis are atopic and suffering from asthma. Interestingly, venom allergy is associated with atopy more frequent in venom-allergic beekeepers, where it was found in about 50% as compared to only 13% in non-venom-allergic beekeepers. It is suggested that during work in bee hives, sensitization may often occur by inhalation of bee dust containing venom proteins in atopic, but not in non-atopic beekeepers [28].

Epidemiologic Aspects

Prevalence of anaphylaxis from Hymenoptera stings in various countries and areas is dependent on climatic and environmental factors and may vary considerably (table 2). A warm and dry climate favors the development of most Hymenoptera species resulting in a higher risk of stings and thus a higher lifetime prevalence, as found e.g. in Mediterranean countries as compared to Great Britain or Scandinavia [25]. In large urban areas, vespid venom anaphylaxis – especially caused by *Vespula* spp. – is definitely more frequent than bee venom anaphylaxis, while the latter prevails in agricultural, especially fruit-growing areas, like in California or in Switzerland [1]. Lifetime prevalence of venom anaphylaxis is of course increasing with age and thus significantly higher in adults [29] than in children [30].

Table 2. Prevalence of anaphylaxis to Hymenoptera stings [1, 25]

Author	Country	Population age	Number questioned	Percent with history of anaphylaxis to venoms
Settipane 1972	USA	boy scouts 11–16 years	2,964	0.8
Golden 1989	USA	adult	269	3.3
Björnsson 1995	Sweden	adult	1,815	1.5
Strupler 1995	Switzerland	adult	8,322	3.5
Kalyoncu 1996	Turkey	mostly adult	786	7.5
Grigoreas 1997	Greece	soldiers	480	3.1
Incorvaia 1997	Italy	conscripts	701	2.7

Fatal reactions to Hymenoptera stings are rare: they range from 0.09 to 0.48 per million inhabitants and year [31, 32]. However, the true number may be underestimated: in one study, specific IgE antibodies to Hymenoptera venoms were detected in 23% of postmortem serum samples from patients who died outdoors from unknown reasons [33]. Between 1961 and 2004, 140 fatal Hymenoptera sting reactions were registered by the federal administration for statistics in Switzerland with about 7.5 million inhabitants, resulting in an average annual fatality rate of 3.18. If these data are extrapolated to Europe with a population of around 500 million, the annual death rate in Europe would amount to about 200.

The *natural history* of Hymenoptera venom anaphylaxis, that is the risk to develop anaphylaxis again when re-stung, has been analyzed in several prospective studies (table 3) [35–37], and in placebo or whole-body extract treated controls of prospective studies on venom immunotherapy [38–40]. It is higher in patients with a history of severe as compared to mild systemic anaphylactic reactions, and in honey bee than in vespid venom-allergic patients – most likely because of the smaller and less constant amount of venom applied by vespids [10, 41]. A short interval between two stings increases the risk of anaphylaxis [25], but severe anaphylaxis may occur again even after intervals of 10–20 years or more.

Diagnosis

History
After a painful sting the elicitor of Hymenoptera venom-induced anaphylaxis is usually clear. However the identification of the responsible species is often difficult.

Table 3. Natural history of Hymenoptera venom allergy

Author	Previous reaction	Patients n	Re-exposure	Percent with systemic reaction to re-exposure			
				bee or vespid	bee	vespid	ant
Re-exposures in untreated patients							
Blaauw 1985 [35]	any systemic	88	challenge	35	50	23	
	mild	30			31	10	
	severe	58			60	33	
Van der Linden 1994 [36]	any systemic	324	challenge		51	25	
	mild						
	bee	17			53 (0% severe)		
	vespid	94				20 (0% severe)	
	severe						
	bee	35			51 (40% severe)		
	vespid	178				28 (14% severe)	
Re-exposures in control groups of controlled studies							
Hunt 1978 [38]	severe systemic	23	challenge	61			
Müller 1979 [39]	severe systemic	12	field sting		75		
Brown 2003 [40]	severe systemic	29	challenge				72

Photos as shown in figure 1, the season and the environment of the sting, as well as whether the sting stayed in the skin may be helpful (see section: Taxonomy and Biology of Responsible Insects).

Skin Tests and Specific IgE Antibodies
The sensitivity of these tests is very high: in the first year after sting anaphylaxis more than 90% of patients have a positive result with both tests; with an increasing interval from the last sting reaction the positivity rate decreases, more rapidly for specific IgE than for intracutaneous skin tests, but even 5 years after the reaction the majority of patients still have positive results [1, 24, 25]. The specificity of both skin tests and

serum venom-specific IgE is however limited: 10–20% of patients without a history of systemic sting reactions have positive tests. Of course they may have been sensitized after the last sting. However, according to one study, only 17% of these history-negative test-positive individuals reacted when re-stung [29]. Moreover, more than 50% may have double positive tests with honey bee and vespid venoms [24]. As mentioned above, cross-reactivity based on the protein structure of venom allergens is limited, but cross-reacting carbohydrate determinants of plant origin may well be responsible for part of these false-positive results.

Other Tests
Cellular tests like the CAST (cellular antigen stimulation test), measuring the leukotriene mediator release from basophils after allergen exposure [42], or the BAT (basophil activation test), analyzing the appearance of activation markers like CD63 on the surface of basophils following allergen exposure [43], may be more specific. However, convincing data in relation to re-exposures are still missing, and these tests are expensive.

Sting provocation tests are often considered to be the gold standard, although they are less reliable in vespids than in honey bees [35–37, 41, 43]. They are commonly used to assure the efficacy of venom immunotherapy, but are generally considered as unethical in untreated patients with a history of venom anaphylaxis.

Prevention and Emergency Treatment

All patients with Hymenoptera venom anaphylaxis should receive oral and written information about the biology of the responsible insects and how to avoid further stings [1, 45]. During the flying season of Hymenoptera they must carry emergency medications, including an adrenaline autoinjector for self-application, and must be instructed about their use in case of a re-sting. Emergency treatment of anaphylaxis to Hymenoptera stings is the same as for anaphylaxis to other elicitors and is discussed in more detail by Ring et al. (see section: Treatment and Prevention).

Immunotherapy

Efficacy and Safety
While in anaphylaxis caused by other frequent elicitors like food and drugs, allergen-specific immunotherapy is not established, immunotherapy with Hymenoptera venoms has been shown to be effective in three prospective controlled trials (table 4) [38–40] and also in a number of studies where patients were submitted to a sting challenge with the responsible insect during venom immunotherapy (table 5) [44]. While over 90% of vespid venom-allergic patients are fully protected and do not develop any

Table 4. Efficacy of venom immunotherapy: controlled prospective studies

Author, year	Immunotherapy with	Number re-exposed	Re-exposure by	Systemic reaction at re-exposure (%)	p verum vs. control
Hunt 1978 [38]	venom (bee or *Vespula*)	19	challenge	1 (5)	
	whole-body extract	11	challenge	7 (64)	<0.01
	placebo	12	challenge	7 (58)	<0.01
Müller 1979 [39]	bee venom	12	field sting	3 (25)	
	whole-body extract	12	field sting	9 (75)	<0.03
Brown 2003 [40]	ant venom	35	challenge	1 (3)	
	placebo	29	challenge	21 (72)	<0.0001

Table 5. Efficacy of venom immunotherapy: Result of sting challenge on maintenance immunotherapy [1, 41, 44]

Author, year	Immunotherapy with venom of	Number challenged	Systemic reaction after challenge (%)
Hoffman, 1981	honey bee, adults	25	5 (20)
Urbanek, 1985	honey bee, children	66	4 (6)
Müller, 1992	honey bee, adults	148	34 (23)
	Vespula, adults	57	5 (9)
Chipps, 1980	mostly *Vespula*, children	42	1 (2)
Golden, 1981	mostly *Vespula*, adults	147	4 (3)

systemic allergic symptoms when re-stung, the full protection rate lies only between 75 and 90% in bee venom-allergic patients. Most of the not fully protected patients do however develop only minor systemic allergic symptoms which are definitely less severe than before treatment. Moreover, an increase of the maintenance dose from the usual 100 µg per injection to 200 µg leads to full protection in most of these patients [46]. Allergic side effects to immunotherapy injections may occur and are more frequent in honey bee than in *Vespula* venom-allergic patients [41–45]. Antihistamine

Table 6. Protocols for venom immunotherapy [51]

Conventional		Ultra-rush		
week	amount of venom, µg	day	min	amount of venom, µg
1	0.01	1	0	0.1
2	0.1		30	1
3	1		60	10
4	2		90	20
5	4		150	30
6	8		210	50
7	10			
8	20	8	0	50
9	40			50
10	60			
11	80	21	0	100
12	100	49	0	100

Afterwards 100 µg monthly for 1 year, then every 6 weeks from year 2 to 5.

premedication during the dose increase phase of venom immunotherapy has been shown to reduce local and systemic allergic side effects significantly in a number of placebo-controlled double-blind studies [47, 48].

Indications

The indication for venom immunotherapy is based on a history of systemic allergic reactions to Hymenoptera stings and positive diagnostic tests, skin tests and/or venom-specific serum IgE antibodies [45, 49]. In the presence of only mild systemic allergic reactions, limited to the skin, immunotherapy is not generally recommended: in the USA not for children, in Europe not for children and adults, unless they are heavily exposed and had repeated such reactions.

Contraindications are the same as for immunotherapy for inhalant allergy, but are relative in nature because of the life-saving potential of venom immunotherapy. Elderly patients, especially with preexisting cardiovascular disease, are at a high risk to develop severe or even fatal anaphylaxis [26]. Therefore, venom immunotherapy is often recommended in patients over 50–60 years of age. Since β-blocker treatment is associated with a significantly increased survival rate in patients with coronary heart disease and chronic heart failure, venom immunotherapy on β-blockers may be indicated for venom anaphylaxis in such patients [50].

Immunotherapy Protocols and Duration

The usual starting dose lies between 0.01 and 0.1 µg of the venom, the usual maintenance dose is 100 µg. The dose may be increased according to conventional protocols with weekly injection, or with rush or ultra-rush protocols [45, 49, 51] (table 6). Rush and especially ultra-rush protocols have the advantage of providing rapid protection, but may be associated with more frequent allergic side effects. After reaching maintenance dose, the recommended interval between injections is 4 weeks in the first year and 6 weeks from the second year. An increase of the maintenance dose to 200 µg or even more is recommended in beekeepers, who often are stung by more than one bee at the time, and in patients with incomplete protection when re-stung during venom immunotherapy [46]. The recommended treatment duration is at least 3–5 years. Even longer treatment is indicated in patients with a history of very severe reactions [26, 50], and in those with concurrent mastocytosis or elevated baseline serum tryptase levels [51, 52].

After stopping venom immunotherapy, most patients remain protected, but relapses may occur, especially after repeated re-exposures [45, 49].

References

1 Müller U: Insect Sting Allergy: Clinical Picture, Diagnosis and Treatment. Stuttgart, Fischer/New York, VCH, 1990.

2 De Groot H: Allergy to bumblebees. Curr Opin Allergy Clin Immunol 2006;6:294–297.

3 Lockey RF: Systemic reactions to stinging ants. J Allergy Clin Immunol 1974;54:132–146.

4 Brown SG, Wu QX, Kelsall GR, et al: Fatal anaphylaxis after jack jumper ant sting in southern Tasmania. Med J Aust 2001;175:644–647.

5 Hoffman DR: Allergic reactions to biting insects; in Levine MI, Lockey RF (eds): Monograph on Insect Allergy. Pittsburgh, Lambert Assoc, 2003, pp 161–174.

6 Golden DB, Breisch NL, Hamilton RG, Guralnick MW, Greene A, Craig TJ, Kagey-Sobotka A: Clinical and entomological factors influence the outcome of sting challenge studies. J Allergy Clin Immunol 2006;117:670–675.

7 Reichmuth DA, Lockey RF: Clinical aspects of ant allergy; in Levine MI, Lockey RF (eds): Monograph on Insect Allergy. Pittsburgh, Lambert Assoc, 2003, pp 133–152.

8 Benton AW, Morse RA, Stewart JD: Venom collection from honey bees. Science 1963;142:228–229.

9 Hoffman DR: Hymenoptera venoms: composition, standardization, stability; in Levine MI, Lockey RF (eds): Monograph on Insect Allergy. Pittsburgh, Lambert Assoc, 2003, pp 37–53.

10 Hoffman DR, Jacobsen RS: Allergens in Hymenoptera venoms. XII. How much protein is in a sting? Ann Allergy 1984;52:276–278.

11 Müller U, Fricker M, Wymann D, Blaser K, Crameri R: Increased specificity of diagnostic tests with recombinant major bee venom allergen phospholipase A$_2$. Clin Exp Allergy 1997;27:915–920.

12 Müller U, Soldatova L, Weber M: Bee venom allergy: comparison of purified natural and recombinant-synthetic venom allergens. J Allergy Clin Immunol 1998;101:33.

13 Grunwald T, Bockisch B, Spillner E, Ring J, Bredehorst R, Ollert M: Molecular cloning and expression and expression in insect cells of honey bee venom allergen acid phosphatase (Api m3). J Allergy Clin Immunol 2006;117:848–854.

14 Kettner A, Hughes GJ, Frutiger S, Astori M, Roggero M, Spertini F, Corradin G: Api m6: a new bee venom allergen. J Allergy Clin Immunol 2001;107:914–920.

15 de Graaf DC, Aerts M, Danneels E, Devreese B: Bee, wasp and ant venomics pave the way for a component resolved diagnosis of sting allergy. J Proteomics 2009;72:145–154.

16 Blank S, Seisman H, Bockish B, Braren I, Ollert MW, Grunwald T, Spillner E: Identification, recombinant expression and characterization of the 100 kDa high molecular weight hymenoptera venom allergens Api m5 and Ves v3. Allergy 2008;63(Suppl 88):13–14.

17 Hemmer W, Focke M, Kolarich D, Jarisch R: Identification by immunoblot of venom glycoproteins displaying IgE-binding N-glycans as cross-reacting allergens in honey bee and yellow-jacket venom. Clin Exp Allergy 2004;34:460–469.

18 Jappe U, Raulf-Heimsoth M, Hoffman M, et al: In vitro Hymenoptera venom allergy diagnosis: improved by screening for cross-reactive carbohydrate determinants and reciprocal inhibition. Allergy 2006;61:1220–1229.

19 Wiese MD, Brown SGA, Chataway TK, Davies NM, Milne RW, Aulfrey SJ, Heddle RJ: *Myrmecia pilosula* (jack jumper) ant venom: identification of allergens and revised nomenclature. Allergy 2007;62:437–443.

20 Dudler T, Schneider T, Annand RR, Suter M, Blaser K: Antigenic surface of bee venom phospholipase A$_2$. J Immunol 1994;152:5514–5522.

21 Soldatova LN, Crameri R, Gmachl M, Kemeny DM, Schmidt M, Müller UR: Superior biologic activity of the recombinant bee venom allergen hyaluronidase expressed in baculovirus-infected insect cells as compared with E. coli. J Allergy Clin Immunol 1998;101:691–698.

22 Henriksen A, King TP, Mirza O, Monsalve RI, Meno K, Ipsen H, Larsen JN, Gajhed M, Spangfort MD: Mayor venom allergen of yellow jackets, Ves v5: structural characterization of a pathogenesis-related superfamily. Proteins 2001;45:438–448.

23 King TP, Lu G, Gonzalez M: Yellow jacket venom allergens hyaluronidase and phospholipase: sequence similarity and antigenic cross-reactivity with their hornet and wasp homologs and possible implications for clinical allergy. J Allergy Clin Immunol 1996;98:588–600.

24 Müller U, Johansen N, Petersen A, Fromberg-Nielsen J, Haeberli G: Hymenoptera venom allergy: analysis of double positivity to honey bee and *Vespula* venom by estimation of IgE antibodies to species-specific major allergens Api m1 and Ves v5. Allergy 2009;64:543–548.

25 Bilo BM, Rueff F, Mosbech H, Bonifazi F, Oude Elberink JNG, Birnbaum J, et al: Diagnosis of Hymenoptera venom allergy. EAACI position paper. Allergy 2005;60:1339–1349.

26 Müller UR: Cardiovascular disease and anaphylaxis. Curr Opin Allergy Clin Immunol 2007;7:337–341.

27 Pumphrey RSH: Lessons for management of anaphylaxis from a study of fatal reactions. Clin Exp Allergy 2000;30:11444–11450.

28 Miyachi S, Lessof MH, Kemeny DM, Green LA: Comparison of the atopic background between allergic and non-allergic beekeepers. Int Arch Allergy Appl Immunol 1979;58:160–166.

29 Golden DBK, Marsh DG, Kagey-Sobotka A, Freidhoff L, Szklo M, Valentine MD, Lichtenstein LM: Epidemiology of insect venom sensitivity. JAMA 1989;262:240–244.

30 Settipane GA, Newstead GJ, Boyd GK: Frequency of Hymenoptera venom allergy in an atopic and normal population. J Allergy Clin Immunol 1972;50:146–150.

31 Nall TM: Analysis of 677 death certificates and 168 autopsies of stinging insects deaths. J Allergy Clin Immunol 1985;75:207.

32 Sasvary Z, Müller UR: Todesfälle an Insektenstichen in der Schweiz 1978–1987. Schweiz Med Wochenschr 1994;124:1887–1894.

33 Schwartz HJ, Squillace DL, Sher TH, Teigland JD, Yunginger JW: Studies in stinging insect hypersensitivity: postmortem demonstration of antivenom IgE antibody in possible sting-related sudden death. Am J Clin Pathol 1986;85:607–610.

34 Reisman RE: Natural history of insect sting allergy: relationship of severity of symptoms of initial sting anaphylaxis to re-sting reactions. J Allergy Clin Immunol 1992;90:335–339.

35 Blaauw PJ, Smithuis LOM: The evaluation of the common diagnostic methods of hypersensitivity for bee and yellow jacket venom by means of an in-hospital insect sting. J Allergy Clin Immunol 1985;75:556–562.

36 Van der Linden PW, Hack CE, Struyvenberg A, van der Zwan JK: Insect sting challenge in 324 subjects with a previous anaphylactic reaction: current criteria for insect venom hypersensitivity do not predict the occurrence and severity of anaphylaxis. J Allergy Clin Immunol 1994;94:1512–1519.

37 Franken HH, Dubois AEJ, Minkema HJ, van der Heide S, de Monchy JG: Lack of reproducibility of a single negative sting challenge response in the assessment of anaphylactic risk in patients with suspected yellow jacket hypersensitivity. J Allergy Clin Immunol 1994;93:431–436.

38 Hunt KJ, Valentine MD, Sobotka AK, Benton AW, Amododio FJ, Lichtenstein LM: A controlled trial of immunotherapy in insect hypersensitivity. N Engl J Med 1978;299:157–161.

39 Müller U, Thurnheer U, Patrizzi R, Spiess J, Hoigné R: Immunotherapy in bee sting hypersensitvity. Allergy 1979;34:369–378.

40 Brown SG, Wiese M, Blackman K, Heddle R: Ant venom immunotherapy: a double blind, placebo-controlled crossover trial. Lancet 2003;361:1101–1106.

41 Müller UR, Helbling A, Berchtold E: Immunotherapy with honey bee and yellow jacket venom is different regarding efficacy and safety. J Allergy Clin Immunol 1992;89:529–535.

42 Maly FE, Marti-Wyss S, Blumer S, Cuhat-Stark I, Wüthrich B: Mononuclear blood cell sulfidoleukotriene generation in the presence of interleukin-3 and whole blood histamine release in honey bee and yellow jacket venom allergy. J Investig Allergol Clin Immunol 1997;7:217–224.

43 Ebo DG, Sainte-Laudy J, Bridts CH, Mertens CH, Hagendorens MM, Schuerwegh AJ, De Clerck LS, Stevens WJ: Flow-assisted allergy diagnosis: current applications and future perspectives. Allergy 2006; 61:1028–1039.

44 Rueff F, Przybilla B, Müller U, Mosbech H: Position paper: The sting challenge test in Hymenoptera venom allergy. Allergy 1996;51:216–225.

45 Bonifazi F, Jutel M, Birnbaum J, Müller U, Bucher C, Forster J, et al: Prevention and treatment of Hymenoptera venom allergy: Guidelines for clinical practice. EAACI position paper. Allergy 1995;60: 1459–1470.

46 Rueff F, Wenderoth A, Przybilla B: Patients still reacting to a sting challenge while receiving conventional Hymenoptera venom immunotherapy are protected by increased venom doses. J Allergy Clin Immunol 2001;108:1027–1032.

47 Brockow K, Kiehn M, Riethmüller C, Vieluf D, Berger J, Ring J: Efficacy of antihistamine pretreatment in the prevention of adverse reactions to Hymenoptera immunotherapy: a prospective, randomized, placebo-controlled trial. J Allergy Clin Immunol 1997;100:458–463.

48 Müller UR, Jutel M, Reimers A, Zumkehr J, Huber C, Kriegel C, Steiner U, Haeberli G, Akdis M, Helbling A, Schnyder B, Blaser K, Akdis C: Clinical and immunologic effects of H1 antihistamine preventive medication during honey bee venom immunotherapy. J Allergy Clin Immunol 2008;122: 1001–1007.

49 Müller UR, Golden DBK, Lockey RF, Shin B: Immunotherapy for Hymenoptera venom hypersensitivity; in Lockey RF, Ledford DK (eds): Allergens and Allergen Immunotherapy. New York, Informa Healthcare, 2008, pp 377–392.

50 Müller U, Haeberli G: Use of β-blockers during immunotherapy for Hymenoptera venom allergy. J Allergy Clin Immunol 2005;115:606–610.

51 Müller U, Haeberli G, Helbling A: Allergic reactions to stinging and biting insects; in Rich RR, Flesher T, et al (eds): Clinical Immunology: Principles and Practice, ed 3. St Louis, Mosby Elsevier, 2008, pp 657–666.

52 Brockow K, Jofer C, Behrendt H, Ring J: Anaphylaxis in patients with mastocytosis: a study on history, clinical features and risk factors in 120 patients. Allergy 2008;63:226–232.

Prof. Dr. Ulrich R. Müller
Medical Department, Allergy Division, Spital Ziegler, Spitalnetz Bern
Morillonstrasse 75–91, CH–3007 Bern (Switzerland)
Tel. +41 31 970 7342, Fax +41 31 970 7537
E-Mail ulrich.mueller@spitalnetzbern.ch

Ring J (ed): Anaphylaxis. Chem Immunol Allergy. Basel, Karger, 2010, vol 95, pp 157–169

Classification and Pathophysiology of Radiocontrast Media Hypersensitivity

Knut Brockow · Johannes Ring

Department of Dermatology and Allergy Biederstein, Technische Universität München (TUM), Munich, and Division of Environmental Dermatology and Allergology, Helmholtz Zentrum München, TUM, Munich, Germany

Abstract

Hypersensitivity reactions to radiocontrast media (RCM) are unpredictable and are a concern for radiologists and cardiologists. Immediate hypersensitivity reactions manifest as anaphylaxis, and an allergic IgE-mediated mechanism has been continuously discussed for decades. Non-immediate reactions clinically are exanthemas resembling other drug-induced non-immediate hypersensitivities. During the past years, evidence is increasing that some of these reactions may be immunological. Repeated reactions after re-exposure, positive skin tests, and presence of specific IgE antibodies as well as positive basophil activation tests in some cases, and positive lymphocyte transformation or lymphocyte activation tests in others, indicate that a subgroup of both immediate and non-immediate reactions are of an allergic origin, although many questions remain unanswered. Recently reported cases highlight that pharmacological premedication is not safe to prevent RCM hypersensitivity in patients with previous severe reactions. These insights may have important consequences. A large multicenter study on the value of skin tests in RCM hypersensitivity concluded that skin testing is a useful tool for diagnosis of RCM allergy. It may have a role for the selection of a safe product in previous reactors, although confirmatory validation data is still scarce. In vitro tests to search for RCM-specific cell activation still are in development. In conclusion, recent data indicate that RCM hypersensitivity may have an allergic mechanism and that allergological testing is useful and may indicate tolerability.

Radiocontrast media (RCM) are highly concentrated solutions of triiodinated benzene derivatives used for performing diagnosis and treatment of vascular disease and enhancement of radiographic contrast [1, 2]. However, adverse reactions after RCM administration are common [3]. The frequency and mechanisms of hypersensitivity reactions differ between monomeric and dimeric as well as between ionic and non-ionic types of RCM. Mild immediate reactions have been reported to occur in 3.8–12.7% of patients receiving ionic monomeric RCM and in 0.7–3.1% of patients receiving non-ionic RCM [4–6]. Severe immediate adverse reactions to ionic RCM have been reported in 0.1–0.4% of intravenous procedures, while reactions to non-ionic iodinated RCM are less frequent (0.02–0.04%) [4–7]. Fatal hypersensitivity

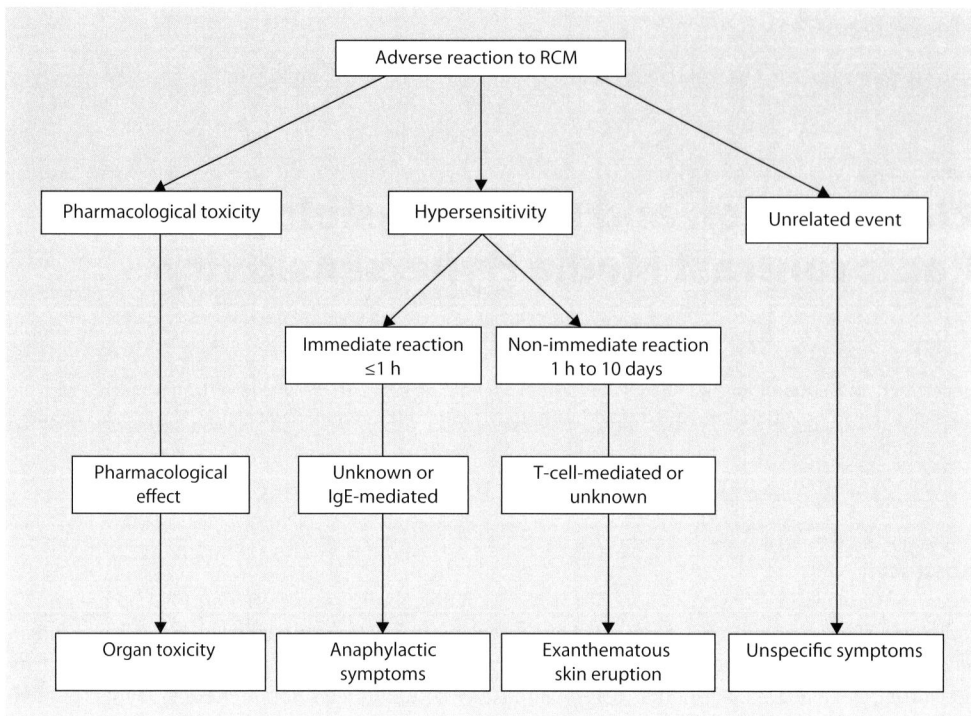

Fig. 1. Classification of adverse side effects after RCM administration [adapted from 2].

reactions are estimated to occur in 1–3 per 100,000 RCM administrations [7]. The frequency of reported non-immediate reactions varies greatly [8]. Skin exanthemas ('skin rash, skin eruptions') accounting for the majority of the RCM-induced non-immediate hypersensitivity reactions have been reported to affect 1–3% of RCM-exposed patients [9, 10]. There seems to be a higher incidence of exanthemas associated with dimeric non-ionic RCM [11]. The main risk factors for immediate as well as non-immediate hypersensitivity reactions are a previous hypersensitivity reaction [10, 12]. However, an immediate reaction is not a risk factor for developing a non-immediate reaction and vice versa.

Classification of Adverse Reactions to Radiographic Contrast Media

Not all symptoms after RCM exposure do resemble a hypersensitivity reaction. Toxic reactions related to the toxicity of RCM, unspecific reactions of unknown origin and or factors unrelated to RCM, such as chronic idiopathic urticaria, may occur (fig. 1) [3]. Hypersensitivity reactions to RCM may both present either under the clinical picture of anaphylaxis with the potential to result in fatalities or as delayed occurring exanthemas, not unlike those to other drugs. They have been classified in regard to the time interval between administration and the first appearance of symptoms as immediate, when they occur within 1 h after RCM administration, or non-immediate, when they occur 1 h up to 10 days after iodinated RCM injection [3]. In the last years, positive skin tests have been described in case reports and in a recent multicenter study in patients with RCM hypersensitivity [13–22]. In addition, laboratory data in favor of an allergic mechanism has been published [19, 23–25]. The present review will be focused on our present understanding of the mechanisms of immediate and non-immediate hypersensitivity reactions to RCM and how this translates into recommendations concerning diagnostic procedures.

Clinical Presentation of Radiocontrast Media Hypersensitivity

Immediate RCM hypersensitivity reactions manifest as anaphylaxis. Pruritus and urticaria, sometimes angioedema, occur in the majority of patients with immediate reaction [4]. For other frequent reactions, such as heat sensation, nausea, and vomiting, however, it remains questionable if these reactions represent real hypersensitivity or rather toxic reactions. Gastrointestinal symptoms such as abdominal pain and diarrhea may also occur. More severe reactions involving the respiratory and cardiovascular systems present with dyspnea, bronchospasm, and/or a sudden drop in blood pressure. Hypotension may be associated with a loss of consciousness (anaphylactic shock) and with reflex tachycardia [4]. The onset of immediate hypersensitivity reactions is very rapid. About 70% of reactions occur within 5 min after injection, and 96% of severe or fatal reactions manifest within 20 min [4, 13]. Several grading systems for the severity of hypersensitivity reactions have been published. The classification system published by Ring and Messmer [26] is helpful for scoring the severity regardless of the mechanism.

The typical clinical manifestation of a non-immediate RCM reaction is a maculopapular exanthema. It occurs from some hours to several days after the RCM administration (table 1) [10, 13]. Other skin reactions are erythema, urticaria, angioedema, fixed drug eruption, macular exanthema, erythema exsudativum multiforme, scaling skin eruption, pruritus and pompholyx [1, 10]. More untypical presentations, such as a graft-versus-host reaction, a symmetrical drug-related intertriginous and flexural exanthema (SDRIFE), or a drug-related eosinophilia with systemic symptoms (DRESS) have been described. Thus, RCM appear not different from other drugs, such as penicillins, in their ability to cause a wide spectrum of exanthemas. Non-immediate RCM hypersensitivity reactions usually have a mild to moderate severity and are self-limiting [13]. Rare cases of severe reactions have been reported such as cutaneous vasculitis, Stevens-Johnson syndrome, toxic epidermal necrolysis and papulopustular eruptions [3]. Systemic symptoms with more immediate-type manifestations such as hypotension, fever, abdominal pain, dyspnea and biphasic reactions do not appear common and have only been rarely reported [3, 22].

Table 1. Clinical manifestations of immediate and non-immediate hypersensitivity reactions to RCM

Immediate reactions	Non-immediate reactions
Urticaria	Exanthema (mostly macular or maculopapular drug eruption)
Angioedema/facial edema	
Abdominal pain, nausea, diarrhea	Urticaria, angioedema
Rhinitis (sneezing, rhinorrhea)	Erythema multiforme minor
Hoarseness, cough	Fixed drug eruption
Dyspnea (bronchospasm, laryngeal edema)	Stevens-Johnson syndrome
Respiratory arrest	Toxic epidermal necrolysis
Hypotension, cardiovascular shock	Graft-versus-host reaction
Cardiac arrest	Drug related eosinophilia with systemic symptoms (DRESS)
	Symmetrical drug-related intertriginous and flexural exanthema (SDRIFE)
	Vasculitis

Pathophysiology of Immediate Reactions

The mechanisms of the allergy-like reactions to RCM are still a matter of speculation (table 2). Anaphylaxis to RCM has been discussed to be due to a direct membrane effect possibly related to the osmolality of the RCM solution or the chemical structure of the RCM molecule (pseudo-allergy) [2], an activation of the complement system [27], a direct bradykinin formation [28], or an IgE-mediated mechanism [3].

A higher histamine release after incubation of high-osmolal ionic monomeric RCM as compared to low-osmolal nonionic RCM has been reported [29]. On the other hand, Stellato et al. [29] reported heterogeneity of human basophils and human mast cells isolated from lung, skin and heart concerning their ability to release histamine and tryptase after incubation of RCM. For mast cells, they found no correlation between osmolality of RCM and histamine release. Similarly, an activation of the complement system has been described with a decrease of CH_{50} in the presence of RCM in vitro [30]. In vivo, the anaphylatoxins C3a and C4a were reported to be increased in a fraction of patients with immediate life-threatening reactions to RCM, without significant differences between RCM-intolerant and -tolerant patients [31]. The increase has been attributed to a secondary activation of the complement system by tryptase. In other studies, complement activation has also been demonstrated in patients who did not develop immediate reactions [32]. These concepts regarding direct histamine release, complement activation and bradykinin formation remain controversial as long as pathologic changes are reported for reactors as well as for non-reactors [32].

Table 2. Arguments for an immunologic mechanism of RCM hypersensitivity

Con	Pro
No sensitization phase	Preclinical sensitization to environmental cross-reactive substance
Immediate hypersensitivity	
Repeated reactions do not always recur and do not always increase in severity	Previous reaction is a strong risk factor for subsequent reaction, some case reports with increasing severity
No increase of plasma leukotrienes after RCM administration	Mast cell mediator release correlates with severity of reaction, positive basophil activation test to RCM in patients
Only anecdotal reports of RCM-specific IgE antibodies	Low levels of IgE antibodies to ioxaglic acid in one study
Low affinity of IgE to RCM	Specific IgE to RCM higher in reactors than in controls in one study
RCM are not able to form haptens	Positive skin tests in patients but not in controls in optimal concentrations
Non-immediate hypersensitivity	
Con	Pro
No sensitization phase	Preclinical sensitization to cross-reactive substance possible, PI concept
RCM are not able to form haptens	PI concept
Not all patients show positive skin tests	Positive skin tests in patients but not in controls in optimal concentrations
Atypical manifestations reported	Maculopapular exanthema and time course resembles drug allergy
Repeated reactions do not always recur or increase in severity	Previous reaction highest risk factor for subsequent reaction, several case reports with breakthrough reactions
	Histopathology shows T-cell pathology and T-cell activation in acute reaction and in skin test
	Enhanced frequency in IL-2-treated patients
	Positive lymphocyte transformation test and lymphocyte activation tests
	Demonstration of RCM-specific T cells
	Generation of RCM-specific T-cell lines and T-cell clones

The evidence that immediate hypersensitivity reactions may indeed be caused by an IgE-mediated allergic mechanism is also mainly indirect. However, some data support the concept that a subgroup of reactions may be IgE-mediated:

Immediate hypersensitivity reactions to RCM are associated with histamine release from basophils and mast cells [27], and extensive mast cell activation in vivo associated with clinical symptoms has been demonstrated by Laroche et al. [31]. Patients with hypersensitivity reactions after contrast medium exposure had increased plasma levels of both histamine and tryptase, and levels correlated with severity. Also other investigators have reported high levels of tryptase in connection with severe or fatal reactions [21, 33].

In some countries such as Japan, pretesting with intravenous injection of 0.5–1 ml of RCM as a means of predicting severe or fatal reactions had been performed. This approach had been abandoned after severe cardiovascular reactions to these minute amounts RCM were described [34]. The possibility to react to low amounts of allergen is regarded to be typical for IgE-mediated reactions.

Several groups have reported positive skin test results for patients with severe immediate reactions to either ionic or non-ionic RCM [13]. Some of these patients were shown to react not only to the culprit contrast medium but also to other RCM [13]. The frequency of positive skin tests has also been investigated in a European multicenter study in patients with RCM hypersensitivity and in 82 controls [13]. The intradermal test (IDT) remained negative in 96.3% of controls, but was positive in 26% of patients. The relatively high percentage of skin-test-positive patients may have been be fostered by a selective recruitment of patients with typical features of RCM hypersensitivity and involvement of allergy departments experienced in drug hypersensitivity. The percentage of positive skin test results was up to 50% in patients that could be tested within 2–6 months after the reaction.

Positive basophil activation tests were reported in patients with immediate RCM hypersensitivity reactions, which may be regarded as another indirect indication for an IgE-mediated allergy [35].

It has been tried to demonstrate contrast medium-specific IgE for decades by immunoassays. Only few groups reported specific IgE antibodies and those only in low levels and, due to methodological problems, only to the older ionic products coupled to a solid phase. Laroche et al. [31] studied specific IgE to the ionic RCM ioxaglate and ioxitalamate in 20 patients with immediate reactions and reported significantly higher levels as compared to control patients. Mita et al. [25] reported ioxaglate-specific IgE in 43% of (16/34) of patients with a history of reaction to this RCM, in 20.6% (14/68) of patients who reacted to ioxaglate when serum was sampled in the next 24 h, but in none of the 10 RCM-tolerant controls. It has to be noted that RCM-specific IgE was not much higher as compared to controls, usually less than 2-fold higher than the cut-off level. In addition, the dissociation constant K_D (18.7 mM) was very low, which may be regarded as an argument against specificity. Unfortunately, assays for the modern non-ionic RCM have not been described, as it is extremely difficult to bind non-ionic RCM to a solid phase, limiting research in this field.

All this evidence taken together indicates that not all immediate hypersensitivity reactions to RCM may be pseudo-allergic reactions, and that diagnostic testing may be of value. In those patients with negative skin tests, the mechanism involved remains unknown. Patients can react to a RCM on first exposure and the reaction does not always recur. This has been seen as an important argument against an allergic mechanism. The lack of a clear sensitization phase, however, is similar to the situation described in anaphylaxis to muscle relaxants [36], where it has been discussed that these previously non-exposed patients may have already been sensitized. The chemical structure(s) responsible for the possible sensitization remain unknown. On the other hand, the positive immediate skin tests reported by several investigators, the fact that up to 50% of patients had a positive skin test when tested 2–6 months after the reaction, the detection of RCM-specific IgE antibodies in sera from immediate reactors to ionic RCM as well as the positive basophil activation test in immediate reactors with positive IDTs to the implicated non-ionic RCM support the concept of an IgE-mediated mechanism at least in a subgroup of patients (table 2).

Pathophysiology of Non-Immediate Reactions

During the past decade, a lot of data on the pathogenesis of non-immediate reactions induced by RCM has indicated that the majority of these reactions are T-cell-mediated reactions (table 2):

The most common clinical picture of non-immediate RCM reactions is a maculopapular exanthema, which resembles other drug-induced T-cell-mediated hypersensitivity reactions. The reported onset of skin eruptions 2–10 days after the first exposure to a RCM and 1–2 days after re-exposure to the same substance is typical for an allergic drug reaction with a sensitization phase.

The histopathology of such exanthematous reactions and of positive skin test sites provides further evidence for a T-cell-mediated mechanism [19, 24]: mostly a dermal lymphocyte-rich infiltrate accompanied by intraepidermal spongiosis and sometimes hydropic degeneration of the basal cell layer have been reported [37]. Positive skin test site biopsies show a perivascular infiltrate consisting mainly of CD4+ and CD8+ (CD45RO+) T cells [19, 24]. The dermal perivascular mononuclear cell infiltrate in most patients with maculopapular exanthemas shows CD4 lymphocytes exceeding CD8 T lymphocytes, a moderate expression of CD25 and expression of HLA-DR and CLA [24]. Eosinophils are common. Skin biopsies obtained at the site of the positive skin tests to the culprit RCM showed similar results to those seen in the initial acute phase biopsy, with high expression of CD69 in lymphocytes [18, 24, 38].

There is an enhanced frequency of RCM-related side effects in interleukin-2-treated patients, which is indicative of a T-cell-mediated pathology. Interleukin-2 has been reported to reduce the threshold for T-cell activation and to increase the possibility for clinical symptoms.

Previous reactors are at high risk for a new reaction. In many cases reported, re-administration of the culprit contrast medium to patients with a previous non-immediate exanthema resulted in a repeat reaction [1]. In some (but not all) cases, a more severe reaction with subsequent RCM exposure has been described. After provocation tests, a re-appearance of the exanthemas after intravenous administration of the culprit contrast medium has been reported in patients with previous contrast medium-induced eruptions [1].

Numerous positive delayed skin tests in patients with contrast medium-induced non-immediate skin reactions have been reported when the patients were tested with the culprit contrast medium [summarized in 1]. In a large European multicenter study, 37% of patients with non-immediate reactions were positive in delayed IDTs and/or patch tests [13]. The majority of the patients also reacted to the culprit contrast medium and also to other, structurally similar RCM. Notably, in more than 30% of those skin test-positive patients a RCM had been administered for the first time. Thus, there is a lack of a sensitization phase. Again it may be hypothesized that these previously non-exposed patients may have already been sensitized. Different patterns of RCM cross-reactivity indicate that several chemical entities could be involved. No positive skin tests have been obtained with other contrast medium excipients, such as ethylenediaminetetraacetic acid (EDTA), and only rarely patients have been found to react to inorganic iodide.

The presence of contrast medium-specific T cells in patients with non-immediate exanthematous skin eruptions has been demonstrated. Peripheral blood mononuclear cells (PBMCs) from patients show an enhanced in vitro proliferation when the culprit contrast medium is added to the culture (mainly in the range 10–100 mg iodide/ml) [19]. Flow cytometric analysis demonstrated increased T-lymphocyte activation markers (CD69, CD25 and human leukocyte antigen D-related) and skin homing receptors (cutaneous lymphocyte-associated antigen, CLA) in CD4+ lymphocytes, and perforin expression was increased in the CD8+ cytotoxic lymphocytes [24]. The early T-cell activation marker CD69 was expressed in about 0.5–3% of T cells after incubation with RCM [23]. The precursor frequency of peripheral RCM-specific T cells was estimated between 0.05 and 0.6% by CFSE staining assays [23]. It has thus been speculated that the reactive cell population consisted of a few drug-specific T cells and a higher number of cytokine-activated bystander T cells amplifying the reaction [39]. High levels of cross-reactivity between different RCM were also found in vitro by CD69 upregulation and lymphocyte proliferation, in patient PBMCs as well as in generated T-cell lines and T-cell clones from patients with RCM hypersensitivity [23]. The in-vitro experiments confirm the principal presence and importance of drug-specific T cells in selected non-immediate reactions to RCM.

An argument against an immunologic reaction in non-immediate hypersensitivity reactions has been the lack of a hapten. Non-ionic RCM are chemically non-reactive

Table 3. Recommended skin test concentrations for RCM

Test	Concentration[1]	Readings	
		immediate reaction	non-immediate reaction
Skin prick test	undiluted	20 min	20 min, 48 h, 72 h[2]
Intradermal test	1/10 diluted	20 min	20 min, 48 h, 72 h[2]
Patch test	undiluted		20 min, 48 h, 72 h[2]

[1] Undiluted RCM with an iodine concentration of 300–320 mg/ml.
[2] If the patient notices a positive reaction (pruritus, erythema) at the skin test site at other time points, additional readings may be performed (e.g. after 24 or 96 h).

and unable to bind covalently to proteins. Recently it has been shown that drugs are also able to stimulate T cells non-covalently in a HLA-restricted pattern [40]. This concept has been termed the p-i concept (pharmacological interaction of drugs with immune receptors) and requires neither drug metabolism nor protein processing. This model would also explain the cross-reactivity observed between different compounds.

Diagnosis

Immediate Hypersensitivity Reactions

As immediately after the reaction, elevated plasma histamine and serum or plasma tryptase levels of histamine and tryptase have been found [31, 34], an anaphylaxis may be confirmed by blood samples for histamine analysis drawn as soon as possible after the reaction and for tryptase drawn 1–2 h after onset of symptoms [31]. Tryptase values have to be compared to baseline levels.

The further allergologic workup is recommended to be performed between 2 and 6 months after the reaction (table 3) [13]. A skin prick test should be performed with undiluted RCM. Afterwards, IDTs with RCM (300–320 mg/ml) diluted 10-fold in sterile saline and reading after 20 min are recommended [13]. As cross-reactivity is frequent, a panel of several different RCM should be tested in an attempt to find a skin test-negative product, which might be tolerated in future RCM examinations.

Unfortunately there is no commercial assay for routine measurement of serum levels of RCM-specific IgE antibodies. The reliability of other in vitro tests, such as the basophil activation test, has not yet been established. Results from individual patients indicate that the basophil activation test may be helpful [36]. However, at the moment it is only added on an experimental scientific basis. Provocation is not generally recommended, as intravenous applications of as low as 0.5–1 ml RCM have led to severe anaphylaxis [41].

Non-Immediate Hypersensitivity Reactions

Hematology and clinical chemistry should be considered in more severe exanthema, as systemic involvement has been described [1]. A skin biopsy may sometimes be needed for differential diagnosis.

The further allergologic workup is recommended should be performed within 6 months after the reaction [13]. Both delayed IDTs and patch tests are frequently positive, when read after 48 and 72 h (in case of local pruritus or erythematous plaques optionally at other time points, e.g. 24 h, 96 h). Since some patients tested positive with only one of these tests, it is recommended to use both tests in parallel to enhance test sensitivity (table 3). Patch tests should be conducted with undiluted RCM, whereas 10-fold diluted products in physiologic saline had been recommended when performing delayed IDTs. IDTs and late readings with undiluted RCM may be discussed in non-severe reactions to increase sensitivity, however this has not been evaluated in a sufficient number of controls. A panel of several different RCM should be tested to identify skin test-negative substances.

RCM-related T-cell activity may be assessed in vitro by lymphocyte transformation test [19, 24]. In addition, CD69 upregulation (lymphocyte activation test) was observed in patients with a positive lymphocyte transformation test [24, 39]. These tests appear to be a promising tool to identify drug-reactive T cells in the peripheral blood of patients with RCM-induced drug-hypersensitivity reactions. However, the sensitivity and specificity remain unknown and, therefore, these tests cannot be recommended for routine use yet, but further research on the specificity and sensitivity is indicated.

Provocation tests with progressive increase of the injected RCM dose over several days has been done to confirm negative skin test results [17]. Safe re-administration of a skin test-negative RCM has so far only been published for individual case reports and in a series of 15 patients with non-immediate skin eruptions [17]. In this study, however, non-serious skin symptoms after exposition of the dimeric agents iodixanol (n = 4) or ioxaglate (n = 1) were described despite negative skin tests for these agents. Thus, it remains unknown if false-negative skin tests are a phenomenon for all RCM or specific for dimeric RCM. Skin test results are currently validated in a European multicenter follow-up study by provocation tests and re-exposure data. Until further results are available, a positive skin test to a given RCM dictates that this RCM should not be chosen for a future exposure, but a negative test does not necessarily guarantee tolerance. Here, graded provocation tests are helpful, depending on the time course of the primary reaction: e.g. 1/10 of the full dose on day 1, 1/2 of this volume on day 2 and the full dose on day 3 at the radiology department [17]. Due to the potential risk involved, provocation tests should be performed only in centers with experience to perform monitoring and emergency treatment. Noteworthy, a previous non-immediate exanthematous reaction does not pose a higher risk for a subsequent immediate anaphylactic reaction.

Prevention

In patients with bronchial asthma or previous RCM-induced immediate adverse reaction, radiologists routinely administer non-ionic RCM because of their lower incidence of total reactions [42]. If a patient with a previous immediate hypersensitivity reaction to a RCM needs a new contrasted examination, the culprit preparation should be avoided. Skin tests (skin prick test and IDT) with RCM and reading after 20 min are recommended [1]. In case of a positive reaction, a skin test-negative product should be chosen by testing a panel of several different RCM [13]. The value of skin tests and in vitro tests for selection of a safe, alternative RCM in patients with previous immediate reaction still has to be further defined. The use of premedication in patients at high risk of immediate RCM reaction is becoming more and more controversial [43, 44]. Corticosteroids and H_1- and H_2-antihistamines are the most frequently used agents [45, 46]. There are different protocols and administration routes. However, severe reactions still develop in patients who receive corticosteroid premedication [47, 48]. The recurrence rate of RCM reaction after corticosteroid administration has been estimated to be almost 10% [47]. It has been concluded that in unselected patients, the usefulness of premedication is doubtful [43]. Sufficient data supporting the use of premedication in patients with a history of allergic reactions are lacking. Physicians dealing with these patients should not rely on the efficacy of premedication [43].

Patients with previous non-immediate skin exanthemas to RCM are at risk for developing new eruptions upon re-exposure to the RCM [1]. Another RCM should be chosen if re-exposure is required. However, due to frequent cross-reactivity between different RCM, a change of product is no guarantee against a repeat reaction. Patch tests and delayed IDT are recommended to confirm an allergic reaction to the culprit RCM [13]. In case of positive skin tests, the substances that are able to elicit test reactions should be avoided. It has not yet been proven whether skin testing is a suitable tool for the selection of an alternative RCM that can be safely used. At present, the administration of skin test-negative RCM in previous reactors should be done with caution since cases of reaction have been observed after administration of skin test-negative dimeric RCM in 5 patients [17]. A fractionated provocation test may be indicated. In current practice, steroid prophylaxis is often given in patients with previous serious non-immediate adverse reactions. An intensive immunosuppressant protocol used intramuscular 6-methylprednisolone (40 mg daily) and oral cyclosporine (100 mg twice daily) 1 week before and 2 weeks after each of four angiograms in a patient with two previous episodes of maculopapular reactions after RCM administration, the last despite steroid premedication [16]. However, no studies have so far been conducted to establish the optimum pretreatment regimen. Repeated non-immediate reactions, including a case of TEN, have been reported despite corticosteroid premedication [16, 49]. There is not enough data to support the safety of pharmacological prevention in patients with non-immediate reactions to RCM.

Acknowledgements

The authors thank Cathrine Christiansen and Werner Pichler for stimulating discussions and support on the way of clarifying the underlying mechanism s of RCM hypersensitivity.

References

1   Brockow K: Contrast media hypersensitivity – scope of the problem. Toxicology 2005;209:189–192.
2   Gueant-Rodriguez RM, Romano A, Barbaud A, et al: Hypersensitivity reactions to iodinated contrast media. Curr Pharm Des 2006;12:3359–3372.
3   Brockow K, Christiansen C, Kanny G, et al: Management of hypersensitivity reactions to iodinated contrast media. Allergy 2004;60:150–158.
4   Katayama H, Yamaguchi K, Kozuka T, et al: Adverse reactions to ionic and nonionic contrast media. A report from the Japanese Committee on the Safety of Contrast Media. Radiology 1990;175:621–628.
5   Wolf GL, Arenson RL, Cross AP: A prospective trial of ionic vs. non-ionic contrast agents in routine clinical practice: comparison of adverse effects. AJR Am J Roentgenol 1989;152:939–944.
6   Palmer FJ: The RACR survey of intravenous contrast media reactions. Final report. Australas Radiol 1988;32:426–428.
7   Caro JJ, Trindade E, McGregor M: The risks of death and of severe nonfatal reactions with high- vs. low-osmolality contrast media: a meta-analysis. AJR Am J Roentgenol 1991;156:825–832.
8   Webb JA, Stacul F, Thomsen HS, Morcos SK: Late adverse reactions to intravascular iodinated contrast media. Eur Radiol 2003;13:181–184.
9   Yasuda R, Munechika H: Delayed adverse reactions to nonionic monomeric contrast-enhanced media. Invest Radiol 1998;33:1–5.
10 Hosoya T, Yamaguchi K, Akutsu T, et al: Delayed adverse reactions to iodinated contrast media and their risk factors. Radiat Med 2000;18:39–45.
11 Sutton AG, Finn P, Grech ED, et al: Early and late reactions after the use of iopamidol 340, ioxaglate 320, and iodixanol 320 in cardiac catheterization. Am Heart J 2001;141:677–683.
12 Katayama H, Yamaguchi K, Kozuka T, et al: Full-scale investigation into adverse reaction in Japan. Risk factor analysis. The Japanese Committee on the Safety of Contrast Media. Invest Radiol 1991;26(suppl 1):33–36.
13 Brockow K, Romano A, Aberer W, et al: Skin testing in patients with hypersensitivity reactions to iodinated contrast media – a European multicenter study. Allergy 2009;64:234–241.

14 Christiansen C, Dreborg S, Pichler WJ, Ekeli H: Macular exanthema appearing 5 days after X-ray contrast medium administration. Eur Radiol 2002; 12(suppl 3):S94–S97.
15 Kvedariene V, Martins P, Rouanet L, Demoly P: Diagnosis of iodinated contrast media hypersensitivity: results of a 6-year period. Clin Exp Allergy 2006;36:1072–1077.
16 Romano A, Artesani M, Andriolo M, et al: Effective prophylactic protocol in delayed hypersensitivity to contrast media: report of a case involving lymphocyte transformation studies with different compounds. Radiology 2002;225:466–470.
17 Vernassiere C, Trechot P, Commun N, et al: Low negative predictive value of skin tests in investigating delayed reactions to radiocontrast media. Contact Dermatitis 2004;50:359–366.
18 Brockow K, Becker EW, Worret WI, Ring J: Late skin test reactions to radiocontrast medium. J Allergy Clin Immunol 1999;104:1107–1108.
19 Kanny G, Pichler W, Morisset M, et al: T-cell-mediated reactions to iodinated contrast media: evaluation by skin and lymphocyte activation tests. J Allergy Clin Immunol 2005;115:179–185.
20 Arnold AW, Hausermann P, Bach S, Bircher AJ: Recurrent flexural exanthema (SDRIFE or baboon syndrome) after administration of two different iodinated radiocontrast media. Dermatology 2007; 214:89–93.
21 Laroche D: Immediate reactions to contrast media: mediator release and value of diagnostic testing. Toxicology 2005;209:193–194.
22 Brockow K, Kiehn M, Kleinheinz A, et al: Positive skin tests in late reactions to radiographic contrast media. Allerg Immunol (Paris) 1999;31:49–51.
23 Lerch M, Keller M, Britschgi M, et al: Cross-reactivity patterns of T cells specific for iodinated contrast media. J Allergy Clin Immunol 2007;119: 1529–1536.
24 Torres MJ, Mayorga C, Cornejo-Garcia JA, et al: Monitoring non-immediate allergic reactions to iodine contrast media. Clin Exp Immunol 2008;152: 233–238.
25 Mita H, Tadokoro K, Akiyama K: Detection of IgE antibody to a radiocontrast medium. Allergy 1998; 53:1133–1140.
26 Ring J, Messmer K: Incidence and severity of anaphylactoid reactions to colloid volume substitutes. Lancet 1977;1:466–469.

27 Ring J, Arroyave CM, Frizler MJ, Tan EM: In vitro histamine and serotonin release by radiographic contrast media. Complement-dependent and -independent release reaction and changes in ultrastructure of human blood cells. Clin Exp Immunol 1978;32:105–118.

28 Lasser EC, Lyon SG: Inhibition of angiotensin-converting enzyme by contrast media. I. In vitro findings. Invest Radiol 1990;25:698–702.

29 Stellato C, de Crescenzo G, Patella V, et al: Human basophil/mast cell releasability. XI. Heterogeneity of the effects of contrast media on mediator release. J Allergy Clin Immunol 1996;97:838–850.

30 Ring J, Endrich B, Intaglietta M: Histamine release, complement consumption, and microvascular changes after radiographic contrast media infusion in rabbits. J Lab Clin Med 1978;92:584–594.

31 Laroche D, Aimone-Gastin I, Dubois F, et al: Mechanisms of severe, immediate reactions to iodinated contrast material. Radiology 1998;209:183–190.

32 Simon RA, Schatz M, Stevenson DD, et al: Radiographic contrast media infusions. Measurement of histamine, complement, and fibrin split products and correlation with clinical parameters. J Allergy Clin Immunol 1979;63:281–8.

33 Brockow K, Vieluf D, Puschel K, et al: Increased postmortem serum mast cell tryptase in a fatal anaphylactoid reaction to non-ionic radiocontrast medium. J Allergy Clin Immunol 1999;104:237–238.

34 Yamaguchi K, Katayama H, Takashima T, et al: Prediction of severe adverse reactions to ionic and nonionic contrast media in Japan: evaluation of pretesting. A report from the Japanese Committee on the Safety of Contrast Media. Radiology 1991;178:363–367.

35 Trcka J, Schmidt C, Seitz CS, et al: Anaphylaxis to iodinated contrast material: nonallergic hypersensitivity or IgE-mediated allergy? AJR Am J Roentgenol 2008;190:666–670.

36 Mertes PM, Laxenaire MC, Lienhart A, et al: Reducing the risk of anaphylaxis during anaesthesia: guidelines for clinical practice. J Investig Allergol Clin Immunol 2005;15:91–101.

37 Hari Y, Frutig-Schnyder K, Hurni M, et al: T-cell involvement in cutaneous drug eruptions. Clin Exp Allergy 2001;31:1398–1408.

38 Kanny G, Marie B, Hoen B, et al: Delayed adverse reaction to sodium ioxaglic acid-meglumine. Eur J Dermatol 2001;11:134–137.

39 Beeler A, Zaccaria L, Kawabata T, et al: CD69 upregulation on T cells as an in vitro marker for delayed-type drug hypersensitivity. Allergy 2008;63:181–188.

40 Pichler WJ: Delayed drug hypersensitivity reactions. Ann Intern Med 2003;139:683–693.

41 Kwak R: A case of shock by pretesting of contrast media (in Japanese). Rinsho Hoshasen 1985;30:407–409.

42 Morcos SK, Thomsen HS, Webb JA: Prevention of generalized reactions to contrast media: a consensus report and guidelines. Eur Radiol 2001;11:1720–1728.

43 Tramer MR, von Elm E, Loubeyre P, Hauser C: Pharmacological prevention of serious anaphylactic reactions due to iodinated contrast media: systematic review. BMJ 2006;333:675.

44 Kopp AF, Mortele KJ, Cho YD, et al: Prevalence of acute reactions to iopromide: postmarketing surveillance study of 74,717 patients. Acta Radiol 2008;49:902–911.

45 Greenberger PA, Patterson R: The prevention of immediate generalized reactions to radiocontrast media in high-risk patients. J Allergy Clin Immunol 1991;87:867–872.

46 Ring J, Rothenberger KH, Clauss W: Prevention of anaphylactoid reactions after radiographic contrast media infusion by combined histamine H_1- and H_2-receptor antagonists: results of a prospective controlled trial. Int Arch Allergy Appl Immunol 1985;78:9–14.

47 Freed KS, Leder RA, Alexander C, et al: Breakthrough adverse reactions to low-osmolar contrast media after steroid premedication. AJR Am J Roentgenol 2001;176:1389–1392.

48 Roberts M, Fisher M: Anaphylactoid reaction to iopamiro (after pretreatment). Australas Radiol 1992;36:144–146.

49 Courvoisier S, Bircher AJ: Delayed-type hypersensitivity to a nonionic, radiopaque contrast medium. Allergy 1998;53:1221–1224.

PD Dr. Knut Brockow
Department of Dermatology and Allergy Biederstein, Technische Universität München
Biedersteiner Strasse 29, DE–80802 Munich (Germany)
Tel. +49 89 41400, Fax +49 89 4140 3171
E-Mail knut.brockow@lrz.tum.de

Ring J (ed): Anaphylaxis. Chem Immunol Allergy. Basel, Karger, 2010, vol 95, pp 170–179

Analgesics

Andrzej Szczeklik

Department of Medicine, Jagiellonian University Medical College, Cracow, Poland

Abstract
Aspirin and other non-steroidal anti-inflammatory drugs (NSAIDs) are often incriminated in hypersensitivity reactions leading to anaphylaxis. Two populations are at the high risk of developing such reactions: patients with asthma and those with urticaria. In a subset of asthmatics, NSAIDs that inhibit cyclooxygenase-1 (COX-1) precipitate non-allergic, hypersensitivity reactions, characterized by violent attacks of dyspnea. These patients suffer from a distinct clinical syndrome, called aspirin-induced asthma (AIA), which includes chronic eosinophilic rhinusinusitis and persistent asthma. In patients with chronic idiopathic urticaria, and less commonly in patients without chronic urticaria, NSAIDs usually acting through inhibition of COX-1 can induce or exacerbate skin eruptions. While alterations in eicosanoid biosynthesis characterized both AIA and aspirin-triggered urticaria, other patients may rarely manifest IgE-mediated reactions.

Copyright © 2010 S. Karger AG, Basel

Aspirin and other non-steroidal anti-inflammatory drugs (NSAIDs) are often incriminated in hypersensitivity reactions. The incidence of anaphylaxis due to NSAIDs varies depending on whether or not asthmatic subjects are included. It is generally agreed that NSAIDs are the second most common offenders next to antibiotics. Of the miscellaneous mechanisms operating, a non-immunological one, that dependent on the pharmacological actions of NSAIDs, is the most common. Two populations are at high risk: patients with asthma and those with urticaria.

Historical Note

No drugs have been a more faithful companion to man throughout his history than salicylates, the forebears of aspirin. About 3,500 years ago the Ebers Papyrus recommended the application of a decoction of leaves of myrtle to the abdomen and back to get rid of rheumatic pains. Hippocrates championed the juices of the poplar tree and willow bark to treat fever and labor pains. These plants and trees are abundant in compounds derived from salicylic acid, which gets its name from them (in Latin *salix* is a willow tree). For thousands of years on all continents they have helped to

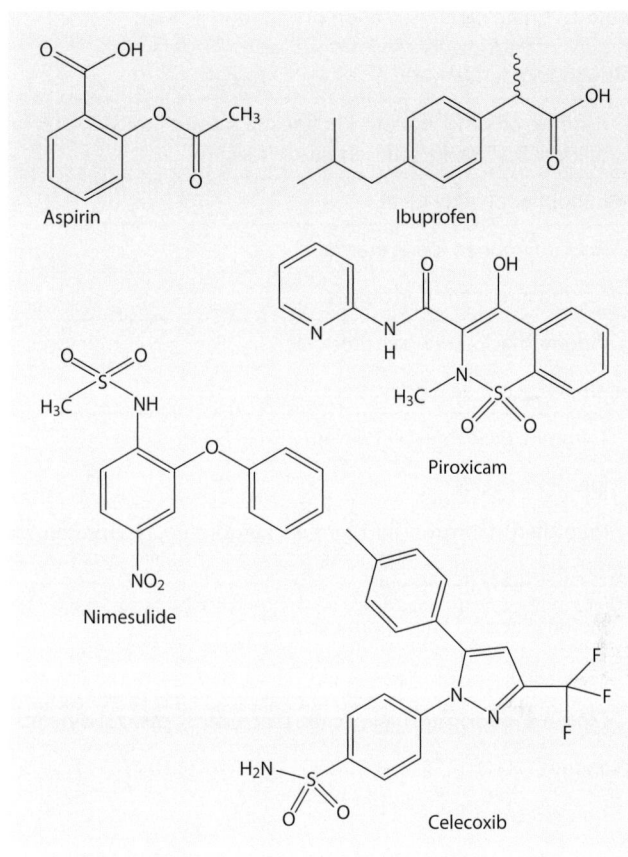

Fig. 1. Non-steroidal anti-inflammatory drugs.

relieve pain, bring down fever and reduce inflammation [1]. In 1899 the laboratories of pharmaceutical firm Bayer brought a simple synthetic derivative of salicylic acid onto the market – aspirin (acetylsalicylic acid). It has since become the most popular drug in the world. The phenomenal success of aspirin has stimulated the production of many drugs that act in a similar way. They are called non-steroidal anti-inflammatory drugs – NSAIDs (fig. 1). Despite the diversity of their chemical structures, these drugs all share to some extent the same therapeutic properties (table 1). In varying doses they alleviate the swelling, redness and pain of inflammation, reduce a general fever and cure a headache. More than that – they also share to a greater or lesser extent a number of similar side effects. The diverse actions of those drugs are based on a single biochemical intervention. In 1971, John Vane and his colleagues [2] discovered that aspirin and similar drugs inhibit cyclooxygenase (COX), the enzyme which generates prostanoids. This mode of action has been generally accepted, which does not exclude the possibility of other pharmacological effects of rather secondary importance.

Table 1. Chemical classification of common NSAIDs

Salicylic acid derivatives

    Aspirin, sodium salicylate, choline magnesium trisalicylate, salsalate, diflunisal, salicylsalicylic acid, sulfasalazine, olsalazine

p-Aminophenol derivatives

    Acetaminophen (paracetamol)

Indole and acylacetic derivatives

    Indomethacin, sulindac, etodolac

Heteroaryl acetic acid derivatives

    Tolmetin, diclofenac, ketorolac

Arylpropionie acids

    Ibuprofen, naproxen, flurbiprofen, ketoprofen, fenoprofen, oxaprozin

Anthranilic acids (fenamates)

    Mefenamic acid, meclofenamic acid

Enolic acids

    Oxicams (piroxicam, meloxicam, tenoxicam), pyrazolidinediones

Alkanones

    Nabumetone

Sulfoanilide compounds

    Nimesulide

Benzotriazines

    Azopropazone

Pyrazolone derivates

    Phenylbutazone, oxyphenbutazone, dipyrone, antipyrine (phenazone)

Three years after introduction of aspirin into therapy, Hirschberg in Poznań, now in Poland, described the first case of a transient, acute angioedema/urticaria, occurring shortly after ingestion of aspirin. Reports of anaphylactic reactions to aspirin soon followed. The other major type of adverse reaction, acute bronchospasm, was described in the second decade of the 20th century. In 1920, Van der Veer reported the first death due to aspirin. The association of aspirin sensitivity, asthma and nasal polyps was first recorded by Widal in 1922. This clinical entity, later named 'the aspirin triad' was popularized in 1968 by Samter and Beers [3], who presented a perceptive description of this syndrome. In the 1970s the link between precipitation of asthmatic attacks and inhibition of arachidonic acid COX by aspirin and other NSAIDs was discovered [4]. In the following decades, other alterations in arachidonic acid metabolism were observed in aspirin-sensitive patients. For a history of aspirin hypersensitivity, especially the early decades of research, the reader is referred to a review [5].

Classification

In some adult patients with asthma or chronic idiopathic urticaria, NSAIDs can elicit or aggravate symptoms of the disease. Thus, two most common clinical presentations of aspirin hypersensitivity are: aspirin-induced asthma (AIA) and aspirin-triggered urticaria/angioedema. They should be clearly differentiated from other adverse reactions to NSAIDs with allergic background, which are limited to a single drug, or the drugs with very similar structure.

Aspirin-Induced Asthma

The term refers to a distinct clinical syndrome characterized by aggressive and continuous inflammatory disease of the airways with chronic eosinophilic rhinosinusitis, asthma and often nasal polyposis [6–8]. Aspirin and other NSAIDs that inhibit COX-1 exacerbate the condition, precipitating violent asthmatics attacks. This is a hallmark of the syndrome. The prevalence of aspirin hypersensitivity in the general population ranges from 0.6 to 2.5%, but is much more frequent in adult asthmatic subjects where it reaches 10–15%, although it is often underdiagnosed.

AIA runs a characteristic clinical course [9]. It is more frequent in women than men, and is unusual in children, beginning in adulthood, on average at the age of 30 years. Rhinorrhea and nasal congestion are usually the first symptoms, subsequently complicated by polyposis. Asthma and aspirin hypersensitivity develop 2–15 years later. Once developed, aspirin intolerance remains through life, although sporadic disappearance of intolerance has been reported. Asthma, characterized by blood and nasal eosinophilia, runs a protracted course despite avoidance of analgesics. In about half the patients, the course of asthma is severe, necessitating use of systemic corticosteroids.

The accurate diagnosis of AIA can be established by oral, inhaled, nasal or intravenous placebo-controlled provocations tests with increasing doses of aspirin [10], There is no reliable in vitro test. Oral challenges are most commonly performed, because the oral route mimics natural exposure and the test does not require special equipment, except simple spirometry. The threshold dose of aspirin which provokes a 20% fall in FEV_1 (positive reaction) will vary with individual patients, depending also on control of asthma. In case of positive reaction, the symptoms are relived by inhalation of 2–4 puffs of short-acting β_2-agonist until FEV_1 returns to normal value. If more severe reactions are observed oral or intravenous corticosteroids (40 mg of prednisolone or equivalent) are administrated. Very severe, anaphylactic reactions (which are most unusual, if the protocol of the test is observed) require immediate intervascular injection of epinephrine. Treatment of adverse respiratory reactions due to aspirin challenges has been reviewed in detail elsewhere [10].

The clinical range of adverse reactions to aspirin and NSAIDs is large and to a certain extent is mimicked by the provocation tests which should be carried out in the specialized centers. On average, the reactions occur 30 min to 3 h after oral administration of the drug. In case of parenteral administration (including ocular drops) it becomes much shorter and the symptoms may develop within a minute. In light cases the reaction will be limited to sporadic urticarial eruptions, or conjunctivitis or rhinitis. In other patients, shortness of breath may occur leading to an open asthmatic attack. Anaphylactic shock is fortunately not common but has been well documented; the bronchial obstruction then becomes very tight and its opening even in the hands of experienced physician in setting of intensive care unit could be very difficult; fatal cases have been reported.

A non-allergic mechanism underlying precipitation of asthmatic attacks by aspirin in hypersensitive patients was proposed over 30 years ago [4]. It was founded on pharmacological inhibition of COX of arachidonic acid and explained a cross-reactivity between different NSAIDs varying in chemical structure. This COX theory was confirmed by several studies [11] and was further refined following discovery of the second COX isoenzyme – COX-2. At least two COX isoenzymes, COX-1 and COX-2, are coded by separate genes. Their role in inflammation, asthma and anaphylaxis has been reviewed previously [12].

Cross-reactions with aspirin and NSAIDs are of practical importance. Typically, AIA patients are sensitive to all NSAIDs that preferentially inhibit COX-1 (table 2). Acetaminophen (paracetamol), a weak inhibitor of COX-1, is regarded as a relatively safe therapeutic alternative for almost all patients with AIA. High doses of the drug ($\geq 1,000$ mg) have been reported to provoke mild, easily reversed bronchospasm in some AIA patients [13]. Some rare, well-documented cases of coexistence of aspirin and paracetamol sensitivity have been described. However, according to a recent meta-analysis, less that 2% of asthmatics are sensitive to both aspirin and paracetamol [14].

Meolxicam and nimesulide, known as preferential inhibitors of COX-2, are usually well tolerated by AIA patients when given at low doses. Higher doses can elicit reactions.

Highly selective COX-2 inhibitors – coxibs (rofecoxib, celecoxib, or less popular – valdecoxib, etoricoxib parecoxiband lumiracoxib) – were found to be well tolerated in a series of placebo-controlled clinical trials [8]. However, rofecoxib and valdecoxib have been withdrawn from the market because of an increased incidence

Table 2. Universal cross-reactions occur between aspirin and the following NSAIDs which preferentially inhibit COX-1

Generic name	Brand name
Indomethacin	Metindol
Piroxicam	Feldene
Metamizole	Pyralgin
Sulindac	Clinoril
Tolmetin	Tolectin
Ibuprofen	Rufen, Motrin, Advil
Naproxen	Naprosyn
Fenoprofen	Nalfon
Meclofenamate	Meclomen
Mefenamic acid	Ponstel
Flurbiprofen	Ansaid
Diflunisal	Dolbid
Ketoprofen	Orudis, Profenid, Ketonal
Diclofenac	Voltaren, Cataflam
Ketoralac	Toradol
Etodolac	Lodine
Nabumetone	Relafen
Oxaprozin	Daypro

of cardiovascular complications. Occasional patients, who are extremely sensitive to aspirin, may develop hypersensitive reactions to celecoxib and other coxibs [15]. In some cases this may be attributable to IgE-mediated reactions.

Prevention and Treatment

Once diagnosed, patients with AIA should avoid aspirin and any other NSAIDs strongly inhibiting COX-1; their education is of utmost importance. They should receive a list of contraindicated and well-tolerated analgesics (table 2). Even topical administration (intravascular or by iontophoresis) of a NSAID may cause an asthma attack and should be avoided.

Paracetamol, coxibs and codeine are usually safe choices for acute pain. Azapropazone and choline magnesium trisalicylate, which are very weak inhibitors of COX-1 and COX-2, are also well tolerated by a large majority of AIA patients. The same applies to nimesulide and meloxicam, although the small degree of residential COX-1 inhibition displayed by these compounds may be enough to trigger reactions at high doses or in highly sensitive patients. Therefore, it is prudent to administer the first dose of these drugs in a physician's office.

In general, treatment of the asthma underlying NSAIDs sensitivity should follow standard asthma guidelines. This type of asthma is often severe and frequently high doses of inhaled corticosteroids and daily doses of oral corticosteroids are necessary. A special treatment option is a chronic desensitization to aspirin [8]. Desensitization and aspirin maintenance is routinely used in some centers for treatment of chronic rhinusinusitis with nasal polyposis. It is the only available procedure which allows AIA patients with ischemic heart disease to use aspirin. During the state of desensitization to aspirin, not only aspirin but almost all strong NSAIDs are tolerated, so desensitization and NSAID maintenance could be used for treatment of rheumatic disease or chronic pain syndromes.

Aspirin-Sensitive Urticaria/Angioedema

Some patients with chronic idiopathic urticaria develop wheals and even angioedema after aspirin or NSAIDs. In others, aspirin causes an obvious increase in the underlying urticaria. The reaction may occur in just 15 min or up to 24 h following aspirin ingestion, but on average it develops within 1–4 h. Most cases resolve within a few hours, but in severe reactions bouts of multiform skin eruptions, covering most of the body, may continue for 10 days after aspirin intake [8, 16, 17].

Patients with chronic idiopathic urticaria, who develop cutaneous reactions in response to aspirin, display certain similarities in eicosanoid profile with AIA. The mechanism of the reactions is often related to COX-1 inhibition [18]. Therefore, aspirin and all drugs that inhibit COX-1 should be avoided in patients who already have had cutaneous reactions to NSAID. Coxibs are usually well tolerated, although occasional adverse reactions have been reported [19, 20]. For treatment of the reactions, antihistamines are usually sufficient, but in more severe cases adrenaline and corticosteroids may be warranted.

Hypersensitivity to Pyrazolones

Pyrazolone derivatives are analgesic substances that have been known for a long time. The use of antipyrine (phenazone) and aminopyrine was sharply curtailed after their bone marrow toxicity was reported. Other derivatives, however, like phenylbutazone, metamizole, sulfinpyrazone and propyphenazone are widely used and can be obtained without prescription in many countries. They are not infrequently a cause of adverse reactions ranging from urticaria, angioedema or asthma to anaphylactic shock. These reactions, based on their mechanism, can clearly be separated into two groups [21, 22]. *In the first group*, which corresponds to AIA: (1) metamizole, aminophenazone, phenylbutazone and sulfinpyrazone as well as several other COX-1 inhibitors, including aspirin, precipitate bronchoconstriction; (2) skin tests with pyrazolone drugs are uniformly negative, and (3) all patients have chronic rhinosinusitis and/or asthma [21, 22]. *In the second group* the reactions are of an allergic type, most likely IgE-mediated [22, 23] and can be life-threatening: (1) They are limited to a single pyrazolone drug or two drugs chemically closely related (e.g. metamizole and aminophenazone); this strict clinical specificity is corroborated by results in experimental animals [24]. (2) Skin tests with the incriminated drug are frequently positive. (3) Other pyrazolones (e.g. phenylbutazone or sulfinpyrazone in case of allergy to metamizole), aspirin and other COX-1 inhibitors can be taken with impunity. (4) Chronic bronchial asthma is present only in about one-fourth of the patients. These allergic reactions may have a genetic predisposition [25]. Azapropazone, a benzotriazone misclassified originally as a pyrazolone, rarely if ever, is the cause of the above pseudo-allergic or allergic reactions [8].

Allergic Anaphylactic Reactions to NSAIDs

Though pharmacological inhibition of COX-1 is the most frequent background mechanism for adverse reactions to aspirin and other NSAIDs, in a few subjects the reactions could have allergic or pseudo-allergic explanations. The average prevalence to the single NSAID-induced anaphylactic reaction varies from 0.1 to 3.6% of subjects who take NSAIDs intermittently or chronically for acute pain. Most drug-induced anaphylaxis episodes are attributed to diclofenac, naproxen, ibuprofen, ketorolac, paracetamol and pyrazolone derivates [8]. Such patients can be challenged with aspirin and structurally different NSAIDs without adverse effects. In cases of anaphylactic shock to celecoxib [26, 27] a suspicion was raised of cross-sensitivity between sulfonamides and the sulfur moiety of celecoxib. However, in another case report no allergy to sulfamethoxazole was found [27].

NSAIDs can induce a number of other adverse reactions, including bleeding disorders, anemia, thrombocytopenia, erythema nodosum, erythema multiforme, fixed drug eruptions, toxic epidermal necrolysis, Stevens-Johnson syndrome, leukocytoclasitc vasculitis, recurrent fever with exanthema and, of course, the well-known gastric cytotoxicity.

Acknowledgements

This chapter was supported by a grant from the Foundation for Development of Polish Pharmacy and Medicine.

References

1 Vane JR, Botting RH (eds): Aspirin and Other Salicylates. London, Chapman & Hall, 1992, pp 3–17.

2 Vane JR: Inhibition of prostaglandin synthesis as a mechanism of action for aspirin-like drugs. Nature New Biol 1971;231:232–234.

3 Samter M, Beers RF Jr: Intolerance to aspirin. Clinical studies and consideration of its pathogenesis. Ann Intern Med 1968;68:975–983.

4 Szczeklik A, Gryglewski RJ, Czerniawska-Mysik G: Relationship of inhibition of prostaglandin biosynthesis by analgesics to asthma attacks in aspirin-sensitive patients. Br Med J 1975;1:67–69.

5 Settipane GA: Landmark commentary: history of aspirin intolerance. Allergy Proc 1990;11:251–252.

6 Szczeklik A, Sanak M: The broken balance in aspirin hypersensitivity. Eur J Pharmacol 2006;533:145–155.

7 Stevenson DD, Szczeklik A: Clinical and pathologic perspectives on aspirin sensitivity and asthma. J Allergy Clin Immunol 2006;118:773–786.

8 Szczeklik A, Niżankowska-Mogilnicka E, Sanak M: Hypersensitivity to aspirin and nonsteroidal anti-inflammatory drugs; in Adkinson NF, Busse WW, Bochner BS, et al (eds): Middleton's Allergy, ed 7. St Louis, Mosby Elsevier, 2009, pp 1227–1243.

9 Szczeklik A, Nizankowska E, Duplaga M: Natural history of aspirin-induced asthma. AIANE Investigators. European Network on Aspirin-Induced Asthma. Eur Respir J 2000;16:432–436.

10 Nizankowska-Mogilnicka E, Bochenek G, Mastalerz L, Swierczyńska M, Picado C, Scadding G, Kowalski ML, Setkowicz M, Ring J, Brockow K, Bachert C, Wöhrl S, Dahlén B, Szczeklik A: EAACI/GA2LEN guideline: aspirin provocation tests for diagnosis of aspirin hypersensitivity. Allergy 2007;62:1111–1118.

11 Szczeklik A: The cyclooxygenase theory of aspirin-induced asthma. Eur Respir J 1990;3:588–593.

12 Szczeklik A, Sanak M: The role of COX-1 and COX-2 in asthma pathogenesis and its significance in the use of selective inhibitors. Clin Exp Allergy 2002;32:339–342.

13 Bavbek S, Dursun AB, Dursun E, Eryilmaz A, Misirligil Z: Safety of meloxicam in aspirin-hypersensitive patients with asthma and/or nasal polyps. A challenge-proven study. Int Arch Allergy Immunol 2007;142:64–69.

14 Jenkins C, Costello J, Hodge L: Systematic review of prevalence of aspirin-induced asthma and its implications for clinical practice. BMJ 2004;328:434–437.

15 Baldassarre S, Schandene L, Choufani G, Michils A: Asthma attacks induced by low doses of celecoxib, aspirin and acetaminophen. J Allergy Clin Immunol 2006;117:215–217.

16 Zembowicz A, Mastalerz L, Setkowicz M, Radziszewski W, Szczeklik A: Safety of cyclooxygenase-2 inhibitors and increased leukotriene synthesis in chronic idiopathic urticaria with sensitivity to nonsteroidal anti-inflammatory drugs. Arch Dermatol 2003;139:1577–1582.

17 Zembowicz A, Mastalerz L, Setkowicz M, Radziszewski W, Szczeklik A: Histological spectrum of cutaneous reactions to aspirin in chronic idiopathic urticaria. J Cutan Pathol 2004;31:323–329.

18 Mastalerz L, Setkowicz M, Sanak M, Szczeklik A: Hypersensitivity to aspirin: common eicosanoid alterations in urticaria and asthma. J Allergy Clin Immunol 2004;113:771–775.

19 Mastalerz L, Sanak M, Gawlewicz A, Gielicz A, Faber J, Szczeklik A: Different eicosanoid profile of the hypersensitivity reactions triggered by aspirin and celecoxib in a patient with sinusitis, asthma and urticaria. J Allergy Clin Immunol 2006;118:957–958.

20 Quiralte J, Blanco C, Castillo R, Delgado J, Carrillo T: Intolerance to nonsteroidal anti-inflammatory drugs: results of controlled drug challenges in 98 patients. J Allergy Clin Immunol 1996;98:678–685.

21 Szczeklik A, Gryglewski RJ, Czerniawska-Mysik G: Clinical patterns of hypersensitivity to nonsteroidal anti-inflammatory drugs and their pathogenesis. J Allergy Clin Immunol 1977;60:276–284.

22 Czerniawska-Mysik G, Szczeklik A: Idiosyncrasy to pyrazolone drugs. Allergy 1981;36:381–384.

23 Himly M, Jahn-Schmid B, Pittertschatscher K, Bohle B, Grubmayr K, Ferreira F, Ebner H, Ebner C: IgE-mediated immediate-type hypersensitivity to the pyrazolone drug propyphenazone. J Allergy Clin Immunol 2003;111:882–888.

24 Schneider CH, Kasper MF, de Weck AL, Rolli H, Angst BD: Diagnosis of antibody-mediated drug allergy. Pyrazolinone and pyrazolidinedione cross-reactivity relationships. Allergy 1987;42:597–603.

25 Kowalski ML, Woszczek G, Bienkiewicz B, Mis M: Association of pyrazolone drug hypersensitivity with HLA-DQ and DR antigens. Clin Exp Allergy 1998;28:1153–1158.

26 Schuster C, Wuthrich B: Anaphylactic drug reaction to celecoxib and sulfamethoxazole: cross-reactivity or coincidence? Allergy 2003;58:1072.

27 Fontaine C, Bousquet PJ, Demoly P: Anaphylactic shock caused by a selective allergy to celecoxib, with no allergy to rofecoxib or sulfamethoxazole. J Allergy Clin Immunol 2005;115:633–634.

Prof. Andrzej Szczeklik
Department of Medicine, Jagiellonian University Medical College
Skawińska 8, PL–31-066 Cracow (Poland)
Tel. +48 12 656 2840, Fax +48 12 656 5786
E-Mail mmszczek@cyf-kr.edu.pl

Ring J (ed): Anaphylaxis. Chem Immunol Allergy. Basel, Karger, 2010, vol 95, pp 180–189

Anaphylaxis to General Anesthetics

D. Anne Moneret-Vautrin[a] · P. Michel Mertes[b]

[a]Department of Internal Medicine, Clinical Immunology and Allergology and [b]Department of Anesthesia and Intensive Care, University Hospital, Nancy, France

Abstract

The incidence of hypersensitivity reactions to anesthetics is estimated 1 in 13,000 anesthetics up to 1 in 3,180. The rate of mortality ranges between 3 and 9%. 90% of reactions appear at anesthesia induction. Cardiovascular collapse and bronchospasm are more frequent in IgE-dependent reactions. The leading causes are neuromuscular blocking agents (50–70% of cases). IgE-dependent reactions are predominant. Previous sensitization by other compounds containing quaternary ions is suspected. Cross-reactions are frequent. Latex allergy is the second cause, followed by antibiotics and β-lactams in general. The incidence of anaphylaxis to vital dyes and chlorhexidine increases. Anaphylaxis to intravenous hypnotics, plasma substitutes, aprotinin, protamine and other drugs can occur. Any suspected hypersensitivity reaction during anesthesia must be extensively investigated to confirm the nature of the reaction, to identify the responsible drug, to study cross-reactivity in cases of anaphylaxis to a neuromuscular blocking agent and to provide recommendations for future anesthetic procedures. Tryptase assay at the time of the reaction has to be implemented by thorough investigations carried out weeks later: prick tests and intradermal tests, quantification of specific IgE to compounds containing quaternary ammonium ions, histamine release test or cytometric analysis of basophile activation.

Anaphylaxis during general anesthesia (GA) is a severe event that can culminate in death [1–3]. The frequency of anaphylactic reactions varies considerably between countries and is poorly appreciated through the ICD codes. Current knowledge is supported by reports of large series that reflect an active policy of systematic investigation of anaphylactic reactions during GA and further potentiated by the fact that data are being gathered through specialized networks for peroperative anaphylaxis such as GERAP in France. The peroperative situation is characterized by the constant contact of the patient with latex (gloves essentially), and the huge number of drugs that are currently used not only for general and locoregional anesthesia but also to prevent infections (antibiotics, disinfectants), to search for sentinel lymph nodes in breast cancer, make the vessels visible (iodinated contrast media), adding drugs for extracorporeal circulation, biological glues, numerous antalgic and non-steroidal anti-inflammatory drugs, etc. The simultaneous or successive use of different administration routes (intravenous, intraperitoneal, intramuscular, subcutaneous, intrathecal) and the handling with latex gloves of peritoneum or of genital mucosa also have to be kept in mind. It can be agreed that anesthetists are the medical practitioners most likely to see severe anaphylactic reactions. In close parallelism, hospital departments of allergy are more and more involved in the diagnosis of peroperative anaphylaxis and both specialities have to share decisions in the field of drug allergy, and to conduct preventive strategies in high-risk patients.

Epidemiology

The reality of the risk of an allergic reaction occurring during anesthesia is established on the basis of the more than 15,000 cases of peroperative hypersensitivity reactions published in the literature during the past 30 years. Most reports on the incidence of anaphylaxis originate in France, Australia, New Zealand, the UK, Spain and Norway. They reflect an active policy of systematic clinical and/or laboratory investigation of hypersensitivity reactions, or result from the analysis of drug-related adverse event databases. Based on these reports, the estimated incidence of all immune and non-immune-mediated immediate hypersensitivity reactions was 1 in 5,000 to 1 in 13,000 anesthetics in Australia, 1 in 4,600 in France, 1 in 1,250 to 1 in 5,000 in New Zealand, and 1 in 3,500 in England [1, 4–7]. The incidence is on the increase in France: 1 in 3,180 [8]. The expected mortality rate ranges between 3 and 9% [1–3].

Specific Clinical Features of Anesthesia Induced Anaphylaxis

They differ to some extent from signs and symptoms that occur during anaphylaxis not associated with anesthesia. Early subjective symptoms such as malaise, pruritus, sensation of heat, and dizziness are absent in the anesthetized patient. Cutaneous signs in a completely wrapped patient may escape the attention of the anesthetist. The increase in heart rate, a decrease in blood pressure and an increase in airway resistance may be initially misinterpreted as a result of a pharmacological dose-related effect of the drugs, or of excessively light anesthesia. Many differential diagnoses have to be considered (table 1).

Anaphylaxis may occur at any time. 90% of reactions appear at anesthesia induction, within minutes or seconds after the intravenous injection of a neuromuscular blocking agent (NMBA) or an antibiotic. A later occurrence suggests an allergy to latex, volume expanders or dyes. Particles from gloves, which accumulate in the uterus during obstetrical maneuvers, can be released into the systemic blood flow following oxytocin injection. Anaphylactic reactions to antibiotics can follow the removal of a tourniquet during orthopedic surgery.

Table 1. Differential diagnosis of perioperative anaphylaxis

Overdose of vasoreactive substance	Malignant hyperthermia
Asthma	Myotonias and masseter spasm
Arrhythmia	Hyperkaliemia
Myocardial infarction	
Pericardial tamponade	
Pulmonary edema	
Pulmonary embolism	
Tension pneumothorax	
Venous embolism	
Sepsis	
Hereditary angioedema	
Mastocytosis	

Table 2. Clinical signs observed in case of IgE-mediated reactions compared with non-IgE–mediated reactions [9]

Clinical signs	IgE-mediated reactions: 491 cases	Non-IgE-mediated reactions
Cutaneous symptoms	326 (66.4%)	206 (93.6%)
Erythema	209	151
Urticaria	101	177
Edema	50	60
Cardiovascular symptoms	386 (78.6%)	70 (31.7%)
Hypotension	127	50
Cardiovascular collapse	249	12
Cardiac arrest	29	–
Bronchospasm	129 (39.9%)	43 (19.5%)

Initial features are mostly pulselessness, difficulty in ventilation, desaturation, and a decreased end-tidal CO_2. Cutaneous symptoms are observed in 66–70% of patients in case of IgE-mediated reactions but in more than 90% in non-IgE-mediated reactions. On the contrary, cardiovascular collapse and bronchospasm are more frequent in IgE-dependent reactions (table 2). Severe anaphylaxis may be a primary cardiac arrest [9].

Clinical manifestations show striking variations of intensity in different patients, ranging from mild hypersensitivity reactions to severe anaphylactic shock and death (table 3). However, IgE-mediated reactions are usually more severe than non-IgE-mediated reactions [9]. In addition, IgE-mediated reactions to NMBAs have been shown to be more severe than reactions to other substances like latex in some series [9].

In mild cases restricted to a single symptom, spontaneous recovery may be observed. In most cases, after adequate treatment, clinical signs regress within an

Table 3. Grade of severity for quantification of immediate hypersensitivity reactions (according to the classification from the French Society for Anesthesiology)

Grade	Symptoms
I	Cutaneous signs: generalized erythma, urticaria, angioedema
II	Measurable but not life-threatening symptoms
	Cutaneous signs, hypotension, tachycardia
	Respiratory disturbance: cough, difficulty to inflate
III	Life-threatening symptoms: collapse, tachycardia or bradycardia, arrhythmias, bronchospasm
IV	Cardiac and/or respiratory arrest

hour without sequelae. However, in some cases, severe bronchospasm can resist to treatment, with a risk of cerebral anoxia or death.

Population at Risk

The potential severity of anaphylaxis during anesthesia underscores the interest of developing a rational approach to reduce its incidence by identifying potential risk factors before surgery. Recommendations concerning the identification of population at risk of peroperative anaphylaxis, who would benefit from preoperative investigation, have been proposed [10].

Patients at risk have been defined as follows: (a) Patients who are allergic to one of the drugs or products likely to be administered or used during the anesthesia procedure and for which the diagnosis had been established by a previous allergy investigation. (b) Patients who have shown clinical signs suggesting an allergic reaction during a previous anesthesia. (c) Patients who have presented the clinical manifestations of allergy when exposed to latex, whatever the circumstances in which this occurred. (d) Children who have had multiple operations, especially those with spina bifida, because of the high frequency of sensitization to latex and of the high incidence of anaphylactic shock caused by latex in such patients [11]. (e) Patients who have experienced clinical manifestations of allergy to avocado, kiwi, banana, chestnut, buckwheat, etc., because of the high frequency of cross-reactivity with latex.

Causal Agents

The overall distribution of the various causal agents is very similar in most reported series. NMBAs represent the most frequently involved substances with a range of 50–70%, followed by latex (12–16.7%) and in recent reports antibiotics (15%) [1–7] (table 4).

Table 4. Substances responsible for IgE-mediated hypersensitivity reactions in France. Results from seven consecutive surveys [9] (% values)

	1984–1989 n = 821	1990–1991 n = 813	1992–1994 n = 1,030	1994–1996 n = 734	1997–1998 n = 486	1999–2000 n = 518	2001–2002 n = 502
NMBAs	81.0	70.2	59.2	61.6	69.2	58.2	54
Latex	0.5	12.5	19.0	16.6	12.1	16.7	22.3
Hypnotics	11.0	5.6	8.0	5.1	3.7	3.4	0.8
Opioids	3.0	1.7	3.5	2.7	1.4	1.3	2.4
Colloids	0.5	4.6	5.0	3.1	2.7	4.0	2.8
Antibiotics	2.0	2.6	3.1	8.3	8.0	15.1	14.7
Other	2.0	2.8	2.2	2.6	2.9	1.3	3.0
Total	100	100	100	100	100	100	100

NMBAs: Immune-Mediated Hypersensitivity Reactions Are Predominant

Most of them are IgE-dependent reactions. Epitopes have been shown to be quaternary ammonium ions [12]. Since the structure of NMBAs includes two substituted ammonium ions per molecule, this bivalency could explain the immediate bridging of two adjacent membrane-specific IgEs not requiring a previous binding to a proteinic carrier [13]. However, the IgE recognition site of the molecule also depends on the molecular structure adjacent to the ammonium ion, and that accounts for the heterogeneity of the cross-reactivity among patients [13, 14]. Indeed, the patterns of cross-reactivity vary considerably between patients. Cross-reactivity to all NMBAs is relatively unusual, but seems to be more frequent with amino steroid NMBAs than with benzylisoquinoline-derived NMBAs.

Differences regarding the relative risk of allergic reactions between NMBAs have been recognized in large epidemiologic surveys. Suxamethonium appears to be more frequently involved, and pancuronium and *cis*-atracurium have the lowest incidence of anesthetic anaphylaxis in large series [1, 3, 6, 9, 11]. A trend concerning an increased frequency of allergic reactions to rocuronium was initially reported in Norway and France but not in USA [15].

To explain the possible differences observed regarding the risk of allergic reactions with the different NMBAs, it has been suggested that the flexibility of the chain between the ammonium ions as well as the distance between the substituted ammonium ions might be of importance in the elicitation of mediator release [16]. Suxamethonium is a linear flexible chain.

In 15–50% of cases, IgE-mediated anaphylaxis to a NMBA has been reported at the first known contact with a NMBA [1, 3, 14]. This suggests a possible cross-reaction with IgE antibodies generated by previous contact with apparently unrelated chemicals: drugs, such as pholcodine, cosmetics, disinfectants and industrial materials [14,

17, 18]. The predominance of females, more than 65% in all large series, remains unexplained.

Non-Immune-Mediated Hypersensitivity Reactions

The rate of non-IgE-mediated immediate hypersensitivity reactions usually varies between 20 and 50% [1–7, 9]. They are assumed to result from direct non-specific mast cell and basophil activation, which causes direct histamine release [19]. Histamine release is predominantly found with the use of the benzylisoquinolines *d*-tubocurarine, atracurium and mivacurium, and the aminosteroid rapacuronium. Severe bronchospasm related to rapacuronium administration has been reported in children and adults. It might be related to the higher affinity of rapacuronium for M2 versus M3 muscarinic receptors [20]. Rapacuronium has been withdrawn from the market in the USA.

Latex. Allergy to natural rubber latex is the second most common cause of anaphylaxis during anesthesia in the general population. In children subjected to numerous operations, particularly those suffering from spina bifida, it is the primary cause of anaphylaxis [11]. The relative frequency of allergy to latex has rapidly increased, rising from 0.5% before 1980 to 20% in France in 2002. A low rate has been reported in countries where a strategy aimed to reduce latex exposure was implemented [6].

Antibiotics. Antibiotics are commonly administered peroperatively. At the present time, allergy to β-lactams represents 12–15% of the peroperative reactions observed in France [9]. Vancomycin, which is increasingly used for prophylaxis, has been incriminated in some cases. The 'red man syndrome' is due to non-specific histamine release induced by a rapid intravenous administration [21].

Hypnotics. Common hypnotics are thiopental, propofol, midazolam, etomidate, ketamine and inhaled anesthetics. The incidence of hypersensitivity reactions with thiopental is rare. Recently, thiopental was involved in less than 1% of allergic reactions in France [9]. Ever since Cremophor EL, used as a solvent for some non-barbiturate hypnotics, has been avoided, many previously reported hypersensitivity reactions have disappeared. In the last French surveys, reactions to propofol accounted for less than 2.5% of allergic reactions, and reactions to midazolam, etomidate or ketamine appear to be really rare [9]. Finally, no immune-mediated immediate hypersensitivity reaction involving isoflurane, desflurane or sevoflurane has been reported despite their wide use.

Opioids. Reactions to morphine, codeine phosphate, meperidine, fentanyl and its derivatives are uncommon. Because of their direct histamine-releasing properties, especially regarding morphine and codeine, distinction between anaphylaxis and non-immune-mediated histamine release is not always easy. Only 12 cases were recorded in the last 2 years' epidemiologic survey in France, 9 of them being related to morphine administration [9].

Local Anesthetics. Local anesthetics used in anesthesiology are currently amide derivatives (lidocaine, mepivacaine, prilocaine, bupivacaine, levobupivacaine, ropivacaine). Inadvertent intravascular injection leading to excessive blood concentrations of the local anesthetic, or systemic absorption of epinephrine that was combined with the local anesthetic, are by far the most common causes of adverse reactions produced by these drugs. They have been involved in less than 0.6% of the peroperative reactions [9].

Colloids. The overall incidence of reactions has been estimated to less than 0.22%. Gelatins and dextrans are more frequently incriminated than albumin or hetastarch. Evidence for IgE-mediated adverse reactions to gelatin has been reported. Adverse reactions to dextrans were estimated to 0.275%, when it was 0.099% for albumin and 0.058% for hydroxyethyl starch solutions, and 0.03% for gelatin solutions [22, 23].

Dyes. Vital dyes have been used for many years in a variety of clinical situations. Patent blue V (also called E131, Acid blue 3, Disulfine blue) and Isosulfan blue (also called Patent blue violet or Lymphazurine), belong to the group of triarylmethane dyes and are the most commonly used [24]. Reports of IgE-dependent anaphylaxis arise. Anaphylactic reactions involving methylene blue seems to be very rare, however, several reports of sensitization to both Patent blue and methylene blue have previously been reported.

Aprotinin. Aprotinin is a naturally occurring serine protease inhibitor, has found widespread applications either by the intravenous route or as a component of biological sealants, because of its ability to decrease blood loss, and, as a consequence, transfusion requirements. Anaphylactic reactions are mediated by IgG and IgE antibodies. The risk of anaphylactic reactions has been estimated between 0.5 and 5.8% when used intravenously during cardiac surgery, and at 5 for 100,000 applications when used as a biologic sealant [25]. Patients previously treated with this drug present an increased risk and any new administration should be avoided for at least 6 months following an initial exposure [25].

Other Agents. Allergic reactions to chlorhexidine have been observed after insertion of central catheters impregnated with this antiseptic, or after intraurethral use or topical application [26]. Only rare cases of anaphylaxis following topical use of povidone-iodine have been reported.

Protamine. Protamine, whose use to reverse heparin anticoagulation has increased over the last two decades, has also been incriminated. Reactions may involve a number of mechanisms including IgE, IgG and complement. The incidence of anaphylactic reactions is estimated at 0.19% (retrospective studies) and 0.69% (prospective studies), respectively [27].

Investigation of an Allergic Reaction

Any suspected hypersensitivity reaction during anesthesia must be extensively investigated using combined per- and postoperative testing to confirm the nature of the reaction, to identify the responsible drug, to detect possible cross-reactivity in cases of anaphylaxis to a NMBA and to provide recommendations for future anesthetic procedures. The diagnostic strategy is based on a detailed history including concurrent morbidity, previous anesthetic history and any known allergies, and on a combination of investigations performed both immediately and days to weeks later. Biological investigations include mediators release assays at the time of the reaction, quantification of specific IgE, immediately or 6 weeks later, skin tests, and other biological assays such as histamine release tests or basophile activation assays.

Histamine and Tryptase during Peroperative Anaphylaxis
Histamine concentrations are maximal almost immediately, decrease thereafter with a half-life of about 20 min, and should be assayed within the first hour of a reaction. The sensitivity of this test for the diagnosis of anaphylaxis was estimated at 75%, the specificity at 51%, the positive predictive value at 75% and the negative predictive value at 51%. Tryptase reaches a peak in the patient's serum 30 min after the first clinical manifestations. Its half-life is 90 min, and the levels usually decrease over time. In a recent series, the sensitivity was estimated at 64%, specificity at 89.3%, positive predictive value at 92–95%, and negative predictive value at 54.3% [9].

Skin Testing
Intradermal or prick tests are usually carried out 4–6 weeks after a reaction. Skin tests to NMBAs may remain positive for years later. Ideally, testing should be carried out by a professional experienced in performing and interpreting tests with anesthetic agents [28]. Detailed recommendations for skin and intradermal test dilutions of anesthetic drugs including NMBAs have been proposed by the French Societies for Anesthesiology and Allergology. They have been confirmed by a prospective study conducted in 120 healthy volunteers tested with all NMBAs available [29].

The estimated sensitivity of skin tests for muscle relaxants is approximately 94–97%. Sensitivity for other substances varies. It is good for synthetic gelatins, β-lactams, but poor for barbiturates, opioids and benzodiazepines dyes, and chlorhexidine.

Specific IgE Assay. Two radioimmunoassays are available in France using a quaternary ammonium compound coupled to Sepharose [30, 31]. The sensitivity of these tests was equivalent at 88%, the specificity reaches 90%. A morphine-based immunoassay has been proposed in Australia [14]. More recently, Ebo et al. [32] investigated a rocuronium ImmunoCAP and set the sensitivity at 85%, the specificity being absolute, provided an assay-specific decision threshold is applied. An ImmunoCAP (Phadia A) is available.

Mediator Release Tests and Basophile Activation Test. Leukocyte histamine release tests were positive in 65% of the allergic patients, for a threshold corresponding to specificity at 100%. The concordance between LHR test and QAS-RIA was 64% [33]. Despite a very good specificity, their diagnostic application remains limited because of the heavy experimental conditions and insufficient sensitivity. They are therefore not used as routine diagnostic tests. Once fully validated, the basophil activation test using flow cytometry will probably represent an interesting diagnostic tool for NMBA anaphylaxis and for cross-sensitization studies [34].

Conclusion

Peroperative anaphylaxis remains a significant adverse event during anesthesia which remains underestimated because it is underreported. NMBAs, latex and antibiotics are the most frequently involved drugs but all other drugs used by the anesthetist are at risk of anaphylaxis. Because no premedication can effectively prevent an allergic reaction, any suspected hypersensitivity reaction must be investigated to confirm the anaphylaxis and to identify the eliciting drug. The possession of a warning card (or wearing of a warning bracelet) is strongly encouraged. A thorough pre-anesthetic history is the most important tool for screening at-risk subjects. Particular attention must be paid to patients who have already experienced such a reaction during anesthesia, those alleging an allergy to muscle relaxants, or those at risk of latex sensitization. In these cases, the choice of the safest possible anesthetic agents should be based on a rigorously performed allergy assessment and the conjugated expertise of the allergists and the anesthetists.

References

1 Laxenaire MC, Mertes PM: Anaphylaxis during anaesthesia. Results of a two-year survey in France. Br J Anaesth 2001;87;549.

2 Mitsuhata H, Hasegawa J, Matsumoto S, Ogawa R: The epidemiology and clinical features of anaphylactic and anaphylactoid reactions in the perioperative period in Japan: a survey with a questionnaire of 529 hospitals approved by Japan Society of Anesthesiology. Masui 1992;41:1825.

3 Light KP, Lovell AT, Butt H, Fauvel N, Holdcroft A: Adverse effects of neuromuscular blocking agents based on yellow card reporting in the UK. Are there differences between males and females? Pharmacoepidemiol Drug Saf 2006;15:151.

4 Watkins J, Ward AM, Thornton JA: Adverse reactions to intravenous induction agents. Br Med J 1978;2:1431.

5 Fisher M, Baldo BA: Anaphylaxis during anaesthesia: current aspects of diagnosis and prevention. Eur J Anaesthesiol 1994;11:263.

6 Harboe TA, Guttormsen B, Irgens A, Dybendal T, Florvaag E: Anaphylaxis during anesthesia in Norway: a 6-year single-center follow-up study. Anesthesiology 2005;102:897.

7 Escolano F, Valero A, Huguet J, Baxarias P, de Molina M, Castro A, Granel C, Sanosa J, Bartolomé B: Prospective epidemiologic study of perioperative anaphylactoid reactions occurring in Catalonia (1996–1997) Rev Esp Anestesiol Reanim 2002; 49:286.

8 Malinovsky JM, Decagny S, Wessel F, Guilloux L, Mertes PM: Systematic follow-up increases incidence of anaphylaxis during adverse reactions in anesthetized patients. Acta Anaesthesiol Scand 2008; 52:175.

9 Mertes PM, Laxenaire MC: Anaphylactic and anaphylactoid reactions occurring during anaesthesia in France. Seventh epidemiologic survey (January 2001–December 2002) (in French). Ann Fr Anesth Reanim 2004;23:1133.

10 Mertes PM, Laxenaire MC, Lienhart A, Aberer W, Ring J, Pichler WJ, Demoly P: Reducing the risk of anaphylaxis during anaesthesia: guidelines for clinical practice. J Investig Allergol Clin Immunol 2005; 15:91.

11 Karila C, Brunet-Langot D, Labbez F, Jacqmarcq O, Ponvert C, Paupe J, Scheinmann P, de Blic J: Anaphylaxis during anesthesia: results of a 12-year survey at a French pediatric center. Allergy 2005;60: 828.

12 Baldo BA, Fisher MM: Substituted ammonium ions as allergenic determinants in drug allergy. Nature 1983;306:262.

13 Moneret-Vautrin DA: Cross-reactions to muscle relaxants in the operating room. Clin Rev Allergy Immunol 1997;15:471.

14 Baldo BA, Fisher MM, Pham NH: On the origin and specificity of antibodies to neuromuscular blocking (muscle relaxant) drugs: an immunochemical perspective. Clin Exp Allergy 2009;39: 325.

15 Bhananker SM, O'Donnell JT, Salemi JR, Bishop MJ: The risk of anaphylactic reactions to rocuronium in the United States is comparable to that of vecuronium: an analysis of food and drug administration reporting of adverse events. Anesth Analg 2005;101:819.

16 Didier A, Cador D, Bongrand P, Furstoss R, Fourneron P, Senft M, Philip-Joet F, Charpin D, Charpin J, Vervloet D: Role of the quaternary ammonium ion determinants in allergy to muscle relaxants. J Allergy Clin Immunol 1987;79:578.

17 Florvaag E, Johansson SG, Oman H, Venemalm L, Degerbeck F, Dybendal T, Lundberg M: Prevalence of IgE antibodies to morphine. Relation to the high and low incidences of NMBA anaphylaxis in Norway and Sweden, respectively. Acta Anaesthesiol Scand 2005;49:437.

18 Harboe T, Johansson SG, Florvaag E, Oman H: Pholcodine exposure raises serum IgE in patients with previous anaphylaxis to neuromuscular blocking agents. Allergy 2007;62:1445.

19 Moss J: Muscle relaxants and histamine release. Acta Anaesthesiol Scand Suppl 1995;106:7–12.

20 Jooste E, Klafter F, Hirshman CA, Emala CW: A mechanism for rapacuronium-induced bronchospasm: M2 muscarinic receptor antagonism Anesthesiology 2003;98:906.

21 Renz C, Lynch J, Thurn J, Moss J: Histamine release during rapid vancomycin administration. Inflamm Res 1998; 47(suppl 1):69.

22 Ring J, Messmer K: Incidence and severity of anaphylactoid reactions to colloid volume substitutes. Lancet 1977;1:466–469.

23 Laxenaire MC, Charpentier C, Feldman L: Anaphylactoid reactions to colloid plasma substitutes: incidence, risk factors, mechanisms. A French multicenter prospective study (in French). Ann Fr Anesth Reanim 1994;13:301.

24 Forschner K, Kleine-Tebbe A, Zuberbier T, Worm M: Type I sensitization towards Patent blue as a cause of anaphylaxis Allergy 2003;58:457.

25 Dietrich W, Ebell A, Busley R, Boulesteix AL: Aprotinin and anaphylaxis: analysis of 12,403 exposures to aprotinin in cardiac surgery. Ann Thorac Surg 2007;84:1144.

26 Garvey LH, Kroigaard M, Poulsen LK, Skov PS, Mosbech H, Venemalm L, Degerbeck F, Husum B: IgE-mediated allergy to chlorhexidine. J Allergy Clin Immunol 2007;120:409.

27 Nybo M, Madsen JS: Serious anaphylactic reactions due to protamine sulfate: a systematic literature review. Basic Clin Pharmacol Toxicol 2008;103:192.

28 Moneret-Vautrin DA, Kanny G: Anaphylaxis to muscle relaxants: rational for skin tests. Allerg Immunol (Paris) 2002;34:233.

29 Mertes PM, Moneret-Vautrin DA: Skin reactions to intradermal neuromuscular blocking agent injections: a randomized multicenter trial in healthy volunteers. Anesthesiology 2007;107:245.

30 Moneret-Vautrin DA, Gueant JL, Kamel L, Laxenaire MC, el Kholty S, Nicolas JP: Anaphylaxis to muscle relaxants: cross-sensitivity studied by radioimmunoassays compared to intradermal tests in 34 cases. J Allergy Clin Immunol 1988;82:745.

31 Guilloux L, Ricard-Blum S, Ville G, Motin J: A new radioimmunoassay using a commercially available solid support for the detection of IgE antibodies against muscle relaxants. J Allergy Clin Immunol 1992;90:153.

32 Ebo DG, Venemalm L, Bridts CH, Degerbeck F, Hagberg H, De Clerck LS, Stevens WJ: Immunoglobulin E antibodies to rocuronium: a new diagnostic tool. Anesthesiology 2007;107:253.

33 Mata E, Gueant JL, Moneret-Vautrin DA, Bermejo N, Gerard P, Nicolas JP, Laxenaire MC: Clinical evaluation of in vitro leukocyte histamine release in allergy to muscle relaxant drugs. Allergy 1992;47:471.

34 Sudheer PS, Hall JE, Read GF, Rowbottom AW, Williams PE: Flow cytometric investigation of perianaesthetic anaphylaxis using CD63 and CD203c. Anaesthesia 2005;60:251.

Prof. D.A. Moneret-Vautrin
Department of Internal Medicine, Clinical Immunology and Allergology, University Hospital
29, avenue de Lattre de Tassigny, FR–54035 Nancy (France)
Tel. +33 383 85 28 63, Fax +33 3 83 85 28 64
E-Mail a.moneret-vautrin@chu-nancy.fr

Ring J (ed): Anaphylaxis. Chem Immunol Allergy. Basel, Karger, 2010, vol 95, pp 190–200

Anaphylactic Reactions to Local Anesthetics

Johannes Ring · Regina Franz · Knut Brockow

Department of Dermatology and Allergy Biederstein, Klinikum rechts der Isar, Technische Universität München, Munich, Germany

Abstract

Local anesthetics (LA) are common elicitors of adverse reactions and the clinical symptoms often correspond to anaphylaxis with tachycardia, hypotension and subjective feelings of weakness, heat or vertigo. The pathomechanism of immediate hypersensitivity reactions to LA is largely unknown – they are commonly regarded as 'pseudo-allergic' or 'non-immune type' anaphylaxis. Immunologically mediated reactions have rarely been observed with positive skin prick tests. Other ingredients in LA preparations have to be considered as elicitors, e.g. preservatives like benzoates or sulfites or latex contaminants in injection bottles. Practical management of patients with a history of LA reaction includes a careful allergy history, skin-prick and intradermal tests. Undiluted LA solutions may elicit false-positive intradermal test reactions. If prick and intradermal tests are negative, the procedure of subcutaneous provocation testing is applied in a placebo-controlled manner. When patients are constantly reacting to placebo, a regimen of 'reverse placebo provocation' with injection of a LA (verum) is applied while the patient is informed about receiving placebo in order to 'rule out psychosomatic involvement'. With this regimen it is possible to eliminate anxiousness and fear, and the patient has proof that he has tolerated the respective LA substance.

Copyright © 2010 S. Karger AG, Basel

Since the introduction of cocaine (methylbenzoylecgonine) into medicine for topical analgesic effects, local anesthetics (LAs) have been a major progress in the history of medicine [1]. They are widely used with an estimate of more than 5 million injections every day worldwide, and although they are generally well tolerated, a certain number of patients suffer from adverse reactions to these substances [2]. The prevalence of these phenomena is not well established. Estimates range from 0.1 to 1% [3]. Larger studies show a much lower figure. In the UK, 70 million lidocaine applications have been registered for dental procedures, while only 249 cases of adverse reactions were reported [4]. The reason for this discrepancy may be seen in the fact that many of these adverse reactions are primarily regarded as 'autonomic', 'vagovasal' and are neglected without further diagnostic steps taken. Sometimes patients are labeled 'allergic' without diagnostic testing; there is some confusion among physicians and patients with regard to LA hypersensitivity.

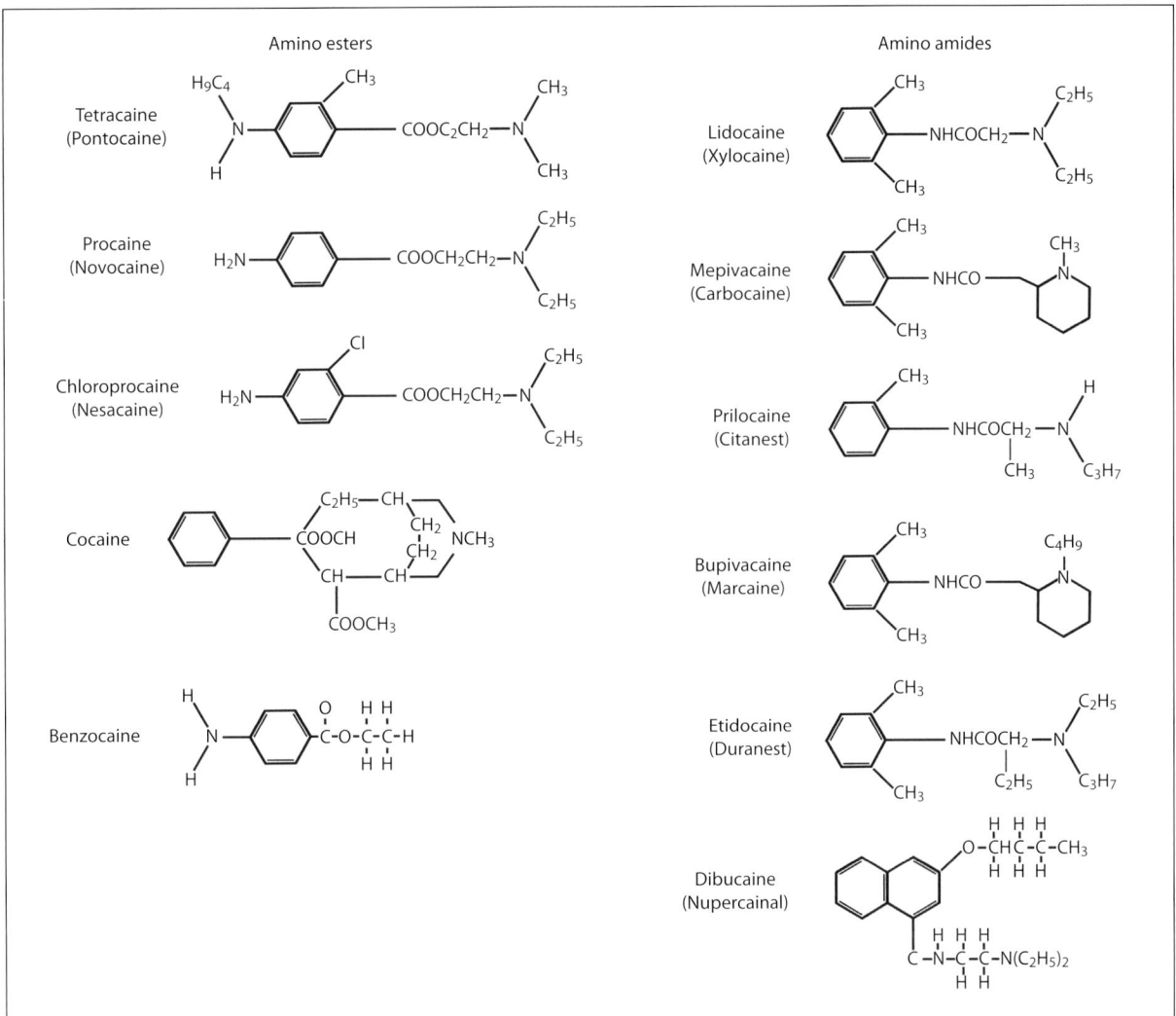

Fig. 1. Chemical structure of ester- and amide-type LAs.

In this chapter it will be stressed that patients suffering from such adverse reactions after application of LAs should undergo an allergy diagnostic work-up in order to give save recommendations for future treatments [5].

Chemical Structure

LAs are small molecular weight chemicals with a lipophilic group (aromatic ring), and a hydrophilic (amine) group and a linkage between both groups. Regarding the chemical structure, they are roughly classified as ester or amide compounds, based

Table 1. Ester and amide-type LAs

Ester-type LA	Amide-type LA
Chloroprocaine	Dibucaine (= cinchocaine)
Cocaine (methylbenzoylecgonine)	Etidocaine
Procaine	Levobupivacaine
Proparacaine	Lidocaine (= lignocaine)
Tetracaine	Mepivacaine
Benzocaine	Prilocaine
Articaine	Ropivacaine
Bupivacaine	Sameridine
	Tonicaine

Table 2. Adverse reactions to LAs: etiopathophysiology

Toxicity (cardiovascular, CNS)
Type I allergy (IgE): rare
Type IV allergy (contact allergy, local and systemic)
Pseudo-allergic (non-immune anaphylaxis)
   (psychoneurogenic, autonomic, vagovasal)
Hypersensitivity to other ingredients (e.g. latex, preservatives)
Pharmacologic effect of other ingredients (e.g. adrenaline)

on the nature of the intermediate linkage (fig. 1). While the ester compounds are the more classical substances, newer agents are mostly of the amide-type and can be further subgrouped into aminoacylamides (e.g. lidocaine, mepivavacaine, bupivacaine, xylocaine) and aminoacylamides (e.g. dibucaine, procainamide) (table 1).

Clinical Symptomatology

Clinical symptomatology as experienced by patients undergoing immediate-type reactions to LAs comprise urticaria [6], angioedema [7], dyspnea, vomiting, chill, tachycardia, arrhythmia, sensation of heat, loss of consciousness, headache, vertigo, nausea and other subjective symptoms. The majority of the reactions start within the first 30 min after the injection. In around 20% of the patients, reactions may occur only after 2 h. From the clinical symptomatology it is often very difficult to differentiate various pathomechanisms, namely true anaphylaxis from autonomic vagovasal reactions, especially when skin symptoms are lacking. Adverse reactions to LAs can be caused by very different pathomechanisms (table 2).

Toxicity

LAs are powerful pharmacologic agents acting directly on the peripheral nerve, but also on the central nervous system (CNS) and the cardiovascular system. Toxic reactions occur after a too high dosage which can happen after large area infiltration LA or after incidental intravasal application of the agent. The typical symptoms are speech disturbance, disorientation, difficulty in focusing the eyes, apprehension, localized muscle twitching, drowsiness or lethargy, sometimes accompanied by a drop in blood pressure, respiratory rate and heart rate. Cardiac toxicity induces a comparable effect to the action of quinidine, with a direct depressive effect on the myocardium and slowing of conduction impulses at the AV node. Lidocaine has been used as an antiarrhythmic for decades.

The well-known adverse reaction formerly often observed after intramuscular injection of clemizol penicillin in the treatment of syphilis with anaphylaxis-like symptoms plus CNS involvement in the absence of immunological sensitization to penicillin was called the Hoigné syndrome or embolic-toxic reaction, and might be explained by intravasal application of LA with subsequent toxic effects [8].

Pharmacologic Effect

LAs are not often used as a single substance, but are mixed preparations with adrenaline and preservatives. This has to be differentiated by the diagnostic procedure [9]. Pharmacologic effects of adrenaline (paleness, tachycardia, hypertension, feeling of fear) have to be differentiated from anaphylactic reactions to the LA substance [10].

Hypersensitivity Reactions

IgE-Mediated Anaphylaxis
True IgE-mediated anaphylactic reactions to LAs are extremely rare [11–13]. Only single cases have been reported in the literature with positive prick tests [14, 15]. A case of a positive open patch test in a patient suffering from contact urticaria after topical application of lidocaine, pilocaine mixture (Emla cream) might represent a true IgE-mediated allergy [16]. The majority of immediate-type reactions are non-immune in nature.

Contact Allergy (Type IV Reactions)
True allergic reactions to LA are not uncommon in the form of contact allergy [17, 18] (type IV) against topically applied LA in suppositories, creams and ointments [1]. A mixture of several caines is part of the international standard patch tests for contact allergy testing [19]. The symptomatology of type IV reactions differs from the above-mentioned anaphylactic type. Local redness and itching usually appear at the site of injection which

may spread and lead to papulovesicular eruptions. Rarely, after LA injection a systemic contact allergic reaction (hematogenous contact dermatitis) may develop [20–22].

In a study performed by Ruzicka et al. [23], 104 patients with positive patch tests to LAs and a history of contact dermatitis were tested with LA in a prick test and in an intradermal setting. All prick tests remained negative. There were 9 persons positive for procaine in the intradermal test and 3 positive for butanilicaine. There was no correlation to history in the patients with skin tests and no correlation between patch test results and results of the intradermal test [23].

Non-Immune Anaphylactic ('Pseudo-Allergic') Reactions
The majority of immediate-type adverse reactions to LA seem to be non-immune in nature, earlier called pseudo-allergic [24]. Following the new nomenclature of the World Allergy Organization, these reactions should now be called 'non-immune anaphylaxis' [25].

Contrary to other elicitors of non-immune anaphylactic reactions (radiocontrast media, neuromuscular blocking agents, non-steroidal anti-inflammatory drugs (NSAIDs)) where there are at least hypothetical concepts regarding the pathomechanism of these reactions via increased mediator release (e.g. histamine release, shift in arachidonic acid metabolism from prostaglandins towards leukotrienes, etc.) [26], there is almost no literature regarding the pathomechanism of these reactions after LA application.

We proposed the term 'psychoneurogenic' for the mechanism of these reactions, since the direct action on the nerve might elicit a reflex cascade via the CNS and then lead to the above-mentioned symptoms. Why these reactions only occur in certain individuals, maybe due to pharmacogenomics and specific hyperexcitability of peripheral nerves, remains open for speculation. There is a high degree of psychosomatic involvement in such reactions.

Results of Skin Test and Provocation Test Procedures

In the diagnostic work-up, allergists usually start with a skin-prick test, followed by an intradermal test, and soon continuing with subcutaneous provocation testing (see below). In a very detailed study performed by Gall et al. [27], 177 patients suffering from 197 anaphylactic reactions after LA application were investigated with a skin-prick test, intradermal test and subcutaneous provocation testing with the suspected agents. They found a total number of 14 positive provocation reactions, three going along with objective symptoms (urticaria twice, local erythema once, and systemic dermatitis after 24 h) and subjective symptoms (as mentioned above) in 11 patients. Five of the patients also reacted to preservatives in the LA preparations (sulfites, benzoates) [27]. Table 3 shows the results of subcutaneous provocation testing in several studies in the literature. There seem to be surprisingly little positive reaction, however, unfortunately, the

Table 3. Specificity of subcutaneous provocation with LA: positive test with causative agent (literature review)

0/90	de Shazo and Nelson [31]	1979
1/25	Le Sellin et al. [2]	1986
0/59	Chandler et al. [11]	1987
0/35	Escolano et al. [12]	1990
0/26	Fisher and Graham [9]	1984
0/50	Incaudo et al. [13]	1978
3/143	Gall et al. [27]	1996
0/108	Astarita et al. [38]	2001
1/236	Berkum et al. [34]	2003
1/36	Wöhrl et al. [5]	2006

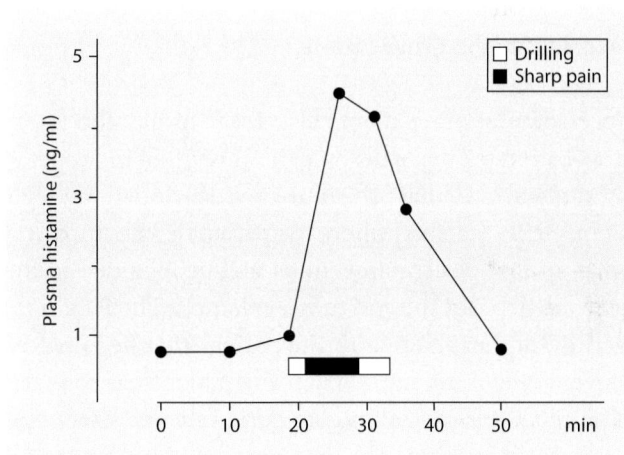

Fig. 2. Increasing plasma histamine concentration in a patient undergoing dental treatment without further medication [from Ring, 1986].

authors did not comment on the frequency of placebo responses in their patients, but rather subtracted people with placebo reactions which may lead to confusion.

Psychosomatic Involvement

It is obvious and a well-known clinical experience that psychosomatic influence is extremely common in LA reactions. Figure 2 shows the example of a patient who,

Table 4. Reverse placebo provocation: procedure and patient information [from Ring, 1985]

Subcutaneous provocation	Information
SCP with LA 1	'one LA'
SCP with LA 2	'another LA'
SCP with NaCl	'another LA'
SCP with LA 1	'NaCl'
SCP with LA 1	'LA 1'

while undergoing a dental procedure, released a significant amount of histamine in the plasma without any actual drug application; just the simple strain of the situation induced a histamine release which can be compared to a mild anaphylactic reaction in true IgE-mediated allergy [28].

Reverse Placebo Provocation

Since some of our patients also react to placebo after intradermal or subcutaneous provocation testing, and since they are often in desperate need of a LA for an impending surgical or dental procedure, we developed the regimen of reverse placebo provocation (RPP) (table 4) where the patient is informed at the beginning of the diagnostic work-up that placebo injections will be included in the regimen and everything will be blinded, but at the end fully explained. The RPP is then started by injecting one LA (verum) and explaining to the patient that he is receiving placebo ('to rule out psychogenic involvement'). When the patient has tolerated the true LA under the label of placebo, it is crucial to give a friendly and exact open explanation embedded in a serious conversation. The patient must never get the feeling of having been fooled or tricked! After that, on the basis of this mutual understanding, a final open provocation with the same LA substance the patient had just tolerated is performed and usually tolerated without reaction.

With the principle of RPP we are able to take away fear and anxiety by proving to the patient that he has tolerated the drug. If we would have stopped after 'placebo-positive', the patient would be left frustrated, would feel that he was not taken seriously and would be anxious before the next LA application.

In 12 patients with a history of severe anaphylactic reactions induced by LAs, RPP was performed: only 3 patients showed mild reactions to LA at doses of 0.3 and 0.5 ml, while they were tolerating the higher doses of 1.0 and 2.0 ml. Nine patients who tolerated the drug were informed of the actual procedure, were re-challenged openly and showed no reaction. The results of placebo provocation strongly support the concept of the involvement of psychoneurogenic reflex mechanisms in the pathophysiology of these reactions. In very severe cases there may be an overlap to panic-fear attacks. Close cooperation with psychologists or psychosomatic medicine is recommended.

Diagnostic Work-Up

The diagnostic work-up in patients with a history of LA anaphylaxis uses the classical steps [29]:

History. This includes the severity grading of the clinical reaction, the time of administration and onset of symptoms, the concomitant use of other drugs, foods or compounds (latex), previous history of drug allergy, atopy in the personal or family history, other underlying conditions such as mastocytosis or C1 esterase inhibitor deficiency. The actual preparation in its galenic identity should be stored or at least listed.

Skin Test. Usually a battery of LAs is tested in the skin-prick test which is almost always negative. Then the intradermal test is performed with a 1:10 dilution of the substances. Undiluted LA preparations may commonly lead to false-positive reactions [30–32] in a rather high percentage of patients.

Subcutaneous Provocation Testing. When prick and intradermal tests are negative, subcutaneous provocation testing is started using 0.1 ml of the undiluted LA solution followed by 0.2, 0.5, 1.0 and 2.0 ml into the extensor side of the patient's upper arm at 30-min intervals. For most of the patients it is possible to find a tolerable LA which is recommended for future applications [33] (table 3). In a long-term follow-up, Wasserfallen and Frei [32] found in 28 patients undergoing skin and subcutaneous provocative testing that over 3 years in 19 cases re-exposure to a tolerated LA was well tolerated without untoward reaction.

In vitro Diagnosis. Unfortunately, there is no reliable in-vitro allergy diagnostic test available for routine use. Gall et al. [27] had used a self-made radioallergosorbent test with coupled LA to polystyrol discs, however, all the patients were negative. In-vitro cellular diagnostic assays have not been described as useful until now.

The field of anaphylactic reactions to LAs is difficult; there is still a need for research regarding the pathophysiology, but also for maybe more efficient and less risky diagnostic procedures.

Conclusion

LA preparations are common elicitors of adverse reactions, i.e. ca. 0.1–1% of applications in dental and other procedures. The clinical symptoms often correspond to anaphylactic reactions with tachycardia, hypotension, and subjective feelings such as weakness, heat or vertigo. LA preparations also are well-known contact sensitizers eliciting allergic contact dermatitis when used in topical preparations.

The pathomechanism of immediate hypersensitivity reactions to LA is largely unknown; they are commonly regarded as 'pseudo-allergic' or 'non-immune'-type reactions in the literature [29, 34]. Rarely, immunologically mediated reactions have been observed with positive skin-prick tests. After intramuscular application 'embolic-toxic' reactions can be observed due to intravasal application of the LA or other ingredients in LA preparations (e.g. epinephrine). Among the group of non-immune anaphylactic reactions, LA reactions are probably not caused by direct mediator release (e.g. histamine) or activation of complement or other systems; they can be classified as 'psychoneurogenic' reactions whereby the immediate pharmacologic action of the agent on the nerve is eliciting a reflex phenomenon with vagovasal component [35]. Other ingredients in LA preparations also have to be considered as elicitors, e.g. preservatives like benzoates or sulfites [36, 37] or latex [35] contaminants in injection bottles with latex closure. The chemical structure of LA seems to have little influence with regard to immediate-type hypersensitivity reactions [38, 39]. However, it plays an important role in type IV contact sensitivity where LA with ester groups seems to be stronger contact sensitizers than those with amide groups [40].

Practical management of patients with a history of LA reaction includes a careful allergy history (cofactors, other elicitors of anaphylaxis), skin-prick tests and intradermal tests with a battery of LAs [41]. Undiluted LA solutions may elicit false-positive immediate-type test reactions in up to 20%. Sometimes patients already react to the intradermal test with systemic symptoms. If prick and intradermal tests are negative, the procedure of subcutaneous provocation testing is started with increasing doses of the LA in a pure solution (ampoules without preservatives) [42]. We start with 0.1 ml with dose increments of 0.2, 0.5, 1.0 and 2.0 ml in the exterior side of the upper arm at 20-min intervals. The test has to be performed in a placebo-controlled manner. Some patients are constantly also reacting to placebo [43]. In this case we perform the regimen of RPP with injection of a LA substance (verum), while the patient is informed to receive a placebo injection in order to 'rule out psychosomatic involvement'. When the patient has tolerated this verum injection under the label of 'placebo', it is crucial to explain the findings in an open and respectful way. The patient never must get the feeling of having been 'deceived'. However, with this regimen we are able to eliminate anxiousness and fear, since we have proven to the patient that he has tolerated this LA substance. Most of the patients will then tolerate the selected LA in future applications.

Acknowledgement

This work has been supported by the Christine Kühne Center for Allergy Research and Education (CK-CARE).

References

1 Thyssen JP, Menné T, Elberberg J, Plaschke P, Johansen D: Hypersensitivity to local anesthetics – update and proposal of evaluation algorithm. Contact Dermatitis 2008;59:69–78.

2 Le Sellin J, Drouet M, Bonneau JC, Sabbah A: Management of suspected allergy to lidocaine (in French). Allerg Immunol (Paris) 1986;18:35–38.

3 Fisher MM, Bowey CJ: Alleged allergy to local anaesthetics. Anaesth Intensive Care 1997;25:611–614.

4 Hodgson TA, Shirlaw PJ, Challacombe SJ: Skin testing after anaphylactoid reactions to dental local anesthetics. A comparison with controls. Oral Surg Oral Med Oral Pathol 1993;75:706–711.

5 Wöhrl S, Vigl K, Stingl G: Patients with drug reactions – is it worth testing? Allergy 2006;61:928–934.

6 Prieto A, Herrero T, Rubio M, et al: Urticaria due to mepivacaine with tolerance to lidocaine and bupivacaine. Allergy 2005;60:261–262.

7 Bircher AJ, Messmer SL, Surber C, Rufli T: Delayed-type hypersensitivity to subcutaneous lidocaine with tolerance to articaine: confirmation by in vivo and in vitro tests. Contact Dermatitis 1996;34:387–389.

8 Hoigné R: Allergische und pseudo-allergische Reaktionen auf Penicillinpräparate (in German). Acta Allergol 1962;17:521.

9 Fisher MM, Graham R: Adverse responses to local anaesthetics. Anaesth Intensive Care 1984;12:325–327.

10 Ravindranathan N: Allergic reaction to lignocaine. A case report. Br Dent J 1975;138:101–102.

11 Chandler MJ, Grammer LC, Patterson R: Provocative challenge with local anesthetics in patients with a prior history of reaction. J Allergy Clin Immunol 1987;79:883–886.

12 Escolano F, Aliaga L, Alvarez J, Alcon A, Olive A: Allergic reactions to local anesthetics (in Spanish). Rev Esp Anestesiol Reanim 1990;37:172–175.

13 Incaudo G, Schatz M, Patterson R, Rosenberg M, Yamamoto F, Hamburger RN: Administration of local anesthetics to patients with a history of prior adverse reaction. J Allergy Clin Immunol 1978;61:339–345.

14 Bonnet MC, du Cailar G, Deschodt J: Anaphylaxis caused by lidocaine (in French). Ann Fr Anesth Reanim 1989;8:127–129.

15 Noormalin A, Shahnaz M, Rosmilah M, Mujahid SH, Gendeh BS: IgE-mediated hypersensitivity reaction to lignocaine – a case report. Trop Biomed 2005;22:179–183.

16 Waton J, Boulanger A, Trechot PH, Schmutz JL, Barbaud A: Contact urticaria from Emla cream. Contact Dermatitis 2004;51:284–287.

17 Adriani J: Etiology and management of adverse reactions to local anesthetics. Int Anesthesiol Clin 1972;10:127–151.

18 Melamed J, Beaucher WN: Delayed-type hypersensitivity (type IV) reactions in dental anesthesia. Allergy Asthma Proc 2007;28:477–479.

19 Andersen KE, White IR, Goossens A: Allergens from the standard series; in Frosch PJ, Menné T, Lepoittevin JP (eds): Contact Dermatitis. Heidelberg, Springer, 2006, pp 453–492.

20 Breit S, Rueff F, Przybilla B: 'Deep impact' contact allergy after subcutaneous injection of local anesthetics. Contact Dermatitis 2001;45:296–297.

21 Orasch CE, Helbling A, Zanni MP, Yawalkar N, Hari Y, Pichler WJ: T-cell reaction to local anaesthetics relationship to angioedema and urticaria after subcutaneous application-patch testing and LTT in patients with adverse reaction to local anaesthetics. Clin Exp Allergy 1999;29:1549–1554.

22 Ring J (ed): Allergy in Practice. Berlin, Springer, 2005.

23 Ruzicka T, Gerstmeier M, Przybilla B, Ring J: Allergy to local anesthetics: comparison patch test with prick and intradermal test results. J Am Acad Dermatol 1987;16:1202–1208.

24 Ring J: Anaphylaktoide Reaktionen. Heidelberg, Springer, 1978.

25 Johansson SGO, Bieber R, Dahl R, Friedmann PS, Lanier BQ, Lockey RF, Motala C, Ortega Martell JA, Platts-Mills TAE, Ring J, Thien F, Van Cauwenberge P, Williams HC: A revised nomenclature for allergy for global use. Report of the Nomenclature Review Committee of the World Allergy Organization, October 2003. J Allergy Clin Immunol 2004;113:832–836.

26 Ring J, Behrendt H: Anaphylaxis and anaphylactoid reactions – classification and pathophysiology. Clin Rev Allergy Immunol 1999;17:387–399.

27 Gall H, Kaufmann R, Kalveram CM: Adverse reactions to local anesthetics: analysis of 197 cases. J Allergy Clin Immunol 1996;97:933–937.

28 Ring J: Pseudo-allergic drug reactions; in Korenblat PE, Wedner HJ (eds): Allergy: Theory and Practice. Philadelphia, Saunders, 1992, pp 243–264.

29 Schatz M, Fung DL: Anaphylactic and anaphylactoid reactions due to anesthetic agents. Clin Rev Allergy 1986;4:215–227.

30 Aldrete JA, O'Higgins JW: Evaluation of patients with history of allergy to local anesthetic drugs. South Med J 1971;64:1118–1121.

31 De Shazo RD, Nelson HS: An approach to the patient with a history of local anesthetic hypersensitivity: experience with 90 patients. J Allergy Clin Immunol 1979;63:387–394.

32 Wasserfallen JB, Frei PC: Long-term evaluation of usefulness of skin and incremental challenge tests in patients with history of adverse reaction to local anesthetics. Allergy 1995;50:162–165.

33 Troise C, Voltolini S, Minale P, Modena P, Negrini AC: Management of patients at risk for adverse reactions to local anesthetics: analysis of 386 cases. J Investig Allergol Clin Immunol 1998;8:172–175.

34 Berkum Y, Ben-Zvi A, Levy Y, Galili D, Shalit M: Evaluation of adverse reactions to local anesthetics: experience with 236 patients. Ann Allergy Asthma Immunol 2003;91:342–345.

35 Pichler WJ (ed): Drug Hypersensitivity. Basel, Karger, 2007.

36 Dooms-Goossens A, de Alam AG, Degreef H, Kochuyt A: Intolerance due to metabisulfite. Contact Dermatitis 1989;20:124–126.

37 Simon RA: Adverse reactions to drug additives. J Allergy Clin Immunol 1984;74:623–630.

38 Astarita C, Gargano D, Romano C, et al: Long-term absence of sensitization to mepivacaine as assessed by a diagnostic protocol including patch testing. Clin Exp Allergy 2001;31:1762–1770.

39 Morais-Almeida M, Gaspar A, Marinho S, Rosado-Pinto J: Allergy to local anesthetics of the amide group with tolerance to procaine. Allergy 2003;58: 827–828.

40 Jacobsen RB, Borch JE, Bindslev-Jensen C: Hypersensitivity to local anaesthetics. Allergy 2005;60:262–264.

41 Soto-Aguilar MC, de Shazo RD, Dawsonn ES: Approach to the patient with suspected local anaesthetic sensitivity. Immunol Allergy Clin North Am 1998;18:851–855.

42 Aberer W, Bircher A, Romano A, et al: Drug provocation testing in the diagnosis of drug hypersensitivity reactions: general considerations. Allergy 2003;58:854–863.

43 Hein UR, Chantraine-Hess S, Worm M, Zuberbier T, Henz BM: Evaluation of systemic provocation tests in patients with suspected allergic and pseudo-allergic drug reactions. Acta Derm Venereol 1999; 79:139–142.

Univ.-Prof. Dr. med. Dr. phil. Johannes Ring
Klinik und Poliklinik für Dermatologie und Allergologie am Biederstein
Klinikum rechts der Isar der Technischen Universität München
Biedersteiner Strasse 29, DE–80802 Munich (Germany)
Tel. +49 89 4140 3170/3217, Fax +49 89 4140 3171, E-Mail johannes.ring@lrz.tum.de

Ring J (ed): Anaphylaxis. Chem Immunol Allergy. Basel, Karger, 2010, vol 95, pp 201–210

Anaphylaxis: Acute Treatment and Management

Johannes Ring[a, b] · Martine Grosber[a, b] · Matthias Möhrenschlager[b] · Knut Brockow[a]

[a]Department of Dermatology and Allergy Biederstein, ZAUM – Zentrum Allergie und Umwelt, Technische Universität München, Munich, Germany, and [b]Christine Kühne Center for Allergy Research and Education (CK-CARE), Hochgebirgsklinik, Davos, Switzerland

Abstract

Anaphylaxis is the maximal variant of an acute life-threatening immediate-type allergy. Due to its often dramatic onset and clinical course, practical knowledge in the management of these reactions is mandatory both for physicians and patients. It has to be distinguished between acute treatment modalities and general recommendations for management of patients who have suffered from an anaphylactic reaction. Acute treatment comprises general procedures like positioning, applying an intravenous catheter, call for help, comfort of the patient as well as the application of medication. The acute treatment modalities are selected depending upon the intensity of the clinical symptomatology as they are categorized in 'severity grades'. First of all it is important to diagnose anaphylaxis early and consider several differential diagnoses. This diagnosis is purely clinical and laboratory tests are of no help in the acute situation. Epinephrine is the essential antianaphylactic drug in the pharmacologic treatment. It should be first applied intramuscularly, only in very severe cases or under conditions of surgical interventions intravenous application can be tried. Furthermore, glucocorticosteroids are given in order to prevent protracted or biphasic courses of anaphylaxis; they are of little help in the acute treatment. Epinephrine autoinjectors can be used by the patient him/herself. Histamine H_1-antagonists are valuable in mild anaphylactic reactions; they should be given intravenously if possible. The replacement of volume is crucial in antianaphylactic treatment. Crystalloids can be used in the beginning, in severe shock colloid volume substitutes have to be applied. Patients suffering from an anaphylactic episode should be observed over a period of 4–10 h according to the severity of the symptomatology. It is crucial to be aware or recognize risk patients as for example patients with severe uncontrolled asthma, or under β-adrenergic blockade. When bronchial symptoms are in the focus, inhaled $β_2$-agonists can be tried, also for laryngeal edema. The use of combined H_1- and H_2-antagonists has been recommended for prophylaxis prior to application of potentially anaphylaxis-eliciting drugs (e.g. radiographic contrast media). Patients who have survived an anaphylactic reaction have to be thoroughly examined and an allergy diagnosis has to be performed with regard to the eliciting agent and the pathogenic mechanism involved. In cases of clear-cut IgE-mediated anaphylaxis, allergen-specific immunotherapy is available for some allergens and helpful as for example for insect venom anaphylaxis. Furthermore, patients should be trained with regard to the nature of anaphylaxis, the major eliciting agents and the principles of behavior and coping with the situation including the handling of epinephrine autoinjectors and the application of antianaphylactic medication. Educational programs for anaphylaxis have been developed.

In the management of anaphylaxis – the most severe manifestation of immediate-type allergy – acute treatment modalities have to be distinguished from general management recommendations. The steps of acute treatment of anaphylaxis are based on recommendation which differ between countries and are condensed in national or international guidelines [1–7]. Many of the recommendations are empiric in nature and not very much evidence-based. Due to the dramatic phenomenology and often 'hectic' circumstances, there are few controlled trials evaluating the efficacy of classic anaphylactic treatment [8–12].

In the following the most important steps and drugs in the acute treatment will be discussed as they appear in various recommendations. Currently a general evaluation of worldwide existing recommendations is being prepared by the World Allergy Organization (WAO) [13]. The acute treatment modalities are selected according to the intensity of the clinical symptomatology as they are categorized in various 'severity scales' [14–21] (also see chapter by Ring et al., section: History and Classification of Anaphylaxis, p. 1).

Basic General Treatment Modalities

When a patient develops anaphylaxis, prior to applying medication, some general management aspects have to be considered: positioning, call for help, intravenous catheter, and medication preparation. Anaphylaxis often occurs in a waiting room while the patient is sitting on a chair [22], and antianaphylactic treatment is started in this position. It is crucial to first put the patient into a supine position, with free airways. If cardiovascular symptoms are central, the legs may be slightly elevated. When bronchospasm is the main clinical feature, upright positioning of the thorax is to be preferred. It is important to apply an intravenous catheter in the early state while circulation is still active and give volume. At the same time or immediately after these first steps, help should be called and possible necessary medication should be prepared [3, 18, 23]. When the anaphylactic episode is elicited by an intravenously applied medication, this infusion has to be stopped [24, 25].

Among the antianaphylactic drugs, epinephrine (adrenaline) is the essential substance. In the acute treatment of the anaphylaxis in addition to the classical ABC (airway, breathing, circulation) rule for cardiopulmonary resuscitation [26, 27], one can apply the AAC rule (antigen off, adrenaline, cortisone) [18]. Other drugs playing a role in the treatment of anaphylaxis include antihistamines (H_1-antagonists),

Table 1. Basic rules in the management of an acute anaphylactic reaction

– Diagnosis and exclusion of differential diagnoses of anaphylaxis
– Stop exposure to the eliciting agent ('allergen off!')
– Place the patient into the right position (supine in cardiovascular reactions, thorax upright when bronchoconstriction is the major symptom)
– Call for help
– Inject epinephrine intramuscularly (0.01 mg/kg, maximum 0.5 mg in adults, 0.3 mg in children)
– If there are breathing difficulties give oxygen (6–8 l/min), by facemask
– Introduce an intravenous catheter and apply volume (crystalloid solutions like saline or Ringer's)
– Monitor patient's heart rate, respiration and blood pressure
– In grade IV start cardiopulmonary resuscitation

corticosteroids, β_2-agonists, possibly glucagon or vasoactive peptides (vasopressin) as well as intravenous fluids for volume replacement [28–30].

When cyanosis occurs, oxygen should be supplemented by a facemask or by an oropharyngeal airway with a flow rate of about 7 liters/min. When indicated or when there is a ventilatory insufficiency, intubation should be performed to support breathing. Patients who are vomiting should be positioned adequately in order to avoid aspiration (table 1).

Epinephrine (Adrenaline)

Epinephrine is the essential antianaphylactic drug. Despite its long-time use – it was discovered over a century ago – there are few evidence-based clinical trials evaluating the therapeutic benefit [8, 9, 11, 12]. Epinephrine as an α_1-adrenergic agent has a strong vasoconstrictive effect in most organs of the body and acts at the same time bronchodilatorily relieving laryngeal obstruction and mucosal edema.

While epinephrine is usually well tolerated in young and healthy individuals, there may be problems in elderly patients with cardiac arrhythmia or previous myocardial infarction episodes [31–33]. Pharmacological effects of epinephrine include rapid rise in blood pressure, pallor, anxiety, tachycardia, headache and tremor as well as vertigo. Most commonly these effects occur after intravenous injection or after overdosing epinephrine. Cardiac arrhythmia or pulmonary edema may develop in serious cases [33, 34].

The initial dose of epinephrine which is generally recommended is 0.01 mg/ kg, possibly increased to a maximum of 0.5 mg in adults and 0.3 mg in children,

Table 2. Medication needed in the treatment of acute anaphylactic reactions

– Epinephrine (adrenaline): Epinephrine is available as solution in ampoules 1:1,000 (containing 1 mg/ml), this can be used for intramuscular injection. For intravenous injection dilute further 1:10 for slow intravenous injection, better infusion! There are epinephrine autoinjectors containing 0.15 mg (children) or 0.3 mg (adults) epinephrine
– Histamine H_1-antagonists: For intravenous infusion diphenhydramine, dimetindene and clemastine are available. There are no controlled studies for the new non-sedating antihistamines in the treatment of anaphylaxis
– Histamine H_2-antagonists such as cimetidine or ranitidine can be helpful when combined with H_1-antihistamines
– β_2-Adrenergic agents: β_2-Agonists can be used as aerosols when airway reactions are predominant
– Additional medication: Additional medication to be used rarely under special circumstances include: Glucagon, atropine derivatives, dopamine, vasopressin (these drugs should be given by experienced physicians in the adequate setting)

respectively. The best recommended route of application is the intramuscular injection into the mid-anterolateral thigh. Single epinephrine dosage may be repeated in 5- to 15-min intervals when the symptomatology continues. In severe cases (grade III or IV) with manifest shock or cardiac/respiratory arrest, intravenous infusion has to be performed: here the epinephrine solution has to be diluted (usually 1:10 from the commercially available preparations), so that 0.1 mg/l is slowly infused (table 2).

Rarely, epinephrine can be injected directly intracardially in grade IV reactions. Subcutaneous epinephrine injection has been recommended over many decades, however it is current understanding that this should be avoided, since the necessary distribution in the body is not well achieved. Since epinephrine is mostly injected by the intramuscular route, the safety of this drug has considerably increased [9, 11, 12, 35, 36].

A major progress in the field is the availability of epinephrine autoinjectors which can be used by the patient him-/herself as a self-medication. Different devices are available which either trigger the injection needle just by pressure on the thigh or which have to be triggered by pressing on a button (like a pencil). The handling of these devices has to be explained and practiced with the patients (see 'Management, Education') [37–40].

Glucocorticosteroids

In many countries, glucocorticosteroids are administered as first drug because of their well-known antiallergic effects. However, the onset of action of corticosteroids takes at least from 30 min to some hours. They therefore are not really active in the very acute phase. However, they exert a beneficial effect in preventing late-phase, or bi-phasic or protracted reactions (see 'Classification') [18, 19]. Corticosteroids, when given, should be administered in an adequate dose of 3–5 mg/kg in a bolus intravenous injection [41].

Antihistamines

H₁-Antagonists
Antihistamines are the best studied drugs with regard to controlled trials or animal experiments [42–50]. H₁-antagonists such as dimetindene, clemastine or diphenhydramine have been available for more than half a century and are standard treatment in mild anaphylactic reactions (grade I). In many patients just developing urticaria or angioedema, adequate positioning, application of an intravenous catheter together with an infusion of fluids and intravenous antihistamines is sufficient when close monitoring for blood pressure, heart rate and breathing is available.

Not all grade I reactions necessarily progress to more severe anaphylactic symptomatology. There is maybe one cause for disagreement between various recommendations in different countries, since in some countries only cardiovascular involvement is a prerequisite for the diagnosis 'anaphylaxis', while other authors also include generalized skin symptoms as first degree of anaphylaxis which may develop into more severe forms, but need not necessarily do so. It is not possible to predict the clinical outcome of an acute urticaria or angioedema! Therefore, antihistamines have their definite place in antianaphylactic management [51]. Unfortunately, only classical antihistamines with sedating side effects are available for intravenous injection. Adequate control trials showing efficacy of modern non-sedating antagonists in anaphylaxis are still missing. Nevertheless, in some countries and by some doctors these modern non-sedating antihistamines as tablets or fluids are recommended for self-medication ('emergency kits' for patients).

H₂-Antagonists
H₂-antagonists alone, such as cimetidine or ranitidine, have a modest effect on cutaneous flush reaction and maybe also on the heart [14, 52]. However, when applied they should be given together with H₁-antagonists. There are some studies showing a beneficial effect of combined H₁- and H₂-antagonist treatment or pretreatment in anaphylaxis [46, 53].

Volume Replacement

Volume replacement is crucial in antianaphylactic treatment. It should be started with crystalloid solution (saline or Ringer's solution). However, in severe shock, higher

Table 3. Technical supplies required for adequate treatment of anaphylaxis

Infusion equipment
Oxygen
Facemasks (also for different ages)
Bag/valves/masks
Volume solutions (0.9% saline, Ringer's lactate, HES)
Airway equipment (pharyngeal airway, laryngeal mask, supplies for intubation)
Pulse oximetry
Automatic defibrillation equipment

quantities (2–3 liters) of colloid volume substitutes have to be applied. Here hydroxyethyl starch (HES) solutions are preferred, since gelatin or dextran preparations have been shown to elicit anaphylactic drug reactions in a certain number of patients [54, 55]. There is still a debate whether hyperoncotic HES solutions (≤30,000 MW) are superior to the isoosmolar HES preparations (table 3) [56].

Additional Drugs

Glucagon. In patients taking β-adrenergic blockers, the response to epinephrine is impaired. Glucagon may reverse this effect and should be given to those patients [57].

Anticholinergic treatment (atropine derivatives) may sometimes be indicated, especially in patients with pronounced bradycardia.

Vasoactive Peptides. More recent studies show a beneficial effect of vasopressin which should be evaluated further in clinical trials [58].

General Management of Patients Having Undergone an Anaphylactic Reaction

It is crucial not only to perform adequate treatment of the acute anaphylactic reactions, but to give clear recommendations for the future to every patient having undergone an anaphylactic reaction (table 4) [24, 53, 59–65]. Patients who have survived an anaphylactic reaction have to be thoroughly examined and allergy diagnosis has to be performed with regard to the eliciting agent and the pathogenic mechanism involved [18, 66–77]. In cases of clear-cut IgE-mediated anaphylaxis, allergen-specific immunotherapy is available for some allergens and helpful as for example for insect venom

Table 4. Management of patients having suffered from and survived from anaphylactic reaction

–	Observation according to intensity of clinical symptomatology (4–24 h)
–	Preliminary 'allergy emergency card' with suspected elicitor
–	Perform allergy diagnosis (after 3–4 weeks including in vitro diagnosis, skin test and if necessary provocation tests)
–	Educate patients in handling the situation of an anaphylactic reaction and the necessary medication including the handling of autoinjectors
–	Prescribe an 'emergency set' for self-medication
–	If possible, refer patient to allergen-specific immunotherapy (e.g. insect venom anaphylaxis)
–	Give individually tailored avoidance recommendations
–	Follow-up of the patient after 6 and 12 months

anaphylaxis [18, 78–87]. Furthermore, patients should be trained with regard to the nature of anaphylaxis, the major eliciting agents and the principles of behavior and coping with the situation including the handling of epinephrine autoinjectors and the application of antianaphylactic medication. Educational programs for anaphylaxis have been developed.

References

1 Joint Task Force on Practice Parameters; American Academy of Allergy, Asthma and Immunology; American College of Allergy, Asthma and Immunology; Joint Council of Allergy, Asthma and Immunology: The diagnosis and management of anaphylaxis: an updated practice parameter. J Allergy Clin Immunol 2005; 115(suppl 2):S483–S523.

2 Kemp SF, Lockey RF: Anaphylaxis: a review of causes and mechanisms. J Allergy Clin Immunol 2002;110:341–348.

3 Pumphrey RS: Lessons for management of anaphylaxis from a study of fatal reactions. Clin Exp Allergy 2000;30:1144–1150.

4 Ranft A, Kochs EF: Therapie anaphylaktischer Reaktionen: Synopsis bestehender Leitlinien und Empfehlungen. Anästhesiol Intensivmedl Notfallmed Schmerzther 2004;39:2–9.

5 Sampson HA, Muñoz-Furlong A, Bock SA, Schmitt C, Bass R, Chowdhury BA, Decker WW, Furlong TJ, Galli SJ, Golden DB, Gruchalla RS, Harlor AD, Hepner DL, Howarth M, Kaplan AP, Levy JH, Lewis LM, Lieberman PL, Metcalfe DD, Murphy R, Pollart SM, Pumphrey RS, Rosenwasser LJ, Simons FE, Wood JP, Camargo CA: Symposium on the definition and management of anaphylaxis: summary report. J Allergy Clin Immunol 2005;115:584–591.

6 Soar J, Pumphrey R, Cant A, Clarke S, Corbett A, Dawson P, et al: Emergency treatment of anaphylactic reactions – guidelines for healthcare providers. Resuscitation 2008;77:157–169.

7 Simons FER: Emergency treatment of anaphylaxis. BMJ 2008;336:1141–1142.

8 Brown MJ, Brown DC, Murphy MB: Hypokalemia from β_2-receptor stimulation by circulating epinephrine. N Engl J Med 1983;309:1414–1419.

9 Gu X, Simons KJ, Simons FER: Administration by sublingual tablet feasible for the first aid treatment of anaphylaxis? A proof-of-concept study. Diophar Drug Dispos 2002;23:213–216.

10 Lin RY, Curry A, Pesola GR, Knight RJ, Lee HS, Bakalchuk L, Tenenbaum C, Westfal RE: Improved outcomes in patients with acute allergic syndromes who are treated with combined H_1- and H_2-antagonists. Ann Emerg Med 2000;36:462–468.

11 Simons FER, Gu X, Jounston L, Simons KJ: Can epinephrine inhalations be substituted for epinephrine injection in children at risk for systemic anaphylaxis? Pediatrics 2000;106:1040–1044.

12 Simons FER, Gu X, Simons KJ: Epinephrine absorption in adults: intramuscular versus subcutaneous injection. J Allergy Clin Immunol 2001;108:871–873.

13 Simons FER, et al: WAO survey on global availability of medications, supplies and equipment for the assessment and management of anaphylaxis by physicians in healthcare settings (in preparation).

14 Capurro N, Levi R: The heart as target organ in systemic allergic reactions. Circ Res 1975;36:520–508.

15 Helbing A, Hurni T, Müller UR, Pichler WJ: Incidence of anaphylaxis with circulatory symptoms: a study over a 3-year period comprising 940,000 inhabitants of the Swiss Canton Bern. Clin Exp Allergy 2004;34:285–290.

16 Johansson SGO, Bieber T, Dahl R, Friedmann PS, Lanier BQ, Lockey RF, Motala C, Martell JAO, Platts-Mills TAE, Ring J, Thien F, Cauwenberge PV, Williams HC: Revised nomenclature for allergy for global use: report of the nomenclature review committee of the World Allergy Organization. J Allergy Clin Immunol 2004;113:832–836.

17 Pavek K, Wegmann A, Nordström L, Schwander D: Cardiovascular and respiratory mechanisms in anaphylactic and anaphylactoid shock reactions. Klin Wochenschr 1982;60:941–947.

18 Ring J: Allergy in Practice. Berlin, Springer, 2005.

19 Ring J, Behrendt H: Anaphylaxis and anaphylactoid reactions. Classification and pathophysiology. Clin Rev Allergy Immunol 1999;17:387–399.

20 Ring J, Messmer K: Incidence and severity of anaphylactoid reactions to colloid volume substitutes. Lancet 1977;1:466–469.

21 Smedegard G, Revenäs B, Arfors KE: Anaphylaxis in the monkey: hemodynamics and blood flow distribution. Acta Physiol Scand 1979;106:191.

22 Lockey RF, Benedict LM, Turkeltaub TB, Bukantz SC: Fatalities from immunotherapy and skin testing. J Allergy Clin Immunol 1987;79:666–677.

23 Lieberman PL: Anaphylaxis; in Adkinson NF Jr, Bochner BS, Busse WW, Holgate ST, Lemanske RF Jr, Simons FER (eds): Middleton's Allergy: Principles and Practice, ed 7. St Louis, Mosby/Elsevier Science, 2009, pp 1027–1049.

24 Hepner DL, Castells MC: Anaphylaxis during the perioperative period. Anesth Analg 2003;97:1381–1395.

25 Laine-Cessac P, Moshinaly H, Gouello JP, Geslin P, Allain P: Severe anaphylactoid reaction after intravenous corticosteroids. Report of a case and review of the literature. Therapie 1990;45:505–508.

26 Duda D, Dick W, Lorenz W: Anaphylactic shock. Resuscitation 1998. 4th Congress of the European Resuscitation Council. Bologna, Monduzzi, 1998, pp 15–19.

27 Eisenberg MS, Mengest TJ: Cardiac resuscitation. N Engl J Med 2001;344:1304–1313.

28 Bellomo R, Chapman M, Finfer S, Hickling K, Myburth J: Low-dose dopamine in patients with early renal dysfunction: a placebo-controlled randomised trial. Australian and New Zealand Intensive Care Society (ANZICS) Clinical Trials Group. Lancet 2000;356:2139–2143.

29 Friedrich JO, Adhikari N, Herridge MS, Beyene J: Meta-analysis: low-dose dopamine increases urine output but does not prevent renal dysfunction or death. Ann Intern Med 2005;142:510–524.

30 Hoffmann BB: Catecholamines, sympathomimetic drugs and adrenergic receptor antagonists; in Hardman JG, Limbird LE, Goodman A (eds): Goodman & Gilman: The Pharmaceutical Basis of Therapeutics. New York, McGraw Hill, 2002, pp 215–268.

31 Hannaway PJ, Hoppler GDK: Severe anaphylaxis and drug induced β-blockage. N Engl J Med 1983; 308:1536.

32 Stoelting RK: Systemic circulation; in Stoetting RK (ed): Pharmacology and Physiology in Anesthetic Practice. Philadelphia, Lippincott, 2006, pp 661–678.

33 Sullivan TJ: Cardiac disorders in penicillin-induced anaphylaxis: association with intravenous epinephrine therapy. JAMA 1982;248:2161–2162.

34 Brown SG, Blackman KE, Stenlake V, Heddle RJ: Insect sting anaphylaxis: prospective evaluation of treatment with intravenous adrenaline and volume resuscitation. Emerg Med J 2004;21:149–154.

35 Lieberman P: Use of epinephrine in the treatment of anaphylaxis. Curr Opin Allergy Clin Immunol 2003; 3:313–318.

36 Simons FE: First-aid treatment of anaphylaxis to food: focus on epinephrine. J Allergy Clin Immunol 2004;113:837–844.

37 Crifo G, Bircher A: Selbstbehandlung mit Notfallmedikamenten. Allergologie 2003;26:1516–1523.

38 Müller U, Mosbech H, Blaauw P, Dreborg S, Malling HJ, Przybilla B, Urbanek R, Pastorello E, Blanca M, Bousquet J, Jarisch R, Youlten L: Emergency treatment of allergic reactions to Hymenoptera stings. Clin Exp Allergy 1991;21:281–288.

39 Wüthrich B, Ballmer-Weber BK: Food-induced anaphylaxis. Allergy 2001;56(suppl 67):102–104.

40 Greenberger PA, Rotskoff BD, Lifschultz B: Fatal anaphylaxis: postmortem findings and associated comorbid diseases. Ann Allergy Asthma Immunol 2007;98:252–257.

41 Stark BJ, Sullivan TJ: Biphasic and protracted anaphylaxis. J Allergy Clin Immunol 1986;78:76–83.

42 Baller H, Huchzermeyer H: Histaminwirkungen am Herzen unter besonderer Berücksichtigung kardialer Nebenwirkungen von H_2-Rezeptorantagonisten. J Mol Med 1989;67:743–755.

43 Clough GF, Boutsiouki P, Church MK: Comparison of the effects of levocetirizine and loratadine on histamine-induced wheal, flare, and itch in human skin. Allergy 2001;56:985–988.

44 Grant JA, Riethuisen JM, Moulaert B, DeVos C: A double-blind, randomized, single-dose, crossover comparison of levocetirizine with ebastine, fexofenadine, loratadine, mizolastine, and placebo: suppression of histamine-induced wheal-and-flare response during 24 hours in healthy male subjects. Ann Allergy Asthma Immunol 2002;88:190–197.

45 Holgate ST, Canonica GW, Simons FE, Taglialatela M, Tharp M, Timmerman H, Yanai K: Consensus Group on New-Generation Antihistamines (CONGA): present status and recommendations. Clin Exp Allergy 2003;33:1305–1324.

46 Ring J, Rothenberger KH, Clauss W: Prevention of anaphylactoid reactions after radiographic contrast media infusions by combined histamine H_1- and H_2-receptor antagonists: results of a prospective controlled trial. Int Arch Allergy Appl Immunol 1985;78:9–14.

47 Simons FE: Comparative pharmacology of H_1-antihistamines: clinical relevance. Am J Med 2002;113(suppl 9A):38–46.

48 Simons FE: H_1-antihistamines: more relevant than ever in the treatment of allergic disorders. J Allergy Clin Immunol 2003;112:42–52.

49 Simons FE: Advances in H_1-antihistamines. N Engl J Med 2004;351:2203–2217.

50 Kalesnikoff J, Galli SJ: New developments in mast cell biology. Nat Immunol 2008;9:1215–1223.

51 Winbery SL, Lieberman PL: Histamine and antihistamines in anaphylaxis. Clin Allergy Immunol 2002;17:287–317.

52 De Soto H, Turk P: Cimetidine in anaphylactic shock refractory to standard therapy. Anesth Analg 1990;69:264–265.

53 Lorenz W, Ennis M, Doenicke A, Dich W: Perioperative uses of histamine antagonists. J Clin Anesth 1990;2:345–360.

54 Celik I, Duda D, Stinner B, Kimura K, Gayek H, Lorenz W: Early and late histamine release induced by albumin, hetastarch and polygeline: some unexpected findings. Inflamm Res 2003;52:408–416.

55 Richter W, Hedin H, Ring J, Kraft D, Messmer K: Anaphylaktoide Reaktionen nach Dextran I. Immunologische Grundlagen und klinische Befunde. Allergologie 1980;3:9.

56 Ickx BE, Bepperling F, Melot C, Schulman C, van der Linden PJ: Plasma substitution effects of a new hydroxyethyls starch HES 130/0.4 compared with HES 200/0.5. Br J Anaesth 2003;91:196–202.

57 Zaloga GP, Delacey W, Holmboe E, Chernow B: Glucagon reversal of hypotension in a case of anaphylactoid shock. Ann Intern Med 1986;105:65–66.

58 Kill C, Wranze E, Wulf H: Successful treatment of severe anaphylactic shock with vasopressin. Two case reports. Int Arch Allergy Immunol 2004;134: 260–261.

59 Greenberger PA, Patterson R: The prevention of immediate generalized reactions to radiocontrast media in high-risk patients. J Allergy Clin Immunol 1991;87:867–872.

60 Lorenz W, Duda D, Dick W, Sitter H, Doenicke A, Black A, Weber D, Menke H, Stinner B, Junginger T, Rothmund M, Ohmann CH, Healy MJ: Incidence and clinical importance of perioperative histamine release: randomised study of volume loading and antihistamines after induction of anaesthesia. Lancet 1994;343:933–940.

61 Stumpf JL, Shehab N, Patel AC: Safety of angiotensin-converting enzyme inhibitors in patients with insect venom allergies. Ann Pharmacother 2006;40:699–703.

62 TenBrook JA, Wolf MP, Hoffmann SN, Rosenwasser LJ, Konstam MA, Salem DN: Should β-blockers be given to patients with heart disease and peanut-induced anaphylaxis? A decision analysis. J Allergy Clin Immunol 2004;113:977–982.

63 Toogood HH: Risk of anaphylaxis in patients receiving β-blocker drugs. J Allergy Clin Immunol 1988;81:1–5.

64 Mueller UR: Cardiovascular disease and anaphylaxis. Curr Opin Allergy Clin Immunol 2007;7:337–341.

65 Mertes PM, Laxenaire MC, Lienhart A, Aberer W, Ring J, Pichler WJ, et al: Reducing the risk of anaphylaxis during anaesthesia: guidelines for clinical practice. J Investig Allergol Clin Immunol 2005;15: 91–101.

66 Brockow K, Vieluf D, Puschel K, Grosch J, Ring J: Increased postmortem serum mast cell tryptase in a fatal anaphylactoid reaction to nonionic radiocontrast medium. J Allergy Clin Immunol 1999;104:237–238.

67 Delage C, Irey HC: Anaphylactic deaths: a clinicopathologic study of 43 cases. J Forensic Sci 1972;17: 525.

68 Endrich B, Ring J, Intaglietta M: Effects of radiopaque contrast media on the microcirculation of the rabbit omentum. Radiology 1979;132:331–339.

69 Marone G, Bova M, Detoraki A, Onorati AM, Rossi FW, Spadaro G: The human heart as a shock organ in anaphylaxis. Novartis Found Symp 2004;257:133–149.

70 Maulitz RM, Pratt DS, Schocket AL: Exercise-induced anaphylactic reaction to shellfish. J Allergy Clin Immunol 1979;63:433.

71 Mehl A, Wahn U, Niggemann B: Anaphylactic reactions in children – a questionnaire-based survey in Germany. Allergy 2005;60:1440–1445.

72 Moneret-Vautrin DA, Morisset M, Flabbee J, Beaudouin E, Kanny G: Epidemiology of life-threatening and lethal anaphylaxis: a review. Allergy 2005; 60:443–451.

73 Ring J, Darsow U: Idiopathic anaphylaxis. Curr Allergy Asthma Rep 2002;2:40–45.

74 Rohrer CL, Pichler WJ, Helbling A: Anaphylaxie: Klinik, Ätiologie und Verlauf bei 118 Patienten. Schweiz Med Wochenschr 1998;128:53–63.

75 Sheikh A, Alves B: Hospital admissions for acute anaphylaxis: time trend study. BMJ 2000;320:1441.

76 Brockow K, Jofer C, Behrendt H, Ring J: Anaphylaxis in patients with mastocytosis: a study on history, clinical features and risk factors in 120 patients. Allergy 2008;63:226–232.

77 Brockow K, Ring J: Food anaphylaxis. Anal Bioanal Chem 2009;395:17–23.

78 Barnard JH: Studies of 400 Hymenoptera sting deaths in the United States. J Allergy Clin Immunol 1973;52:259–264.

79 Berchtold E, Maibach R, Müller U: Reduction of side effects from rush-immunotherapy with honey bee venom by pretreatment with terfenadine. Clin Exp Allergy 1991;22:59–65.

80 Bresser H, Sander CH, Rakoski J: Insektenstich-notfälle in München. Allergo J 1995;4:373–376.

81 Hepner MJ, Ownby DR, Anderson JA, Rowe MS, Sears-Ewald D, Brown EB: Risk of systemic reactions in patients taking β-blocker drugs receiving immunotherapy injections. J Allergy Clin Immunol 1990;86:407–411.

82 Hermann K, Ring J: The renin-angiotensin system in patients with repeated anaphylactic reactions during Hymenoptera venom hyposensitization and sting challenge. Int Arch Allergy Immunol 1997;11:251–256.

83 Ludolph-Hauser D, Ruëff F, Fries C, Schöpf P, Przybilla B: Constitutively raised serum concentrations of mast cell tryptase and severe anaphylactic reactions to Hymenoptera stings. Lancet 2001;357:361–362.

84 Müller U, Haeberli G: Use of β-blockers during immunotherapy for Hymenoptera venom allergy. J Allergy Clin Immunol 2005;115:606–610.

85 Nielsen L, Johnsen CR, Mosbech H, Poulsen LK, Malling HJ: Antihistamine premedication in specific cluster immunotherapy: a double-blind, placebo-controlled study: J Allergy Clin Immunol 1996;97:1207–1213.

86 Przybilla B, Ruëff F, Fuchs T, Pfeiffer C, Rakoski J, Stolz W, Vieluf D: Insekten-giftallergie. Leitlinie der Deutschen Gesellschaft für Allergologie und klinische Immunologie. Allergo J 2004;13:186–190.

87 Smith PL, Kagey-Sobotka A, Blecker ER, Traystman R, Kaplan AP, Gralink H, Valentine MD, Permut S, Lichtenstein LM: Physiologic manifestations of human anaphylaxis. J Clin Invest 1980;60:1072.

Univ.-Prof. Dr. med. Dr. phil. Johannes Ring
Klinik und Poliklinik für Dermatologie und Allergologie am Biederstein
Klinikum rechts der Isar der Technischen Universität München
Biedersteiner Strasse 29, DE–80802 Munich (Germany)
Tel. +49 89 4140 3170/3217, Fax +49 89 4140 3171, E-Mail johannes.ring@lrz.tum.de

Ring J (ed): Anaphylaxis. Chem Immunol Allergy. Basel, Karger, 2010, vol 95, pp 211–222

Epinephrine (Adrenaline) in Anaphylaxis

F. Estelle R. Simons[a] · Keith J. Simons[b]

[a]Department of Pediatrics and Child Health, Department of Immunology, Faculty of Medicine, and [b]Faculty of Pharmacy, Department of Pediatrics and Child Health, Faculty of Medicine, University of Manitoba, Winnipeg, Man., Canada

Abstract

Epinephrine (adrenaline) is universally recommended as the initial drug of choice for the treatment of anaphylaxis. No other medication has similar life-saving pharmacologic effects in multiple organ systems, including prevention and relief of both upper and lower airway obstruction, and of shock. Failure to inject epinephrine promptly contributes to anaphylaxis fatalities. It is most effective when given immediately after the onset of anaphylaxis symptoms. The initial recommended adult dose is 0.3–0.5 mg, injected intramuscularly in the anterolateral aspect of the mid-thigh. Injected by other routes, epinephrine appears to have a less satisfactory therapeutic window; for example, onset of action is potentially delayed when it is injected subcutaneously, and risk of adverse effects potentially increases when it is injected intravenously. The possibility of randomized, controlled trials of epinephrine in anaphylaxis should be considered. For ethical reasons, these trials will not be placebo-controlled. They might involve comparison of one epinephrine dose versus another, or one route of epinephrine administration versus another. For first-aid treatment of people with anaphylaxis in the community, novel epinephrine formulations are being developed. These include epinephrine autoinjectors that are safer and easier to use, and epinephrine formulations that can be administered through non-invasive routes.

Copyright © 2010 S. Karger AG, Basel

For nearly a century, epinephrine (adrenaline) has been the cornerstone of the acute management of anaphylaxis [1–6], a sudden-onset multi-systemic allergic reaction that can cause death. The World Health Organization lists epinephrine as an essential medication for anaphylaxis [7]. Where national guidelines are available for the acute management of anaphylaxis, they universally recommend injection of epinephrine as the initial medication of choice [8].

In this review, we will describe the pharmacologic activity of epinephrine in anaphylaxis, the evidence base for its use, epinephrine dosing and routes of administration, epinephrine autoinjector use in first-aid treatment, reasons for failure to inject epinephrine promptly, reasons for occasional apparent lack of response, and future directions in epinephrine research.

Table 1. Pharmacologic activities of epinephrine[1] relevant to anaphylaxis

Strength of recommendation for use as initial treatment of first choice in anaphylaxis[2]	B (adults and children) C (infants)
Pharmacologic effects	at α_1-receptor ↑ vasoconstriction ↑ peripheral vascular resistance ↑ blood pressure ↓ mucosal edema, e.g. in larynx at β_1-receptor ↑ heart rate ↑ force of cardiac contraction at β_2-receptor ↑ bronchodilation ↑ vasodilation ↓ release of pro-inflammatory mediators
Potential undesirable pharmacologic effects when given in usual doses by any route	anxiety, fear, pallor, tremor, restlessness, palpitations, headache

[1] Epinephrine is widely used in clinical medicine for its multiple pharmacologic effects; particularly for its potent vasoconstrictor effects. For example, in a dilute solution of 1:100,000, it provides a surgical tourniquet and facilitates a blood-free operating field. It is administered by nebulizer and face mask for post-intubation croup and for viral croup.

[2] *Strength of recommendation A:* based on a meta-analysis or at least one randomized controlled trial. *Strength of recommendation B:* based on at least one well-designed study, including case control and comparative studies. *Strength of recommendation C:* based on expert reports or opinion (levels of evidence and strength of recommendation. Oxford (UK): Centre for Evidence-Based Medicine. Available at: http://www.cebm.net/levels_of_evidence.asp (accessed December 8, 2008).

Pharmacologic Activity

Epinephrine is an endogenous catecholamine, and a direct-acting sympathomimetic α-adrenergic and β-adrenergic agonist [5, 6, 9]. It has cyclic adenosine monophosphate-mediated pharmacologic effects on many target organ systems (table 1). Through α_1-adrenergic receptors, it increases vasoconstriction and peripheral vascular resistance, leading to a decrease in mucosal edema and an increase in blood pressure. These α_1-adrenergic properties give it a life-saving advantage over all other medications used in anaphylaxis. Through β_1-adrenergic receptors, it is a powerful cardiac stimulant, and increases both the rate and force of cardiac contractions. Through β_2-adrenergic receptors, it has bronchodilator and vasodilator effects, and also decreases the release of mediators of inflammation such as histamine and tryptase from mast cells and basophils. Its effects on the vasculature and on down-regulation of mediator release are bidirectional. Achieving high epinephrine concentrations rapidly in plasma and tissue appears to be critically important, because low concentrations potentially cause vasodilation, decreased blood pressure, and increased mediator release [5, 9].

Therapeutic Window

Epinephrine has a narrow benefit-to-risk ratio. Along with its therapeutic effects, when administered in recommended doses by any route, it potentially causes transient anxiety, fear, restlessness, palpitations, pallor, tremor, and headache. Although usually perceived as adverse effects, such symptoms indicate that a pharmacologically active dose of the medication has been absorbed. The desirable pharmacologic effects of epinephrine cannot be separated from the undesirable pharmacologic effects [10].

With regard to epinephrine's potential adverse cardiac effects, it is important to remember that in anaphylaxis, the heart is a target organ. Mast cells located between myocardial fibers, in perivascular tissue, and in the arterial intima are activated through IgE and other mechanisms to release chemical mediators of inflammation, including histamine, leukotriene C_4, and prostaglandin D_2. Coronary artery spasm, myocardial injury, and cardiac dysrhythmias have been documented in some patients *before* epinephrine has been injected for treatment of anaphylaxis, as well as in patients with anaphylaxis who have *not* been treated with epinephrine [11, 12].

Serious adverse effects of epinephrine potentially occur when it is given in an excessive dose, or too rapidly, for example, as an intravenous bolus or a rapid intravenous infusion. These include ventricular dysrhythmias, angina, myocardial infarction, pulmonary edema, sudden sharp increase in blood pressure, and cerebral hemorrhage. The risk of epinephrine adverse effects is also potentially increased in patients with hypertension or ischemic heart disease, and in those using β-blockers (due to unopposed epinephrine action on vascular $α_1$-adrenergic receptors), monoamine oxidase inhibitors, tricyclic antidepressants, or cocaine. Even in these patients, there is no absolute contraindication for the use of epinephrine in the treatment of anaphylaxis [1, 5, 6].

Epinephrine: Evidence Base for Use in Anaphylaxis

The current evidence base for the injection of epinephrine in the initial acute treatment of anaphylaxis includes: clinical experience during nearly a century of use, observational studies, epidemiological studies, fatality studies, and randomized controlled trials in people at risk for anaphylaxis although not actually experiencing it at the time of the study. Moreover, the pharmacology of epinephrine has been extensively studied in vitro, and in randomized controlled trials in animal models of anaphylaxis.

Epinephrine, like glucocorticoids, H_1-antihistamines, and other medications used in the initial acute management of anaphylaxis, was introduced before the era of prospective, randomized controlled trials and evidence-based medicine [13]. A recent Cochrane Systematic Review did not identify evidence from randomized controlled trials to support the efficacy of epinephrine in the emergency management of anaphylaxis; however, it noted that: (1) based on current evidence, the benefits of injecting appropriate doses of epinephrine likely far outweigh the risks, and (2) anesthetists, who treat anaphylaxis relatively often and usually have sophisticated monitoring in place before, during and after the event, universally report a rapid and predictable response to epinephrine [14].

Given the unexpected occurrence of anaphylaxis, the rapidity with which symptoms evolve after exposure to the trigger, and the observation that delay in epinephrine injection is associated with fatality [15, 16], randomized controlled trials of epinephrine in anaphylaxis will not be easy to conduct; however, it is time to consider the possibility of performing such trials. Future directions with regard to studies of the optimal dose and optimal route of administration of epinephrine in anaphylaxis *that do not involve a placebo control* will be outlined at the end of this review [17].

Epinephrine Dosing

Epinephrine is administered by a variety of different routes in anaphylaxis, except for the oral route, which is not feasible because of rapid inactivation of epinephrine in the gastrointestinal tract by catechol-*O*-methyltransferase and monoamine oxidase [9]. The initial intramuscular epinephrine doses of 0.3–0.5 mg currently recommended for adults with anaphylaxis are low compared with the doses required for resuscitation following cardiac arrest [1, 2, 4, 18].

Rationale for Intramuscular Injection
In anaphylaxis, epinephrine appears to have an optimal benefit-to-risk ratio when it is administered promptly by intramuscular injection [1–6].

In randomized, controlled, appropriately-blinded trials conducted in children at risk for anaphylaxis but not actually experiencing it when the study was being performed, the time to peak plasma epinephrine concentrations, accompanied by prompt pharmacologic effects, was 8 ± (SEM) 2 min after intramuscular injection of 0.3 mg in the anterolateral aspect of the mid-thigh (in the vastus lateralis muscle) [19]. In contrast, after subcutaneous injection of a similar dose in the deltoid region of the arm, the time to peak plasma epinephrine concentrations was significantly longer, 34 ± 14 min (range 5–120 min). The total amount of epinephrine eventually absorbed did not differ significantly in the two groups. Faster absorption of epinephrine after intramuscular injection in the thigh compared to subcutaneous injection in the arm was also documented in a randomized, blinded, placebo-controlled, six-way crossover study in adults [20].

It is not surprising that intramuscular injection of epinephrine into the vastus lateralis produces a prompt peak plasma epinephrine concentration, because of the large size and excellent vascularization of this muscle. It is also not surprising that subcutaneous injection of epinephrine potentially leads to delayed absorption, because of the potent α_1-adrenergic agonist vasoconstrictor effects in the skin and subcutaneous tissue, as evidenced by skin blanching at the injection site [19, 20].

Rationale for Intravenous Injection

In an anesthetized, ventilated canine model of anaphylactic shock defined as hypotension with blood pressure maintained at 50% of baseline, epinephrine infusion produces an improvement in blood pressure, associated with positive inotropy [21].

Anaphylactic patients with impending shock, for example, those with incontinence, sudden loss of hearing or vision, dizziness, or collapse, and those with profound or persistent hypotension, require slow intravenous infusion of a dilute epinephrine solution [0.1 mg in 1 ml (1:10,000)]. Continuous hemodynamic monitoring and dose titration by trained and experienced healthcare professionals are essential. Maximum infusion rates of 5–15 μg/min are recommended in adults [2, 18, 22].

In healthcare settings, the risk of harmful effects is higher with intravenous epinephrine than with epinephrine administered through other routes of injection [2, 6]. Dosing errors have been attributed to the common practice of using ratios such as 1:10,000 to express the epinephrine concentrations; therefore, use of mass concentration such as 0.1 mg in 1 ml is recommended [23].

Rarely, patients are refractory to epinephrine treatment [24], and require other potent vasopressors [1, 2, 18, 22]. In those patients who are refractory to epinephrine because they are taking a β-adrenergic blocker, glucagon should be administered intravenously [5, 18].

Epinephrine Autoinjector Use in First-Aid Treatment

Optimal use of epinephrine autoinjectors for first-aid treatment of anaphylaxis in community settings is hampered by several issues. In most countries, these include the availability of only two pre-measured epinephrine doses and only a few different needle lengths, and the need to replace outdated autoinjectors at 12- to 18-month intervals due to degradation of the epinephrine solution they contain.

Dilemmas in Dosing

Physicians face a dilemma with regard to prescribing an optimal epinephrine dose in an autoinjector for first-aid treatment of people at risk for anaphylaxis in a community setting, because only two pre-measured epinephrine doses, 0.15 and 0.3 mg, are currently available to treat everyone, and people range in size from small infants to large or overweight adults [10, 25].

For infants or young children, to facilitate precise dosing of 0.01 mg/kg, additional pre-measured doses of epinephrine would be ideal. Currently, for children weighing up to 22.5 kg (the average body mass for a 7-year-old), an epinephrine autoinjector dose of 0.15 mg (a 1.5-fold underdose for a 22.5 kg child) is recommended [5]. The decision to prescribe a 0.3-mg dose (a 1.3-fold overdose for a 22.5 kg child) is often guided by the presence of one or more of the following: history of a previous life-threatening reaction; concurrent diagnosis of asthma (which increases the risk of fatality); known history of peanut, tree nut, milk, egg, fish, or shellfish trigger for anaphylaxis; poor access to emergency medical services; or, living in a chaotic or dysfunctional family setting. It should be noted that the absence of a history of a previous life-threatening reaction does not eliminate the possibility of such a reaction in the future [5].

For overweight adolescents and adults, autoinjectors containing a 0.5-mg dose of epinephrine are needed; however, this dose is not available in most countries. Moreover, in many overweight people, attempts to inject epinephrine intramuscularly from most currently available autoinjectors are likely doomed to failure, because the attached needle is too short to penetrate the poorly vascularized adipose tissue layer over the vastus lateralis [26].

Lack of appropriate dose options and needle length options should not deter physicians from prescribing epinephrine autoinjectors for the first-aid out-of-hospital treatment of anaphylaxis.

How Many Epinephrine Doses Are Needed?

Up to 20% of anaphylaxis episodes in adults, and up to 6% of episodes in children, are biphasic or protracted, and involve recurrent or persistent symptoms without any ongoing or additional exposure to the anaphylaxis trigger. Administering too little epinephrine too late during treatment of the initial symptoms of an anaphylaxis episode is one of the factors reported to increase the risk of biphasic or protracted anaphylaxis [27].

Retrospective studies involving a review of emergency department records [28], or a cross-sectional survey [29], indicate that 16–19% of people who require an initial dose of epinephrine in food-triggered anaphylaxis in community settings subsequently required a second dose.

Currently, many physicians advise their patients at risk for anaphylaxis in the community to carry two epinephrine doses with them at all times [30]. In school settings, it has been proposed that one epinephrine autoinjector should be available for each child at risk, along with several extra autoinjectors available as back-up for all children at risk [31].

Although a 5- to 15-min interval between epinephrine injections is often recommended, this interval has not been established in randomized controlled trials, and consequently remains somewhat controversial; in reality, the optimal time interval depends mainly on the clinical response to the initial epinephrine dose [1, 2].

Simons · Simons

Stability of Epinephrine Solution

Epinephrine is an inherently unstable chemical in aqueous solution, even at a low pH and in the presence of an antioxidant such as sodium metabisulfite, up to 1 mg/ml. With the passage of time, the epinephrine dose gradually decreases due to degradation into inactive compounds. If the expiry date has passed, the epinephrine dose correlates inversely with the number of months or years past that date, and will likely be lower than the dose stated on the label even if the solution appears clear and colorless. Nevertheless, if this is the only source of epinephrine available for injection, it should be used in preference to not administering epinephrine at all [32].

Alternative Routes of Epinephrine Administration for First-Aid Treatment

Although epinephrine autoinjectors are widely dispensed for first-aid treatment of anaphylaxis in some countries, they are neither available nor affordable in many others [33]. In these situations, physicians sometimes equip patients at risk for anaphylaxis in the community with an epinephrine ampule and a disposable 1-ml syringe. Some physicians also recommend this approach for infants, for whom, as noted previously, no appropriate epinephrine dose is available in an autoinjector formulation.

People without professional medical training have difficulty in drawing up medications from an ampule rapidly and accurately. In a prospective study, 18 parents, 18 resident physicians, 18 general duty nurses, and 18 emergency department nurses were asked to draw up an infant epinephrine dose from a 1-ml ampule. Although the parents received detailed instructions in a relaxed supportive atmosphere, the doses they drew up varied 40-fold and were usually incorrect; moreover, it took them 142 ± 13 s (range 83–248) to get the epinephrine into the syringe, in contrast to 52 ± 2 s (range 30–83) for physicians, 40 ± 2 s (range 26–71) for general duty nurses, and 29 ± 0.09 s (range 27–33) for emergency department nurses [34].

Some physicians recommend epinephrine metered-dose inhalers as an alternative to epinephrine autoinjectors. While a few inhalations might relieve mild or moderate respiratory symptoms, for relief of life-threatening airway obstruction or shock, adults need to inhale 20–30 puffs and children need to inhale 10–20 puffs, which is hard to do [35]. Epinephrine metered-dose inhalers contain chlorofluorocarbon propellants. For environmental reasons, they might not be manufactured in the future.

Reason for Failure to Inject Epinephrine Promptly

Physicians often face dilemmas with regard to prescribing epinephrine and giving advice about how to use it to those at risk, or the caregivers of children at risk.

Published clinical scenarios outline the available options in making these decisions [36]. It is impossible to predict the outcome of a future anaphylaxis episode with certainty based on the history of a previous episode [37]. Therefore, when in doubt, erring on the side of caution is generally advised: prescribe one or more epinephrine autoinjectors, and advise the person at risk or the caregiver of a child at risk to inject epinephrine promptly in an anaphylaxis episode [36].

Many people who have experienced anaphylaxis in the community and are therefore at risk for recurrence have never received a prescription for an epinephrine autoinjector from an emergency department physician [38, 39] or from their primary care physician. Some of those who have received a prescription for an epinephrine autoinjector do not follow through and get it filled [40]. Even if they do get the epinephrine autoinjector dispensed, they may fail to carry it with them at all times [41]. Adherence to instructions to carry epinephrine can be improved with regular input from a healthcare professional [42]; however, healthcare professionals need to master the complexities of epinephrine autoinjector use [43] before instructing others. People who have survived a mild anaphylaxis episode that was not treated at all, or was treated only with an antihistamine or an asthma puffer, sometimes fail to inject epinephrine because they erroneously assume that their subsequent reactions will also be mild [44].

Reasons for Occasional Lack of Response to Epinephrine

Rarely, anaphylaxis progresses so rapidly that the initial first-aid dose of epinephrine which, as noted previously, is low relative to the initial epinephrine dose of 1 mg used in resuscitation, is ineffective even if given promptly. More commonly, anaphylaxis progresses because epinephrine is given too late, or administered in a suboptimal dose for the patient's body mass (weight), or through a suboptimal route [5].

Context of Epinephrine Use as First-Aid Treatment

Preparedness for first-aid treatment of anaphylaxis in the community involves not only a prescription for epinephrine autoinjectors, but also an Anaphylaxis Emergency Action Plan, appropriate medical identification, and anaphylaxis education.

Anaphylaxis Emergency Action Plan
Epinephrine autoinjectors should be prescribed in the context of a written Anaphylaxis Emergency Action Plan that is developed with the input of the person at risk for anaphylaxis, or the caregiver(s) of the child at risk [45]. The Plan should remind the person at risk about the common symptoms and signs of anaphylaxis, stress the importance of prompt epinephrine injection, and clearly state that H_1-antihistamines

and asthma puffers are not life-saving in anaphylaxis [45, 46]. The Plan should also emphasize that Emergency Medical Services should be called immediately after epinephrine injection, and the person with anaphylaxis should be transported to the nearest hospital, for monitoring and further treatment as necessary. Randomized controlled trials of Anaphylaxis Emergency Action Plans are needed [47].

Medical Identification

People known to be at risk for anaphylaxis should wear up-to-date medical identification such as a bracelet or other jewelry, or carry an Anaphylaxis Wallet Card listing their confirmed trigger factor(s), relevant co-morbidities such as asthma, and concurrent medications [45].

Anaphylaxis Education

At-risk people and the caregivers of children at risk should have access to anaphylaxis education in the form of individualized instruction or small group sessions with a healthcare professional, or an online program with a self-evaluation component. These sessions should provide basic information about prevention of anaphylaxis episodes in the community by trigger avoidance, and immunomodulation, where relevant, as well as about recognition of anaphylaxis and emergency preparedness for anaphylaxis recurrence. Ideally, they should provide an opportunity for supervised practice with an epinephrine autoinjector trainer until technique is perfected, and for regular review of technique with a healthcare professional. Supervised practice with an actual epinephrine autoinjector (not a trainer) has been recommended. Randomized controlled trials of anaphylaxis education programs have not yet been performed [45].

Future Directions

There are no new medications available for the acute treatment of anaphylaxis [17]. Epinephrine, with its multiple relevant life-saving pharmacologic actions, is likely to remain the initial drug of choice in anaphylaxis for the foreseeable future.

There is universal agreement that prompt injection of epinephrine is fundamentally important in the initial acute management of anaphylaxis; therefore, placebo-controlled trials of epinephrine in anaphylaxis are clearly unethical; indeed, underuse of epinephrine in anaphylaxis treatment in emergency departments remains a concern [48]. Nevertheless, it might be possible to conduct randomized, controlled trials comparing two different dosages of epinephrine, for example, the two initial intramuscular doses of 0.3 versus 0.5 mg that are commonly recommended for adults, or two different routes of administration, for example, intramuscular versus subcutaneous injection. In all patients in such trials, other standard-of-care treatments should be initiated promptly. These include supplemental oxygen, airway management, intravenous fluids, and positioning the patient comfortably with lower extremities elevated. Continuous monitoring of blood pressure, cardiac rate and rhythm, oxygen saturation, and other relevant outcomes should be performed [17].

For treatment of anaphylaxis in the community, obvious limitations of currently available epinephrine autoinjectors include not only the restricted range of pre-measured doses and of needle lengths as discussed previously, but also the weight and bulkiness that potentially leads to reluctance to carry them, and the intrinsic design flaws that potentially lead to needle-stick injuries [49]. Autoinjectors that have improved safety features and are easier to use, are currently being developed. In addition, several research groups are developing new needle-free epinephrine formulations, including those that might be suitable for sublingual administration [50].

Ongoing epinephrine research relevant to human anaphylaxis is critically important. In its absence, the use of epinephrine in anaphylaxis treatment in the 21st century will continue to be based mostly on clinical experience, or worse, on expedience, instead of on clinical science.

References

1 Kemp SF, Lockey RF, Simons FER: Epinephrine: the drug of choice for anaphylaxis. A statement of the World Allergy Organization. Allergy 2008;63:1061–1070.

2 Soar J, Pumphrey R, Cant A, Clarke S, Corbett A, Dawson P, Ewan P, Foex B, Gabbott D, Griffiths M, Hall J, Harper N, Jewkes F, Maconochie I, Mitchell S, Nasser S, Nolan J, Rylance G, Sheikh A, Unsworth DJ, Warrell D: Emergency treatment of anaphylactic reactions – guidelines for healthcare providers. Resuscitation 2008;77:157–169.

3 Liberman DB, Teach SJ: Management of anaphylaxis in children. Pediatr Emerg Care 2008;24:861-869.

4 Sampson HA, Munoz-Furlong A, Campbell RL, Adkinson NF Jr, Bock SA, Branum A, Brown SGA, Camargo CA Jr, Cydulka R, Galli SJ, Gidudu J, Gruchalla RS, Harlor AD Jr, Hepner DL, Lewis LM, Lieberman PL, Metcalfe DD, O'Connor R, Muraro A, Rudman A, Schmitt C, Scherrer D, Simons FER, Thomas S, Wood JP, Decker WW: Second symposium on the definition and management of anaphylaxis: summary report – Second National Institute of Allergy and Infectious Disease/Food Allergy and Anaphylaxis Network symposium. J Allergy Clin Immunol 2006;117:391–397.

5 Simons FER: First-aid treatment of anaphylaxis to food: focus on epinephrine. J Allergy Clin Immunol 2004;113:837–844.

6 McLean-Tooke APC, Bethune CA, Fay AC, Spickett GP: Adrenaline in the treatment of anaphylaxis: what is the evidence? Br Med J 2003;327:1332–1335.

7 WHO Model List of Essential Medicines, ed 15, March 2007, available from http://www.who.int/medicines/publications/essentialmedicines/en (accessed December 17, 2008).

8 Alrasbi M, Sheikh A: Comparison of international guidelines for the emergency medical management of anaphylaxis. Allergy 2007;62:838–841.

9 Westfall TC, Westfall DP: Adrenergic agonists and antagonists; in Brunton LL, Lazo JS, Parker KL (eds): Goodman & Gilman's The Pharmacological Basis of Therapeutics, ed 11. New York, McGraw-Hill, 2006, pp 237–247.

10 Simons FER, Gu X, Silver NA, Simons KJ: EpiPen Jr versus EpiPen in young children weighing 15–30 kg at risk for anaphylaxis. J Allergy Clin Immunol 2002;109:171–175.

11 Marone G, Bova M, Detoraki A, Onorati AM, Rossi FW, Spadaro G: The human heart as a shock organ in anaphylaxis. Novartis Found Symp 2004;257:133–149.

12 Mueller UR: Cardiovascular disease and anaphylaxis. Curr Opin Allergy Clin Immunol 2007;7:337–341.

13 Simons FER: Anaphylaxis: evidence-based long-term risk reduction in the community. Immunol Allergy Clin North Am 2007;27:231–248.

14 Sheikh A, Shehata Y, Brown SGA, Simons FER: Adrenaline for the treatment of anaphylaxis: Cochrane systematic review. Allergy 2009;64:204–212.

15 Bock SA, Munoz-Furlong A, Sampson HA: Further fatalities caused by anaphylactic reactions to food, 2001–2006. J Allergy Clin Immunol 2007;119:1016–1018.

16 Pumphrey RSH, Gowland MH: Further fatal allergic reactions to food in the United Kingdom, 1999–2006. J Allergy Clin Immunol 2007;119:1018–1019.

17 Simons FER: Emergency treatment of anaphylaxis. Br Med J 2008;336:1141–1142.

18 Simons FER, Camargo CA: Anaphylaxis: Rapid recognition and treatment; in Basow DS (ed): UpToDate. Waltham, UpToDate, 2008.

19 Simons FER, Roberts JR, Gu X, Simons KJ: Epinephrine absorption in children with a history of anaphylaxis. J Allergy Clin Immunol 1998;101:33–37.

20 Simons FER, Gu X, Simons KJ: Epinephrine absorption in adults: intramuscular versus subcutaneous injection. J Allergy Clin Immunol 2001;108:871–873.

21 Mink SN, Simons FER, Simons KJ, Becker AB, Duke K: Constant infusion of epinephrine, but not bolus treatment, improves haemodynamic recovery in anaphylactic shock in dogs. Clin Exp Allergy 2004; 34:1776–1783.

22 Brown SGA, Blackman KE, Stenlake V, Heddle RJ: Insect sting anaphylaxis; prospective evaluation of treatment with intravenous adrenaline and volume resuscitation. Emerg Med J 2004;21:149–154.

23 Wheeler DW, Carter JJ, Murray LJ, Degnan BA, Dunling CP, Salvador R, Menon DK, Gupta AK: The effect of drug concentration expression on epinephrine dosing errors: a randomized trial. Ann Intern Med 2008;148:11–14.

24 Smith PL, Kagey-Sobotka A, Bleecker ER, Traystman R, Kaplan AP, Gralnick H, Valentine MD, Permutt S, Lichtenstein LM: Physiologic manifestations of human anaphylaxis. J Clin Invest 1980;66:1072–1080.

25 Simons FER, Peterson S, Black CD: Epinephrine dispensing patterns for an out-of-hospital population: a novel approach to studying the epidemiology of anaphylaxis. J Allergy Clin Immunol 2002;110:647–651.

26 Song TT, Nelson MR, Chang JH, Engler RJM, Chowdhury BA: Adequacy of the epinephrine auto-injector needle length in delivering epinephrine to the intramuscular tissues. Ann Allergy Asthma Immunol 2005;94:539–542.

27 Lieberman P: Biphasic anaphylactic reactions. Ann Allergy Asthma Immunol 2005;95:217–226.

28 Oren E, Banerji A, Clark S, Camargo CA Jr: Food-induced anaphylaxis and repeated epinephrine treatments. Ann Allergy Asthma Immunol 2007;99: 429–432.

29 Jarvinen KM, Sicherer SH, Sampson HA, Nowak-Wegrzyn A: Use of multiple doses of epinephrine in food-induced anaphylaxis in children. J Allergy Clin Immunol 2008;122:133–138.

30 Kelso JM: A second dose of epinephrine for anaphylaxis: how often needed and how to carry. J Allergy Clin Immunol 2006;117:464–465.

31 Norton L, Dunn Galvin A, Hourihane JO'B: Allergy rescue medication in schools: modeling a new approach. J Allergy Clin Immunol 2008;122:209–210.

32 Simons FER, Gu X, Simons KJ: Outdated EpiPen and EpiPen Jr auto-injectors: past their prime? J Allergy Clin Immunol 2000;105:1025–1030.

33 Simons FER: Lack of worldwide availability of epinephrine autoinjectors for outpatients at risk of anaphylaxis. Ann Allergy Asthma Immunol 2005;94: 534–538.

34 Simons FER, Chan ES, Gu X, Simons KJ: Epinephrine for the out-of-hospital (first aid) treatment of anaphylaxis in infants: is the ampule/ syringe/needle method practical? J Allergy Clin Immunol 2001;108:1040–1044.

35 Simons FER, Gu X, Johnston L, Simons KJ: Can epinephrine inhalations be substituted for epinephrine injection in children at risk for systemic anaphylaxis? Pediatrics 2000;106:1040–1044.

36 Sicherer SH, Simons FER: Quandaries in prescribing an emergency action plan and self-injectable epinephrine for first-aid management of anaphylaxis in the community. J Allergy Clin Immunol 2005;115:575–583.

37 Pumphrey R: Anaphylaxis: can we tell who is at risk of a fatal reaction? Curr Opin Allergy Clin Immunol 2004;4:285–290.

38 Clark S, Bock SA, Gaeta TJ, Brenner BE, Cydulka RK, Camargo CA: Multicenter study of emergency department visits for food allergies. J Allergy Clin Immunol 2004;113:347–352.

39 Clark S, Long AA, Gaeta TJ, Camargo CA Jr: Multicenter study of emergency department visits for insect sting allergies. J Allergy Clin Immunol 2005; 116:643–649.

40 Johnson TL, Parker AL: Rates of retrieval of self-injectable epinephrine prescriptions: a descriptive report. Ann Allergy Asthma Immunol 2006;97:694–697.

41 Sampson MA, Munoz-Furlong A, Sicherer SH: Risk-taking and coping strategies of adolescents and young adults with food allergy. J Allergy Clin Immunol 2006;117:1440–1445.

42 Webb LM, Lieberman P: Anaphylaxis: a review of 601 cases. Ann Allergy Asthma Immunol 2006;97: 39–43.

43 Mehr S, Robinson M, Tang M: Doctor – how do I use my EpiPen? Pediatr Allergy Immunol 2007;18: 448–452.

44 Sicherer SH, Furlong TJ, Munoz-Furlong A, Burks AW, Sampson HA: A voluntary registry for peanut and tree nut allergy: characteristics of the first 5,149 registrants. J Allergy Clin Immunol 2001;108:128–132.

45 Simons FER: Anaphylaxis, killer allergy: long-term management in the community. J Allergy Clin Immunol 2006;117:367–377.

46 Simons FER: Advances in H_1-antihistamines. N Engl J Med 2004;351:2203–2217.

47 Nurmatov U, Worth A, Sheikh A: Anaphylaxis management plans for the acute and long-term management of anaphylaxis: a systematic review. J Allergy Clin Immunol 2008;122:353–361.

48 Gaeta TJ, Clark S, Pelletier AJ, Camargo CA: National study of US emergency department visits for acute allergic reactions, 1993–2004. Ann Allergy Asthma Immunol 2007;98:360–365.

49 Simons FER, Lieberman PL, Read EJ Jr, Edwards ES: Hazards of unintentional injection of epinephrine from auto-injectors: a systematic review. Ann Allergy Clin Immunol 2009;102:267–272.

50 Rawas-Qalaji MM, Simons FER, Simons KJ: Sublingual epinephrine tablets versus intramuscular injection of epinephrine: dose equivalence for potential treatment of anaphylaxis. J Allergy Clin Immunol 2006;117:398–403.

Dr. F. Estelle R. Simons
Department of Pediatrics and Child Health, Department of Immunology
Faculty of Medicine, University of Manitoba
Room FE125, 820 Sherbrook Street, Winnipeg R3A 1R9 (Canada)
Tel. +1 204 787 2537, Fax +1 204 787 5040, E-Mail lmcniven@hsc.mb.ca

Author Index

Akdis, C.A. 22
Akdis, M. 22

Behrendt, H. 1
Brockow, K. 110, 157, 190, 201

de Weck, A. 1

Ferrer, M. 125
Franz, R. 190

Galdiero, M.R. 98
Galli, S.J. 45
Gamboa, P.M. 125
García-Figueroa, B.E. 125
Genovese, A. 98
Grosber, M. 201

Kalesnikoff, J. 45
Kaplan, A.P. 67
Karasuyama, H. 85

Marone, G. 98
Mertes, P.M. 180

Metcalfe, D.D. 110
Möhrenschlager, M. 201
Moneret-Vautrin, D.A. 180
Mukai, K. 85
Müller, U.R. 141

Obata, K. 85
Ozdemir, C. 22

Ring, J. XI, 1, 157, 190, 201
Rossi, F.W. 98

Sanz, M.L. 125
Simons, F.E.R. 211
Simons, K.J. 211
Spadaro, G. 98
Szczeklik, A. 170

Tsujimura, Y. 85

Worm, M. 12

Subject Index